# Substance Use Disorders

*Editor*

MELISSA B. WEIMER

# MEDICAL CLINICS OF NORTH AMERICA

www.medical.theclinics.com

*Consulting Editor*
JACK ENDE

January 2022 • Volume 106 • Number 1

ELSEVIER

1600 John F. Kennedy Boulevard • Suite 1800 • Philadelphia, Pennsylvania, 19103-2899

http://www.theclinics.com

**MEDICAL CLINICS OF NORTH AMERICA Volume 106, Number 1**
**January 2022 ISSN 0025-7125, ISBN-13: 978-0-323-84876-3**

Editor: Katerina Heidhausen
Developmental Editor: Arlene Campos

Medical Clinics of North America (ISSN 0025-7125) is published bimonthly by Elsevier Inc., 360 Park Avenue South, New York, NY 10010-1710. Months of publication are January, March, May, July, September, and November. Business and editorial offices: 1600 John F. Kennedy Boulevard, Suite 1800, Philadelphia, PA 19103-2899. Periodicals postage paid at New York, NY, and additional mailing offices. Subscription prices are USD $316.00 per year (US individuals), $956.00 per year (US institutions), $100.00 per year (US Students), $396.00 per year (Canadian individuals), $1,004.00 per year (Canadian institutions), $200.00 per year for (foreign students), $100.00 per year for (Canadian students), $439.00 per year (foreign individuals), and $1,004.00 per year (foreign institutions). To receive student/resident rate, orders must be accompanied by name of affiliated institution, date of term, and the signature of program/residency coordinator on institution letterhead. Orders will be billed at individual rate until proof of status is received. Foreign air speed delivery is included in all Clinics' subscription prices. All prices are subject to change without notice. **POSTMASTER:** Send address changes to *Medical Clinics of North America*, Elsevier Health Sciences Division, Subscription Customer Service, 3251 Riverport Lane, Maryland Heights, MO 63043. **Customer Service: Telephone: 1-800-654-2452** (U.S. and Canada); **1-314-447-8871** (outside U.S. and Canada). **Fax: 314-447-8029. E-mail: journalscustomerserviceusa@ elsevier.com** (for print support); **journalsonlinesupport-usa@elsevier.com** (for online support).

*Reprints.* For copies of 100 or more of articles in this publication, please contact the Commercial Reprints Department, Elsevier Inc., 360 Park Avenue South, New York, NY 10010-1710. Tel.: 212-633-3874; Fax: 212-633-3820; E-mail: reprints@elsevier.com.

*Medical Clinics of North America* is also published in Spanish by McGraw-Hill Interamericana Editores S. A., P.O. Box 5-237, 06500 Mexico, D.F., Mexico.

*Medical Clinics of North America* is covered in *MEDLINE/PubMed (Index Medicus), Current Contents, ASCA, Excerpta Medica, Science Citation Index, and ISI/BIOMED.*

Printed in the United States of America.

## PROGRAM OBJECTIVE

The goal of the *Medical Clinics of North America* is to keep practicing physicians up to date with current clinical practice by providing timely articles reviewing the state of the art in patient care.

## TARGET AUDIENCE

All practicing physicians and other healthcare professionals.

## LEARNING OBJECTIVES

Upon completion of this activity, participants will be able to:
1. Review the history and definitions of addiction as a medical concept, as well as the history of addiction treatments and disparities.
2. Explain risks, diagnosis, and treatment options for commonly used substances.
3. Discuss the use and implementation of screening tools for adult alcohol and drug use.

## ACCREDITATION

The Elsevier Office of Continuing Medical Education (EOCME) is accredited by the Accreditation Council for Continuing Medical Education (ACCME) to provide continuing medical education for physicians.

The EOCME designates this journal-based CME activity for a maximum of 14 *AMA PRA Category 1 Credit*(s)™. Physicians should claim only the credit commensurate with the extent of their participation in the activity.

All other healthcare professionals requesting continuing education credit for this enduring material will be issued a certificate of participation.

## DISCLOSURE OF CONFLICTS OF INTEREST

The EOCME assesses conflict of interest with its instructors, faculty, planners, and other individuals who are in a position to control the content of CME activities. All relevant conflicts of interest that are identified are thoroughly vetted by EOCME for fair balance, scientific objectivity, and patient care recommendations. EOCME is committed to providing its learners with CME activities that promote improvements or quality in healthcare and not a specific proprietary business or a commercial interest.

**The planning committee, staff, authors, and editors listed below have identified no financial relationships or relationships to products or devices they or their spouse/life partner have with commercial interest related to the content of this CME activity:**
Audrey Abelleira, PharmD; Gregory Acampora, MD; Ryan S. Alexander, MD, MPH; Julia H. Arnsten, MD, MPH; Sarah M. Bagley, MD, MSc; William C. Becker, MD; Bethany Canver, MD; Carolyn A. Chan, MD; Regina Chavous-Gibson, MSN, RN; Shawn M. Cohen, MD; Chinazo O. Cunningham, MD, MS; Susanna A. Curtis, MD, PhD; Michael J. Durkin, MD, MPH; Sarah Evers-Casey, MPH, CTTS-M; Caroline G. Falker, MD; Samuel Gnanakumar; Leah Hamilton, PhD; Miriam T.H. Harris, MD, MSc; Thomas Hickey, MS, MD; Stephen R. Holt, MD, MS; Danielle S. Jackson, MD, MPH; Ayana Jordan, MD, PhD; Jordana Laks, MD, MPH; Frank T. Leone, MD, MS; Ximena A. Levander, MD, MCR; Sharon Levy, MD, MPH; Stephen Y. Liang, MD, MPHS; Laura R. Marks, MD, PhD; Jennifer McNeely, MD, MS; Ryan McNeil, PhD; Kenneth L. Morford, MD; Mitchell Nazario, PharmD Leah F. Nelson, MD, MS; Nathanial S. Nolan, MD, MPH; Yngvild Olsen, MD, MPH, DFASAM; Merlin Packiam; Linda Peng, MD; Alyssa Peterkin, MD; Kelley Saia, MD; Steve Shoptaw, PhD; Deepika E. Slawek, MD, MPH, MS; Natalie Stahl, MD, MPH; Kimberly L. Sue, MD, PhD Max Jordan Nguemeni Tiako, MD, MS; Wendee M. Wechsberg, PhD, MS; Melissa B. Weimer, DO, MCR, FASAM; Zoe M. Weinstein, MD, MS; Elissa R. Weitzman, ScD, MSc

**The planning committee, staff, authors and editors listed below have identified financial relationships or relationships to products or devices they or their spouse/life partner have with commercial interest related to the content of this CME activity:**
Daniel Ciccarone, MD, MPH: Consultant: Celero Systems, Inc.

## UNAPPROVED/OFF-LABEL USE DISCLOSURE

The EOCME requires CME faculty to disclose to the participants;
1. When products or procedures being discussed are off-label, unlabelled, experimental, and/or investigational (not US Food and Drug Administration [FDA] approved); and
2. Any limitations on the information presented, such as data that are preliminary or that represent ongoing research, interim analyses, and/or unsupported opinions. Faculty may discuss information about pharmaceutical agents that is outside of FDA-approved labelling. This information is intended solely for CME

and is not intended to promote off-label use of these medications. If you have any questions, contact the medical affairs department of the manufacturer for the most recent prescribing information.

## TO ENROLL

To enroll in the *Medical Clinics of North America* Continuing Medical Education program, call customer service at 1-800-654-2452 or sign up online at http://www.theclinics.com/home/cme. The CME program is available to subscribers for an additional annual fee of USD 324.00.

## METHOD OF PARTICIPATION

In order to claim credit, participants must complete the following;

1. Complete enrolment as indicated above.
2. Read the activity.
3. Complete the CME Test and Evaluation. Participants must achieve a score of 70% on the test. All CME Tests and Evaluations must be completed online.

## CME INQUIRIES/SPECIAL NEEDS

For all CME inquiries or special needs, please contact elsevierCME@elsevier.com.

# MEDICAL CLINICS OF NORTH AMERICA

**FORTHCOMING ISSUES**

*March 2022*
**Update in Preventive Cardiology**
Douglas S. Jacoby, *Editor*

*May 2022*
**Disease-Based Physical Examination**
Paul Aronowitz, *Editor*

*July 2022*
**Communication Skills and Challenges in Medical Practice**
Heather Hofmann, *Editor*

**RECENT ISSUES**

*November 2021*
**Update in Endocrinology**
Silvio Inzucchi and Elizabeth H. Holt, *Editors*

*September 2021*
**An Update in ENT for Internists**
Erica Thaler, Jason Brant, and Karthik Rajasekaran, *Editors*

*July 2021*
**Dermatology**
Jeffrey P. Callen, *Editor*

**SERIES OF RELATED INTEREST**

*Primary Care: Clinics in Office Practice*
*Psychiatrics Clinic*

# Contributors

## CONSULTING EDITOR

**JACK ENDE, MD, MACP**
The Schaeffer Professor of Medicine, Perelman School of Medicine, University of Pennsylvania, Philadelphia, Pennsylvania

## EDITOR

**MELISSA B. WEIMER, DO, MCR, FASAM**
Associate Professor of Medicine and Public Health, Program in Addiction Medicine, Yale Department of Medicine, Yale School of Medicine and Public Health, New Haven, Connecticut

## AUTHORS

**AUDREY ABELLEIRA, PharmD**
VA Connecticut Healthcare System, West Haven, Connecticut

**GREGORY ACAMPORA, MD**
MGH/Harvard Center for Addiction Medicine, Pain Management Center at MGH, Assistant Professor of Psychiatry, Harvard Medical School, Massachusetts General Hospital, Boston, Massachusetts

**RYAN S. ALEXANDER, DO, MPH**
Program in Addiction Medicine, Section of General Internal Medicine, Yale School of Medicine, New Haven, Connecticut

**JULIA H. ARNSTEN, MD, MPH**
Professor of Medicine, Psychiatry, and Epidemiology, Chief, General Internal Medicine Division, Department of Medicine, Albert Einstein College of Medicine/Montefiore Medical Center, Bronx, New York

**SARAH M. BAGLEY, MD, MSc**
Grayken Center for Addiction, Clinical Addiction Research and Education (CARE) Unit, Section of General Internal Medicine, Department of Medicine, Boston University School of Medicine, Boston Medical Center, Division of General Pediatrics, Department of Pediatrics, Boston, Massachusetts

**WILLIAM C. BECKER, MD**
Core Investigator, Pain Research, Informatics, Multimorbidities and Education Center, VA Connecticut Healthcare System, Associate Professor, Program in Addiction Medicine, Yale School of Medicine, New Haven, Connecticut

**BETHANY CANVER, MD**
Program in Addiction Medicine, Section of General Internal Medicine, Department of Medicine, New Haven, Connecticut

**CAROLYN A. CHAN, MD**
Program in Addiction Medicine, Section of General Internal Medicine, Department of Medicine, New Haven, Connecticut

**DANIEL CICCARONE, MD, MPH**
Justine Miner Professor of Addiction Medicine, Department of Family and Community Medicine, University of California, San Francisco, San Francisco, California

**SHAWN M. COHEN, MD**
Program in Addiction Medicine, Section of General Internal Medicine, Yale School of Medicine, New Haven, Connecticut

**CHINAZO O. CUNNINGHAM, MD, MS**
Professor of Medicine, Family & Social Medicine, and Psychiatry, Department of Medicine, Albert Einstein College of Medicine/Montefiore Medical Center, Bronx, New York

**SUSANNA A. CURTIS, MD, PhD**
Assistant Professor of Medicine, Department of Medicine, Albert Einstein College of Medicine/Montefiore Medical Center, Bronx, New York

**MICHAEL J. DURKIN, MD, MPH**
Division of Infectious Diseases, Washington University in St. Louis School of Medicine, St Louis, Missouri

**SARAH EVERS-CASEY, MPH CTTS-M**
Comprehensive Smoking Treatment Program, Perelman School of Medicine, Philadelphia, Pennsylvania

**CAROLINE G. FALKER, MD**
VA Connecticut Healthcare System, West Haven, Connecticut

**LEAH HAMILTON, PhD**
Section on Alcohol, Tobacco, and Drug Use, Department of Population Health, NYU Grossman, School of Medicine, Kaiser Permanente Washington Health Research Institute, Seattle, Washington

**MIRIAM T.H. HARRIS, MD, MSc**
Grayken Center for Addiction, Clinical Addiction Research and Education (CARE) Unit, Section of General Internal Medicine, Department of Medicine, Boston University School of Medicine, Boston Medical Center, Boston, Massachusetts

**THOMAS HICKEY, MS, MD**
VA Connecticut Healthcare System, Assistant Professor, Department of Anesthesiology, Yale School of Medicine, West Haven, Connecticut

**STEPHEN R. HOLT, MD, MS**
Program in Addiction Medicine, Section of General Internal Medicine, Yale School of Medicine, New Haven, Connecticut

**DANIELLE S. JACKSON, MD, MPH**
Assistant Professor, Department of Psychiatry, Rutgers University-RWJMS, Piscataway, NJ

**AYANA JORDAN, MD, PhD**
Department of Psychiatry, Yale School of Medicine, New Haven, Connecticut

**JORDANA LAKS, MD, MPH**
Grayken Center for Addiction, Clinical Addiction Research and Education (CARE) Unit, Section of General Internal Medicine, Department of Medicine, Boston University School of Medicine, Boston Medical Center, Boston, Massachusetts

**FRANK T. LEONE, MD MS**
Comprehensive Smoking Treatment Program, Penn Lung Center, Philadelphia, Pennsylvania; Abramson Cancer Center, University of Pennsylvania, Philadelphia, Pennsylvania

**XIMENA A. LEVANDER, MD, MCR**
Assistant Professor, Department of Medicine, Division of General Internal Medicine and Geriatrics, Addiction Medicine Section, Oregon Health & Science University, Portland, Oregon

**SHARON LEVY, MD, MPH**
Associate Professor, Harvard Medical School, Director, Adolescent Substance Use and Addiction Program, Boston Children's Hospital, Associate Professor of Pediatrics, Harvard Medical School, Boston, Massachusetts

**STEPHEN Y. LIANG, MD, MPHS**
Division of Infectious Diseases, Division of Emergency Medicine, Washington University in St. Louis School of Medicine, St Louis, Missouri

**LAURA R. MARKS, MD, PhD**
Division of Infectious Diseases, Washington University in St. Louis School of Medicine, St Louis, Missouri

**JENNIFER MCNEELY, MD, MS**
Section on Alcohol, Tobacco, and Drug Use, Departments of Population Health, and Medicine, Division of General Internal Medicine and Clinical Innovation, and Medicine, NYU Grossman School of Medicine, New York, New York

**RYAN MCNEIL, PhD**
Program in Addiction Medicine, Section of General Internal Medicine, Department of Medicine, New Haven, Connecticut

**KENNETH L. MORFORD, MD**
Assistant Professor of Medicine, Department of Internal Medicine, Section of General Internal Medicine, Program in Addiction Medicine, Yale School of Medicine, New Haven, Connecticut

**MITCHELL NAZARIO, PharmD**
National PBM Clinical Program Manager, VHA Pharmacy Benefits Management (12PBM), Hines, Illinois

**LEAH F. NELSON, MD, MS**
Addiction Medicine Fellow, Adolescent Substance Use and Addiction Program, Boston Children's Hospital, Boston, Massachusetts

**MAX JORDAN NGUEMENI TIAKO, MD, MS**
Department of Internal Medicine, Brigham and Women's Hospital, Harvard Medical School, Boston, Massachusetts

**NATHANIAL S. NOLAN, MD, MPH**
Division of Infectious Diseases, Washington University in St. Louis School of Medicine, St Louis, Missouri

**YNGVILD OLSEN, MD, MPH, DFASAM**
Assistant Professor of Medicine, Part-Time, Department of Medicine, Division of Addiction Medicine, Johns Hopkins School of Medicine, Baltimore, Maryland

**LINDA PENG, MD**
Assistant Professor of Medicine, Department of Medicine, Division of General Internal Medicine and Geriatrics, Addiction Medicine Section, Oregon Health & Science University, Portland, Oregon

**ALYSSA PETERKIN, MD**
Grayken Center for Addiction Medicine, Section of General Internal Medicine, Department of Medicine, Boston University School of Medicine, Boston Medical Center, Boston, Massachusetts

**KELLEY SAIA, MD**
Department of Obstetrics and Gynecology, Boston Medical Center, Boston, Massachusetts

**STEVE SHOPTAW, PhD**
Professor and Vice Chair for Research, Department of Family Medicine, University of California, Los Angeles, Los Angeles, California

**DEEPIKA E. SLAWEK, MD, MPH, MS**
Assistant Professor of Medicine, Department of Medicine, Albert Einstein College of Medicine/Montefiore Medical Center, Bronx, New York

**NATALIE STAHL, MD, MPH**
Yale Program in Addiction Medicine, Yale School of Medicine, New Haven, Connecticut

**KIMBERLY L. SUE, MD, PhD**
Program in Addiction Medicine, Section of General Internal Medicine, Department of Medicine, Medical Director, National Harm Reduction Coalition, New Haven, Connecticut

**WENDEE M. WECHSBERG, PhD, MS**
Substance Use, Gender, and Applied Research Program, RTI International, Research Triangle Park, North Carolina; Gillings School of Global Public Health, The University of North Carolina at Chapel Hill, Chapel Hill, North Carolina; Department of Psychology, North Carolina State University, Raleigh, North Carolina; Department of Psychiatry and Behavioral Sciences, Duke University School of Medicine, Durham, North Carolina

**MELISSA WEIMER, DO, MCR, FASAM**
Associate Professor of Medicine and Public Health, Program in Addiction Medicine, Yale Department of Medicine, Yale School of Medicine and Public Health, New Haven, Connecticut

**ZOE M. WEINSTEIN, MD, MS**
Grayken Center for Addiction Medicine, Section of General Internal Medicine, Department of Medicine, Boston University School of Medicine, Boston Medical Center, Boston, Massachusetts

**ELISSA R. WEITZMAN, ScD, MSc**
Associate Professor, Harvard Medical School, Associate Scientist, Boston Children's Hospital, Boston, Massachusetts

# Contents

Foreword : Toward a New Paradigm for Understanding Substance-Use Disorders     xvii

Jack Ende

Preface: Addiction Care Matters: A Practical Guide to Substance Use Disorder
Prevention, Screening, and Treatment     xix

Melissa B. Weimer

What Is Addiction? History, Terminology, and Core Concepts     1

Yngvild Olsen

Medicine's acceptance of addiction as a medical concept has waxed and
waned over time. Addiction, as a disease, fits with modern disease definitions and scientific advances in elucidating the interactions between
neurobiology and environment. Definitions of addiction need to acknowledge the complex interactions of brain circuits, genetics, environmental
factors, and individual life experiences. Addiction aligns with SEVERAL
diagnostic categories of substance use disorders that THEMSELVES do
not rely on tolerance and withdrawal as SOLE defining characteristics.
Shifts in social and political views of addiction continue to propel and
mirror changes in addiction treatment approaches and terminology within
the medical community.

Screening for Unhealthy Alcohol and Drug Use in General Medicine Settings     13

Jennifer McNeely and Leah Hamilton

Unhealthy alcohol and drug use are among the top 10 causes of preventable death in the United States, but they are infrequently identified and addressed in medical settings. Guidelines recommend screening adult
primary care patients for alcohol and drug use, and routine screening
should be a component of high-quality clinical care. Brief, validated
screening tools accurately detect unhealthy alcohol and drug use, and
their thoughtful implementation can facilitate adoption and optimize the
quality of screening results. Recommendations for implementation include
patient self-administered screening tools, integration with electronic health
records, and screening during routine primary care visits.

Disparities in Addiction Treatment: Learning from the Past to Forge an Equitable
Future     29

Danielle S. Jackson, Max Jordan Nguemeni Tiako, and Ayana Jordan

The Half-Century long problem of addiction treatment disparities. We
cannot imagine addressing disparities in addiction treatment without first
acknowledging and deconstructing the etiology of this inequity. This article
examines the history of addiction treatment disparities beginning with
early twentieth-century drug policies. We begin by discussing structural
racism, its contribution to treatment disparities, using opioid use disorder

as a case study to highlight the importance of a structural competency framework in obtaining care. We conclude by discussing diversity in the workforce as an additional tool to minimizing disparities. Addiction treatment should be aimed at addressing care delivery in the context of the social, economic, and political determinants of health, which require appreciation of their historical origins to move toward equitable treatment.

**The Spectrum of Alcohol Use: Epidemiology, Diagnosis, and Treatment**        43

Shawn M. Cohen, Ryan S. Alexander, and Stephen R. Holt

In the United States, alcohol is the most common substance used and the spectrum of unhealthy alcohol use is highly prevalent. Complications of unhealthy alcohol use affect nearly every organ system. One of the most frequent and potentially life-threatening of these complications is alcohol withdrawal syndrome for which benzodiazepines remain first-line therapy. Pharmacologic treatment of alcohol use disorder, the most severe form of unhealthy alcohol use, is underutilized despite the availability of multiple effective medications. Although behavioral therapies are an important component of treatment, they are often overemphasized at the expense of pharmacotherapy. While abstinence may be an appropriate goal for many, it should not be pursued at the expense of reductions in alcohol use which have been shown to improve outcomes and be long lasting.

**Current Best Practices for Acute and Chronic Management of Patients with Opioid Use Disorder**        61

Alyssa Peterkin, Jordana Laks, and Zoe M. Weinstein

This comprehensive review on opioids summarizes the scope of the current opioid epidemic, the diagnosis and treatment of opioid use disorder, and the medical and psychiatric complications of opioid use.

**Understanding Stimulant Use and Use Disorders in a New Era**        81

Daniel Ciccarone and Steve Shoptaw

Extending from the triple wave epidemic of opioid-related overdose deaths, a fourth wave of high mortality involving methamphetamine and cocaine use has been gathering force. This article provides a review of the published literature on stimulants including epidemiology, pharmacology, neurobiology, medical and psychiatric consequences, withdrawal management, and medical and behavioral treatments.

**Tobacco Use Disorder**        99

Frank T. Leone and Sarah Evers-Casey

Tobacco use disorder is highly prevalent; more than a billion individuals use tobacco worldwide. Popular views on the addictive potential of tobacco often underestimate the complex neural adaptations that underpin continued use. Although sometimes trivialized as a minor substance, effects of nicotine on behavior lead to profound morbidity over a lifetime of exposure. Innovations in processing have led to potent forms of tobacco and delivery devices. Proactive treatment strategies focus on pharmacotherapeutic interventions. Innovations on the horizon hold promise to help clinicians address this problem in a phenotypically tailored manner. Efforts are needed to prevent tobacco use for future generations.

## Benzodiazepines and Related Sedatives        113

Linda Peng, Kenneth L. Morford, and Ximena A. Levander

Benzodiazepine and related sedative use has been increasing. There has been a growing number of unregulated novel psychoactive substances, including designer benzodiazepines. Benzodiazepines have neurobiological and pharmacologic properties that result in a high potential for misuse and physical dependence. Options for discontinuing long-term benzodiazepine use include an outpatient benzodiazepine taper or inpatient withdrawal management at a hospital or detoxification facility. The quality of evidence on medications for benzodiazepine discontinuation is overall low, whereas cognitive behavioral therapy has shown the most benefit in terms of behavioral treatments. Benzodiazepines may also have significant adverse effects, increasing the risk of overdose and death.

## Clinical Approaches to Cannabis: A Narrative Review        131

Deepika E. Slawek, Susanna A. Curtis, Julia H. Arnsten, and Chinazo O. Cunningham

Cannabis use in the United States is growing at an unprecedented pace. Most states in the United States have legalized medical cannabis use, and many have legalized nonmedical cannabis use. In this setting, health care professionals will increasingly see more patients who have questions about cannabis use, its utility for medical conditions, and the risks of its use. This narrative review provides an overview of the background, pharmacology, therapeutic use, and potential complications of cannabis.

## Prevention of Substance Use Disorders        153

Leah F. Nelson, Elissa R. Weitzman, and Sharon Levy

Methods to prevent substance use disorders (SUDs) act on the individual risk factors for addiction. Most adults with SUD initiated substance use during their teenage years, so preventive interventions during adolescence are critical. Antisubstance use messaging, routine screening, and pathways for referral to treatment can be extended into all settings whereby trusted adults interact with adolescents such as sports, mentoring programs, child protective services, and juvenile justice settings. Pediatric primary care is an ideal place to incorporate preventive counseling and screening for substance use. Evidence-based technologic interventions for primary, secondary, and tertiary prevention are needed.

## Perioperative Buprenorphine Management: A Multidisciplinary Approach        169

Thomas Hickey, Audrey Abelleira, Gregory Acampora, William C. Becker, Caroline G. Falker, Mitchell Nazario, and Melissa B. Weimer

Buprenorphine formulations (including buprenorphine/naloxone) are effective treatments of pain and opioid use disorder (OUD). Historically, perioperative management of patients prescribed buprenorphine involved abstinence from buprenorphine sufficient to allow for unrestricted mu-opioid receptor availability to full agonist opioid (FAO) treatment. Evidence is mounting that a multimodal analgesic strategy, including simultaneous administration of buprenorphine and FAO, nonopioid adjuncts such as acetaminophen and nonsteroidal anti-inflammatory drugs, and regional anesthesia, is a safe and effective perioperative strategy for the patient prescribed long-term buprenorphine treatment of OUD. This strategy will likely simplify management and more seamlessly provide continuous buprenorphine treatment of OUD after hospital discharge.

## Infectious Complications of Injection Drug Use 187

Laura R. Marks, Nathanial S. Nolan, Stephen Y. Liang, Michael J. Durkin, and Melissa B. Weimer

The opioid overdose epidemic is one of the leading causes of death in adults. Its devastating effects have included not only a burgeoning overdose crisis but also multiple converging infectious diseases epidemics. The use of both opioids and other substances through intravenous (IV) administration places individuals at increased risks of infectious diseases ranging from invasive bacterial and fungal infections to human immunodeficiency virus (HIV) and viral hepatitis. In 2012, there were 530,000 opioid use disorder (OUD)-related hospitalizations in the United States (US), with $700 million in costs associated with OUD-related infections. The scale of the crisis has continued to increase since that time, with hospitalizations for injection drug use-related infective endocarditis (IDU-IE) increasing by as much as 12-fold from 2010 to 2015. Deaths from IDU-IE alone are estimated to result in over 7,260,000 years of potential life lost over the next 10 years. There have been high-profile injection-related HIV outbreaks, and injection drug use (IDU) is now the most common risk factor for hepatitis C virus (HCV). As this epidemic continues to grow, clinicians in all aspects of medical care are increasingly confronted with infectious complications of IDU. This review will describe the pathogenesis, clinical syndromes, epidemiology, and models of treatment for common infectious complications among persons who inject drugs (PWIDs).

## Harm Reduction in Health Care Settings 201

Carolyn A. Chan, Bethany Canver, Ryan McNeil, and Kimberly L. Sue

Harm reduction is an approach to reduce the risk of harms to an individual using substances without requiring abstinence. This review discusses substance-specific interventions for opioids, alcohol, and stimulants that can minimize harms for individuals who use these substances. Topics discussed include overdose prevention, infection prevention, and low-barrier substance use disorder treatment.

## Gender Dynamics in Substance Use and Treatment: A Women's Focused Approach 219

Miriam T.H. Harris, Jordana Laks, Natalie Stahl, Sarah M. Bagley, Kelley Saia, and Wendee M. Wechsberg

Gender impacts substance use initiation, substance use disorder development, engagement with treatment, and harms related to drug and alcohol use. Using the biopsychosocial model of addiction, this review provides a broad summary of barriers and facilitators to addiction services among women. It also reviews substance use among pregnant and parenting women and approaches to care. Given the increasing rates of substance use among women, there is a need to implement and scale-up gender-responsive addiction programming and pursue advocacy at the policy level that addresses the root drivers of substance use inequities among women.

# Foreword

# Toward a New Paradigm for Understanding Substance-Use Disorders

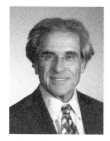

Jack Ende, MD, MACP
*Consulting Editor*

I use the term paradigm cautiously, as it is a word that is much overused of late, as in the term "paradigm shift." But is that not what the past few decades of research have yielded in the field of addiction medicine?

Previously considered a character flaw, addiction was thought to be a disorder as in something that could be corrected by force of will, we now appreciate the molecular, biochemical, and neuroanatomic structural changes that accompany these disorders, and that account for the challenges we face as clinicians working with patients with substance use disorders, including those who wish to change.

There can be no better instrument in the struggle to help substance use disorder patients than knowledge of the pathophysiology, clinical presentation, and evidence-based approaches to recovery. This issue of *Medical Clinics of North America* provides just that. Along with important articles on the socioeconomic determinants of substance use disorders, which should never be forgotten, there are clinical articles dealing with alcohol, tobacco, stimulants, sedatives, cannabis, and opioid use. These disorders are common. We encounter them in our office practices and on our inpatient services. As Guest Editor Dr Melissa Weimer points out, there is a shortage of addiction medicine specialists. Much of the challenge, therefore, of diagnosis and treatment of substance-use disorders falls to primary care physicians, and certainly screening and early detection reside within the province of primary care. We all need to be as well-versed in these disorders as we can. The new paradigm of

Med Clin N Am 106 (2022) xvii–xviii
https://doi.org/10.1016/j.mcna.2021.10.003
0025-7125/22/© 2021 Published by Elsevier Inc.

substance-use disorders situates these disorders as medical conditions. Let the learning begin.

Jack Ende, MD, MACP
The Schaeffer Professor of Medicine
Perelman School of Medicine
University of Pennsylvania
Philadelphia, PA 19104, USA

*E-mail address:*
jack.ende@pennmedicine.upenn.edu

# Preface

# Addiction Care Matters: A Practical Guide to Substance Use Disorder Prevention, Screening, and Treatment

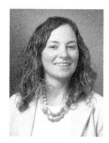

Melissa B. Weimer, DO, MCR, FASAM
*Editor*

Earlier today I was asked by both a colleague and a health reporter how our hospital initiates medications, such as methadone and buprenorphine, for patients with opioid use disorder (OUD). A few months ago, I was asked by a different colleague how outpatient clinics provide extended-release naltrexone to individuals with alcohol use disorder and treatment options other than mutual support groups. A few months before that I was asked by a hospital administrator for a validated screening instrument to assess patients at risk for unhealthy alcohol use. I am an internist and addiction medicine specialist, so I expect to be asked questions about my specialty, and I enjoy sharing knowledge and seeing positive changes that benefit individuals with substance use disorders (SUD). What confuses me, though, is what took so long? Also, what happens when I am not around, or a health system doesn't have a specialist in addiction? Many of the prevention strategies, treatments, and models of care for SUD are not new. Methadone, for example, has greater than 50 years of evidence demonstrating it reduces mortality and opioid use. If you asked the average health care professional how to initiate methadone for a hospitalized patient with OUD, many may not know, and most will likely question its inherent safety and legality. It is beyond time that our health care workforce be prepared and knowledgeable about the basics of SUD and addiction treatment.

SUDs remain major causes of preventable death worldwide; however, unlike other causes of preventable death like cardiovascular disease and diabetes, local and national resources are rarely mobilized in the same way to address SUD. In this issue of *Medical Clinics of North America*, many of the nation's leading experts in the field

Med Clin N Am 106 (2022) xix–xx
https://doi.org/10.1016/j.mcna.2021.10.001
0025-7125/22/© 2021 Published by Elsevier Inc.

of addiction medicine, addiction psychiatry, and public health describe how treatment of SUD is an essential component of general medical care, and the absence of prevention, screening, and treatment is a matter of social and racial inequity. This special issue of the *Medical Clinics of North America* can serve as a practical and accessible resource for the many health care professionals who want to live in a world where individuals with SUD receive the quality of care and treatment they need and deserve, and on par with other health conditions. This compilation will not be enough to make one an addiction medicine specialist, but it will provide a strong foundation for many of the key principles of addiction prevention, screening, and treatment.

This issue details the clinical areas that are important for the current and future generations of practicing health care professionals to know to treat individuals who may be living with SUD. One article is dedicated to understanding the basics of addiction and the history of addiction in the United States. Two articles discuss screening and prevention efforts, which are essential components of general medical practice that are generally overlooked. Each major SUD receives its own article. There are dedicated articles on racial disparities in addiction treatment, pain treatment for patients with OUD, infectious complications of injection drug use, harm reduction in health care settings, and addiction in women.

I care for hospitalized patients with SUDs, and each day I encounter individuals who have gone years without being asked about their substance use, evaluated for their substance use, or offered treatment for their SUD. Clinicians are continually making complex decisions for the care of their patients. In these situations, they must have the most basic information about the conditions that they treat—addiction treatment is no exception. SUDs and their treatment are relevant to all clinicians, and this important issue of *Medical Clinics of North America* hopes to address some of these learning gaps.

Melissa B. Weimer, DO, MCR, FASAM
Yale Department of Medicine
Yale School of Medicine and Public Health
Harkness Hall A, Suite 217
367 Cedar Street
New Haven, CT 06510, USA

*E-mail address:*
melissa.weimer@yale.edu

# What Is Addiction? History, Terminology, and Core Concepts

Yngvild Olsen, MD, MPH, DFASAM

## KEYWORDS

- Addiction • Substance use disorders • Definition • Terminology

## KEY POINTS

- Addiction is a treatable, chronic medical disease involving complex interactions of brain circuitry, genetics, environment, and an individual's life experiences.
- Patients with addiction have identifiable, characteristic signs and symptoms.
- Substance use disorder of a specified severity is the diagnostic term applied to someone with an addiction.
- Stigmatizing terminology associated with addiction and substance use disorders are increasingly falling out of favor.
- Nonjudgmental comprehensive treatment of people with addiction and substance use disorders need to fully replace historical punitive approaches as standard of care.

## HISTORY

The use of substances to produce euphoria is as old as recorded history itself. People consumed alcohol in China more than 12,000 years ago for its rewarding effects.[1] Ancient Sumerians drank the opium-laced juice of the poppy plant to feel joy.[2] Indigenous people in South America started chewing coca leaves for energy 3000 years ago.[3] In a prescientific world, people viewed alcohol and other psychoactive compounds as imbued with divine properties. They also understood the dual nature of substance use for some people. The Greek philosopher and botanist Theophrastus (c. 371–c. 287 BCE) noted the "occasionally lethal" use of opium."[4] Anecdotes in religious texts from different civilizations depict individuals, families, and communities facing calamitous consequences from excessive drinking.[1]

Across history, society blamed lack of appropriate moral values, absence of piety, or flaws in character or personality for substance use and its associated, frowned-

Institutes for Behavior Resources, Inc/REACH Health Services, 2104 Maryland Avenue, Baltimore, MD 21218, USA
E-mail address: Yngvild.olsen@gmail.com
Twitter: @YngvildOlsen (Y.O.)

Med Clin N Am 106 (2022) 1–12
https://doi.org/10.1016/j.mcna.2021.08.001
0025-7125/22/© 2021 Elsevier Inc. All rights reserved.

upon behaviors that fell outside norms of the day. The word "addiction" occasionally appears in the historical context to describe the phenomenon of uncontrolled, compulsive use of a substance or engagement in a behavior to the detriment of the individual and those surrounding them. Stemming from the Latin verb *addicere*, meaning a divine, powerful "speaking to" or a passive act of "enslavement," people with addiction were "moral transgressors" or "sinners," alternately to be shamed and shunned or purified and saved.[5]

This is the background of addiction as a medical concept starting in the late 1700s. Based on detailed observations of patients and family members, physicians Benjamin Rush in the United States and Thomas Trotter in England advocated for conceptualizing excessive and destructive alcohol use as a medical disease, not merely as bad character. More commonly referred to as "inebriety," Drs Rush and Trotter and others described the medical and psychiatric consequences of excessive alcohol use, the progressive course of the disease, its intergenerational nature, persistence of cravings, and the inability to moderate the use of alcohol, despite repeated attempts to do so.[6]

Slowly, the medical community during the 1800s came to accept the disease concept of addiction. Alongside, however, American society was differentially responding to the individual and social consequences of expanding consumption of alcoholic beverages; the introduction of morphine, cocaine, and heroin; and now-recognized racism toward individuals who used opium. Viewing addiction through a nonmedical, often strongly religious lens allowed temperance movements to flourish. Some of these groups became politically active, calling for legal prohibition of alcohol and other substances, including the regular doses of morphine taken to treat opium addiction.[7] Unfortunately, many supported removals of those with addiction to jails, poor houses, or insane asylums, anywhere but within view.

Toward the end of the 1800s, medical and nonmedical communities in the United States solidly landed in the same place, albeit in parallel tracks, with the growth of specialty institutions for the treatment of "inebriety." Between 1878 and 1902, the number of specialized residential treatment facilities increased from 32 to more than 100.[8] Until 1925, ambulatory clinics operated across the country to treat people with problems related to heroin, opium, or cocaine use. The facilities that came out of the medical community were often founded by physicians, included "hospital" or "clinic" in their names, and offered a range of purported cures, including exotic herbal detoxification remedies, regular doses of morphine, or other medicinal-based therapies prescribed by specialist physicians. These specialists also notably adopted the term "addiction" to describe the primary and chronic nature of "inebriety" to alcohol and other substances, meaning a treatable disease not stemming from any other observable cause but characterized by periods of stability interspersed with episodes of recurrence.[9] In the parallel track, the nonmedical institutions typically had "home" in their names, did not use medical staff, and often relied on religious observance and shared work as the basis of treatment, framing addiction as a problem of social mores, a sin, or a crime.

Just as quickly as the medical community's adoption of addiction treatment expanded, so it disappeared. Coupled with the failure of unregulated, poorly researched, and ineffective "cures," the criminalization of substance use and addiction in the first decades of the twentieth century ushered in a long period of mostly punitive approaches to people who use drugs or have the disease. Originally meant to regulate access to opiates but revised in response to pressure from alcohol prohibition proponents, those who held racist views of people smoking opium or injecting cocaine, and those who believed that addiction should be curable, the Harrison Narcotic Tax Act of 1914 set the stage for game-changing Supreme Court decisions in 1919 and 1922. Across a handful of cases, the Court made it illegal to possess morphine, opium, heroin, or cocaine without a doctor's prescription. Concurrently, it declared that such a prescription was a violation of the Harrison Act, essentially outlawing the treatment of an opioid addiction with any opioid agonist. Between 1914 and 1938, the federal government indicted more than 25,000 physicians under the Harrison Act.[10] In fear, mainstream medicine abandoned its prior acceptance of addiction as a primary, treatable, chronic disease. Individuals with addiction became criminals, and addiction treatment became jail or prison. Even within the realm of psychiatry, views of addiction as secondary to personality and character defects with willful bad behavior that would respond only to disciplinary measures predominated for decades.[1] Despite advancements in the scientific understanding of addiction and the American Board of Medical Specialties' recognition of addiction medicine as a multispecialty subspecialty in 2016,[11] the conceptualizations of addiction as a criminal offense, social problem, or character defect still echo today.

## CONTROVERSIES AND DEFINITIONS

As in the past, debates over addiction terminology and its phenomenology continue. Critics of the word "addiction" point to its overuse with a meaning that has become inordinately diffuse and applied to anyone who ever uses a substance with any frequency.[12] Others cite the stigma attached to its corollary, "addict," as reason to avoid the term.[13] Some even dispute the concept of addiction as a disease, pointing to a lack of autonomy and free will perceived as inherent in this framing.[14] At its core, some of the concerns involve the idea of disease itself. Addiction medicine specialists understand that not everyone who uses a substance has a disease. Modern society understands that disease is not just the opposite or absence of health.[15] Importantly, disease definitions do not necessarily equate with full disability, complete loss or lack of individual responsibility or choice, or necessarily purely biologically focused approaches. For some, concepts of disease, spirituality, and religion can, and do, coexist, whether the disease in question is addiction, diabetes,[16] end-stage renal disease,[17] or heart disease.[18] For a person with a chronic disease, accepting, managing, and learning how to live with, and despite, their illness requires making choices and acting on one's own behalf.

Acknowledging the existence of different viewpoints, an analysis of current definitions of disease finds common criteria[19–22]:

- Identifiable, characteristic set of signs and symptoms
- Interruption, cessation, or disorder of a body part, system, or organ structure or function
- Cause and pathology may be known or unknown and may involve several variables including infection, inflammation, environmental factors, genetics

Current scientific understanding of addiction meets the criteria for disease. First, the Diagnostic and Statistical Manual, Version 5 clearly outlines identifiable and characteristic signs and symptoms (**Box 1**).[23] Second, although still requiring further research, scientists have identified the interruptions occurring and persisting in 3 central parts of the brain—the basal ganglia, the extended amygdala, and the prefrontal cortex—in individuals with addiction (**Fig. 1**).[24] Third, although the exact mechanisms involved still need elucidating, robust evidence points to the significant contributions of genetics and environmental factors in the cause of addiction.[25] Finally, attempts at replacing addiction as a singular, universally understood, concise term that encapsulates the complex neurobiology, physiology, genetic and environmental contributions, negative

---

**Box 1**
**Diagnostic criteria for substance use disorder**

1. The substance is often taken in larger amounts or over a longer period than was intended

2. There is a persistent desire or unsuccessful efforts to cut down or control the substance use

3. A great deal of time is spent in activities necessary to obtain, use, or recover from the effects of the substance

4. Craving or a strong desire or urge to use the substance

5. Recurrent substance use resulting in a failure to fulfill major role obligations at work, school, or home

6. Continued substance use despite having persistent or recurrent social or interpersonal problems caused or exacerbated by the effects of the substance

7. Important social, occupational, or recreational activities are given up or reduced because of substance use

8. Recurrent substance use in situations in which it is physically hazardous

9. Continued substance use despite knowledge of having a persistent or recurrent physical or psychological problem that is likely to have been caused or exacerbated by the substance

10. Tolerance, as defined by either of the following:

A need for markedly increased amounts of the substance to achieve intoxication or the desired effect.

A markedly diminished effect with continued use of the same amount of the substance

11. Withdrawal, as manifested by either of the following:

The characteristic withdrawal syndrome for that substance

The substance, or a closely related one, is taken to relieve or avoid withdrawal symptoms

Source: American Psychiatric Association. Substance-Related and Addictive Disorders. In: Diagnostic and Statistical Manual of Mental Disorders: DSM-5. Arlington, VA: American Psychiatric Association, 2013.

---

consequences, and risky actions associated with multiple substances, gambling, and potential other destructive patterns of behavior have come up short.

Based on this reasoning, the American Society of Addiction Medicine (ASAM) defines addiction as "a treatable, chronic medical disease involving complex interactions among brain circuits, genetics, the environment, and an individual's life experiences."[26] ASAM is not alone in defining addiction as a medical disease that affects the brain. The Surgeon General, in a 2016 report, defines addiction as "a chronic brain disease that has the potential for both recurrence (relapse) and recovery."[27]

## RESEARCH

Although genetics account for an estimated 40% to 60% of the risk of developing an addiction, as other chronic diseases, societal and environmental factors play key roles. Adolescents growing up in neighborhoods self-reported as highly disorganized, based on variables including levels of crime, drug selling, violence, graffiti, abandoned buildings, and social disconnectedness, had almost 3 times the odds of meeting diagnostic criteria for a substance use disorder (SUD) compared with age-matched respondents from neighborhoods of low-level disorganization.[28] Living in areas with large numbers of alcohol outlets significantly increases the incidence of alcohol use

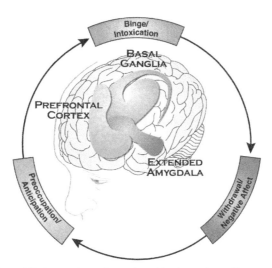

**Fig. 1.** Stages of the addiction cycle and associated brain regions. (Source: US Department of Health and Human Services (HHS), Office of the Surgeon General, Facing Addiction in America: The Surgeon General's Report on Alcohol, Drugs, and Health. Washington, DC: HHS, November 2016.)

disorder among genetically predisposed individuals.[29] Persistent poverty during childhood and moving into poverty during adolescence almost double the chances of developing drug use disorders in adulthood.[30] Poverty resulting from severe economic recessions has been associated with higher risk of alcohol problems.[31]

These nonbiological factors are understood as "social determinants of health." Research on adverse childhood experiences, adverse childhood experiences (ACEs), further underscores the impact of environmental trauma. ACEs include, before age 18 years, different forms of abuse, neglect, parental discord, and witnessing household substance misuse, criminality, or active mental illness. In a graded fashion, these confer increasing risks of substance use and addiction. People with 5 or more ACEs have 10 times the odds of ever injecting drugs, 6.5 times the odds of ever having a drug problem, and 7.7 times the odds of developing an addiction compared with similar individuals with no such adversity early in life.[32]

The effects of racism and other forms of discrimination on substance use cannot be ignored. Acts of racial discrimination may serve as a trigger for substance use in adolescence.[33] Young transgender women who reported avoiding getting mental health care because of discrimination had almost 3 times the odds of nonmedical prescription opioid use compared with individuals without such experience.[34] College-age women reporting experiences of discrimination based on race and sexual orientation were almost twice as likely to smoke cannabis and drink alcohol during a month.[35] Even as views of addiction have evolved, societal response to people of color who use drugs or have an addiction has been a disproportionally criminal rather than a therapeutic one, and huge gaps in addiction treatment access exist.[36]

Certainly, not everyone who uses drugs develops an addiction. The exact mechanisms for how social determinants of health and systemic discrimination contribute to the disease is still an area of active research. To date, studies point to gene-environment interactions, epigenetic modifications, and neuroendocrine changes as possible pathways[37,38]; this may be particularly the case when substance use occurs, as it often does, during the preteen and adolescent years, periods of rapid and critical brain development. Neuroscientists point especially to the delayed full development of the prefrontal cortex occurring at age 25 years relative to the rest of the brain maturing years earlier, and this may have special implications for the underdeveloped ability to exert control over substance taking during adolescence—a prefrontal cortical function—compared with the motivation for reward and pleasure, driven by the basal ganglia. In addition, chronic exposure to social and environmental stressors is recognized as contributing to prolonged activation of the hypothalamic-pituitary-adrenal (HPA) axis and increased allostatic load, the physical impact of the body constantly trying to adapt to toxic stress. The HPA axis, located in the extended amygdala, is also heavily involved in the negative affect component of addiction. Dysregulation or functional alterations in any of the 3 main brain regions involved in the addiction cycle—the basal ganglia, extended amygdala, and the prefrontal cortex—before substance exposure may impart vulnerability to addiction. With the right mix of factors, genetic and otherwise, substance exposure may further alter a predisposed brain, leading to disease.

## DIAGNOSIS CONSIDERATIONS

Despite the tremendous scientific advances made in understanding addiction, there is still no commercially available diagnostic imaging test. Nor are there any routine genetic or other biomarker tests obtainable via blood, urine, saliva, or other biological tissue sampling for diagnostic purposes. Drug testing can provide information about recent substance use, but these results alone do not constitute a diagnosis.

Instead, the diagnosis that clinicians make is a clinical one, falling along the spectrum of substance-related and addictive disorders, as detailed in the Diagnostic and Statistical Manual of Mental Disorders, Fifth Edition (DSM-5).[23] The diagnoses described herein are based on clusters of cognitive, behavioral, and physiologic symptoms that are observable and measurable over time and are problematic for and/or distressing to the individual, even if they are not always fully self-aware of these issues. The DSM-5 categorizes substance-related disorders across 10 separate classes of substances based on their different pharmacologic mechanisms of action, recognizing a uniform set of brain changes.

As for the word "addiction," the DSM-5 notes that "it is not applied as a diagnostic term in this classification, although it is in common usage in many countries to describe severe problems related to compulsive and habitual use of substances."[23] The National Institute for Drug Abuse (NIDA) uses both "disease" and "disorder" in their explanation of drug addiction, stating that "addiction is a lot like other diseases, such as heart disease. Both disrupt the normal, healthy functioning of an organ in the body, both have serious harmful effects, and both are, in many cases, preventable and treatable." NIDA explains that "addiction is defined as a chronic, relapsing disorder….," further noting that "It is considered a brain disorder, because it involves functional changes to brain circuits involved in reward, stress, and self-control. Those changes may last a long time after a person has stopped taking drugs."[39]

The DSM-5 manual distinguishes states of intoxication and withdrawal from substance-specific use disorders that are diagnosed according to a common set of 11 criteria occurring within a 12-month period. Each SUD is further categorized across a severity spectrum of mild, moderate, or severe, based on the number of diagnostic criteria met.

This range of SUDs and severity levels provides for a common, universally recognized, and accepted language through which to talk about the disease of addiction.

It is used by clinicians, patients, family members, insurance companies, health technology firms, regulators, medical boards, and credentialing entities. Perhaps more importantly, the DSM-5 points out that tolerance and withdrawal "occurring during appropriate medical treatment with prescribed medications (eg, opioids analgesics, sedatives, stimulants) are specifically not counted when diagnosing a substance use disorder."[23]

Tolerance and withdrawal make up the well-described phenomenon of physical dependence. Physical dependence is the predictable, expected adaptation of brain and body to chronic exposure of a drug or medication.[40] It develops not only to opioids, alcohol, nicotine, and caffeine but also to classes of medications such as beta-blockers, antidepressants, neuroleptics, and steroid-based medications. Despite their inclusion as diagnostic criteria, tolerance and withdrawal are not the defining characteristics of any SUD or addiction. As stated in the DSM-5, "individuals whose only symptoms are those that occur as a result of medical treatment (ie, tolerance and withdrawal as part of medical care when the medications are taken as prescribed) should not receive a diagnosis solely on the basis of these symptoms."[23]

This statement has profound implications for the diagnosis and treatment of SUDs, particularly opioid use disorder (OUD). Since the introduction of methadone in 1965 as a treatment of heroin addiction, followed by buprenorphine in 2002, opponents of these medical therapies have erroneously represented the use of opioid agonist medications as "substituting one addiction for another" and incompatible with recovery. Those in opposition have included some mutual support groups, drug court judges, operators of recovery homes and programs, and some state legislators and regulators. The stigma and discrimination that has followed methadone and buprenorphine as legitimate, well-researched, life-saving therapies for OUD has caused significant harm and continues to this day.

The opioid crisis of the last 2 decades brought a broader swath of health care professionals into this problem as well. As the epidemic burgeoned, initially driven by a surge in prescribed opioids, many physicians became increasingly concerned that the potential for tolerance to and withdrawal from opioids meant patients were developing addiction to these analgesics. Without adequate education on addiction or knowledge of the DSM-5 statements on physical dependence, prescribers abruptly stopped prescribing opioids to patients with chronic pain, sometimes harmfully labeling patients as "addicts" or worse. Not surprisingly, stigmatizing labels in medicine are associated with poorer patient outcomes.

## DISCUSSION

In addition to an evolution in research and diagnosis, several events over the past 20 years have propelled a shift away from criminalization of addiction and a return to acknowledging and addressing it as a medical condition. Terminology and definitions continue to play a role in the understanding and approach to those with the disease.

In 2000, the federal government passed the Drug Addiction Treatment Act of 2000 (DATA 2000), overturning the Harrison Narcotic Tax Act of 1914 after 86 years. DATA 2000, and subsequent revisions, allow office-based practitioners meeting certain qualifications to prescribe an approved opioid agonist medication to patients with OUD outside of the tightly regulated opioid treatment program system established in 1972 for methadone. In 2002, the Food and Drug Administration approved buprenorphine, a partial opioid agonist, for the treatment of OUD.

These events brought about new nomenclature. Office-based opioid treatment became OBOT, referring to not only ambulatory OUD treatment in a general medical or specialty practice but also an accredited type of specialty treatment program by the Commission on Accreditation of Rehabilitation Facilities.[41] Terminology that previously included only references to methadone, such as methadone maintenance treatment, evolved into medication-assisted treatment (MAT) and medication-assisted recovery and now medications for opioid use disorder (MOUD). The DSM-5 added the concept of remission to describe cessation of signs and symptoms of an SUD over specified lengths of time, allowing for medications that cause physical dependence as part of the definition.

Recovery is a related term that has proliferated along with societal acceptance of addiction as a treatable, chronic disease. Recovery is less well defined than remission, in large part due to its deep roots and long history in communities of people with shared lived experience. As physicians and organized medicine hastily retreated from addiction in the 1920s and 1930s, the movement of mutual aid and support grew more prominent and structured; this included the founding of Alcoholics Anonymous (AA) in 1935 and the printing of a related book ("The Big Book") in 1939. Since that time, other mutual aid societies have emerged with different groups of focus, philosophies, and principles, but all based on a core concept of people who share lived experience helping and supporting each other. Recovery is the hoped-for result of this support. Various entities have attempted to define recovery, particularly for research purposes, and this has proved challenging. As a longitudinal, multilayered, multidimensional phenomenon, individual stories of addiction recovery differ sufficiently to make standardization difficult. In 2010, the federal Substance Abuse and Mental Health Administration (SAMHSA) convened a stakeholder group to develop a common, unified working definition of recovery from addiction or mental illness that still stands (see Sidebar).

The SAMHSA stakeholder group arose from a much larger, multiyear national initiative on recovery-oriented systems of care (ROSC) begun in 2005.[42] This effort coincided with growing public and political pressure to respond to the opioid-related overdose deaths affecting suburban, White communities historically not affected by opioids. The ROSC initiative explicitly called for stigma reduction as a major area for activity. Although the inequity with earlier epidemics that predominantly affected communities of color is stark, a response based on a public health approach furthered the shift away from criminalization.

The ROSC initiative promoted treatment approaches that mirrored other modern chronic disease models such as that for diabetes. Importantly, it also dovetailed with federal efforts to integrate behavioral health and general medical care. The ROSC model, arguably more than any other national effort, fostered a shift from an acute care model of addiction treatment to one that encompasses the continuum of services from prevention to early intervention/harm reduction, treatment, and recovery. Its elements helped form the current principles and treatment approaches for people with SUDs. These principles recognize the value of multidisciplinary teams, including physicians, other practitioners, nurses, behavioral health professionals, and peers. Evidence-based treatment has deliberately moved away from ineffective punitive, paternalistic, and judgmental approaches. Instead, as with other chronic diseases, best practice involves individualized, patient-centered, comprehensive, continuous care using motivational interviewing techniques and collaborative decision-making. Research also supports trauma-informed and strengths-based approaches as standards of care.

Based on the strength of the evidence, entities such as the National Academies of Medicine and SAMHSA promote the chronic disease model of addiction, including the incorporation of opioid agonist medications as standard of care for treatment of OUD.[43,44] More precise, nonjudgmental language that best reflects current research and generally accepted medical practice follows. Just as medical terminology does not describe taking insulin for diabetes as "insulin-assisted diabetes treatment," medicine should avoid similar phrases in addiction care. Therefore, "medications for opioid use disorder" (MOUD) and "medications for addiction treatment" (MAT) replace "medication-assisted treatment." More precise language is not only accurate but also acknowledges the availability of effective pharmacotherapies for alcohol and tobacco use disorders. Stigmatizing terms such as "clean" and "dirty" to describe people with addiction or drug test results are out of favor. No health professional describes a patient with controlled hypertension as "clean" or a HbgA1C of 12 as "dirty." The highest levels of government, including the Office of National Drug Control Policy, and the media have recognized the devastating impact of stigmatizing addiction terminology and offered alternatives.[45,46]

Some of these changes have not been without controversy even within the addiction field. Concerns focus on medication-only approaches, particularly for severe SUDs, given that no medication alone addresses all comorbidities or the social determinants of health that complicate the development and experience of addiction. Instead, patients may need multimodal interventions that take a holistic approach to remission and recovery; incorporate a long-term, continuity of care view; and account for individual trajectories of disease. To avoid repeating the mistakes of the past, this will mean not only change in language but also change at all levels of medical education, health services, and collaborations.

## SUMMARY

Addiction is a complex disease for a complex time; treatments, policies, and public health approaches need to match.

## CLINICS CARE POINTS

This begins with the health care system embracing scientific understanding of addiction as a treatable, chronic medical condition, recognizing substance use disorders as the diagnostic spectrum for the disease, and supporting evidence-based identification, treatment, and recovery practices. Health care practitioners should recall that tolerance and withdrawal alone do not characterize the disease or diagnosis. In treating patients with a substance use disorder, attention to social determinants of health and application of medically oriented approaches and terminology are critical for optimal outcomes.

## DISCLOSURE

The author has nothing to disclose.

## SIDEBAR

Recovery: a process of change through which individuals improve their health and wellness, live a self-directed life, and strive to reach their full potential.

Source: Substance Abuse and Mental Health Services Administration. https://www.samhsa.gov/find-help/recovery

## REFERENCES

1. Nathan PE, Conrad M, Skinstad AH. History of the concept of addiction. Annu Rev Clin Psychol 2016;12:29–51.

2. Olsen Y, Sharfstein JM. The opioid epidemic: what everyone needs to know. New York, NY: Oxford University Press; 2019. p. 3.

3. Biondich AS, Joslin JD. Coca: the history and medical significance of an ancient andean tradition. Emerg Med Int 2016;2016:4048764.

4. Gussow L. Opium, from ancient sumeria to paracelsus to kerouac. Emerg Med News 2013;35(4):25.

5. Rosenthal RJ, Faris SB. The etymology and early history of 'addiction'. Addict Res Theor 2019;27(5):437–49.

6. White W. The seeds of addiction medicine & personal recovery movements. In: Slaying the dragon. The history of addiction treatment and recovery in America. 2nd edition. Bloomington, IL: Chestnut Health Systems/Lighthouse Institute; 2014. p. 1–8.

7. Musto DF. The American disease. In: Origins of narcotic control. 3rd edition. New York, NY: Oxford University Press; 1999.

8. White W. The rise and fall of inebriate homes and asylums. In: Slaying the dragon. The history of addiction treatment and recovery in America. 2nd edition. Bloomington, IL: Chestnut Health Systems/Lighthouse Institute; 2014. p. 33.

9. Crothers TD. Chapter III. Opium inebriety. In: The drug habits and their treatment. A clinical summary of some of the general facts recorded in practice. Chicago: G.P. Engelhard & Company; 1902. p. 61–74.

10. White W. The treatment of addiction to narcotics and other drugs: 1880-1925. In: Slaying the dragon. The history of addiction treatment and recovery in America. 2nd edition. Bloomington, IL: Chestnut Health Systems/Lighthouse Institute; 2014. p. 152.

11. ABMS officially recognizes addiction medicine as a subspecialty. 2016. Available at: https://www.abms.org/news-events/abms-officially-recognizes-addiction-medicine-as-a-subspecialty. Accessed April 24, 2021.

12. Kranzler HR, Li TK. What is addiction? Alcohol Res Health 2008;31(2):93–5.

13. Ashford RD, Brown AM, McDaniel J, et al. Biased labels: an experimental study of language and stigma among individuals in recovery and health professionals. Subst Use Misuse 2019;54(8):1376–84.

14. Foddy B. Addiction and its sciences-philosophy. Addiction 2011;106(1):25–31.

15. Scully JL. What is a disease? EMBO Rep 2004;5(7):650–3.

16. Gutierrez J, Devia C, Weiss L, et al. Health, community, and spirituality: evaluation of a multicultural faith-based diabetes prevention program. Diabetes Educ 2014; 40(2):214–22.

17. Burlacu A, Artene B, Nistor I, et al. Religiosity, spirituality and quality of life of dialysis patients: a systematic review. Int Urol Nephrol 2019;51(5):839–50.

18. Hemmati R, Bidel Z, Nazarzadeh M, et al. Religion, spirituality and risk of coronary heart disease: a matched case-control study and meta-analysis. J Relig Health 2019;58(4):1203–16.

19. Miller-keane encyclopedia and dictionary of medicine, nursing, and allied health. 7th edition. Available at: https://medical-dictionary.thefreedictionary.com/disease. Accessed February 18, 2019.

20. Farlex partner medical dictionary. 2012. Available at: https://medical-dictionary.thefreedictionary.com/disease. Accessed February 18, 2019.

21. The American Heritage® medical dictionary. 2007. Available at: https://medical-dictionary.thefreedictionary.com/disease. Accessed February 18, 2019.

22. Collins dictionary of medicine. 2004. Available at: https://medical-dictionary.thefreedictionary.com/disease. Accessed February 18, 2019.

23. American Psychiatric Association. Substance-related and addictive disorders. In: Diagnostic and statistical manual of mental disorders: DSM-5. Arlington, VA: American Psychiatric Association; 2013. p. 481–589.

24. U.S. Department of health and human services (HHS), office of the Surgeon general, facing addiction in America: the Surgeon General's report on alcohol, drugs, and health. Washington, DC: HHS; 2016.

25. Volkow ND, Koob GF. Drug addiction: the neurobiology of motivation gone awry. In: Miller SC, Fiellin DA, Rosenthal RN, et al, editors. The ASAM principles of addiction medicine. 6th edition. Philadelphia: Wolters Kluwer; 2019. p. 11–4.

26. American Society of Addiction Medicine. Definition of addiction. 2019. Available at: https://www.asam.org/Quality-Science/definition-of-addiction. Accessed February 22, 2021.

27. U.S. Department of health and human services (HHS), office of the surgeon general, facing addiction in America: the Surgeon General's report on alcohol, drugs, and health. Washington, DC: HHS; 2016. p. 1–6.

28. Winstanley EL, Steinwachs DM, Ensminger ME, et al. The association of self-reported neighborhood disorganization and social capital with adolescent alcohol and drug use, dependence, and access to treatment. Drug Alcohol Depend 2008;92(1–3):173–82.

29. Slutske WS, Deutsch AR, Piasecki TM. Neighborhood density of alcohol outlets moderates genetic and environmental influences on alcohol problems. Addiction 2019;114(5):815–22.

30. Manhica H, Straatmann VS, Lundin A, et al. Association between poverty exposure during childhood and adolescence, and drug use disorders and drug-related crimes later in life. Addiction 2021;6(7):1747–56.

31. Kerr WC, Kaplan MS, Huguet N, et al. Economic recession, alcohol, and suicide rates: comparative effects of poverty, foreclosure, and job loss. Am J Prev Med 2017;52(4):469–75.

32. Dube SR, Felitti VJ, Dong M, et al. Childhood abuse, neglect, and household dysfunction and the risk of illicit drug use: the adverse childhood experiences study. Pediatrics 2003;111(3):564–72.

33. Gerrard M, Stock ML, Roberts ME, et al. Coping with racial discrimination: the role of substance use. Psychol Addict Behav 2012;26(3):550–60.

34. Restar AJ, Jin H, Ogunbajo A, et al. Prevalence and risk factors of nonmedical prescription opioid use among transgender girls and young women. JAMA Netw Open 2020;3(3):e201015.

35. Vu M, Li J, Haardörfer R, et al. Mental health and substance use among women and men at the intersections of identities and experiences of discrimination: insights from the intersectionality framework. BMC Public Health 2019;19(1):108.

36. Mendoza S, Rivera AS, Hansen HB. Re-racialization of addiction and the redistribution of blame in the white opioid epidemic. Med Anthropol Q 2019;33(2):242–62.

37. Cadet JL. Epigenetics of stress, addiction, and resilience: therapeutic implications. Mol Neurobiol 2016;53(1):545–60.

38. Juster RP, Russell JJ, Almeida D, et al. Allostatic load and comorbidities: a mitochondrial, epigenetic, and evolutionary perspective. Dev Psychopathol 2016;28(4pt1):1117–46.

39. National Institutes on Drug Abuse (NIDA). Drug misuse and addiction. 2020. Available at: https://www.drugabuse.gov/publications/drugs-brains-behavior-science-addiction/drug-misuse-addiction. Accessed April 4, 2021.

40. O'Brien CP. Chapter 24: drug use disorders and addiction. In: Brunton LL, Hilal-Dandan R, Knollmann BC, editors. Goodman & Gilman's: the pharmacological basis of therapeutics. 13th edition. New York, NY: McGraw-Hill Education; 2018.
41. Commission on Accreditation of Rehabilitation Facilities. New CARF standards address variability of care in office-based opioid treatment settings. 2019. Available at: http://www.carf.org/New-OBOT-standards. Accessed April 4, 2021.
42. Substance Abuse and Mental Health Services Administration. Recovery-Oriented Systems of Care (ROSC) resource guide. 2010. Available at: https://www.samhsa.gov/sites/default/files/rosc_resource_guide_book.pdf. Accessed April 4, 2021.
43. National Academies of Sciences, Engineering, and Medicine. Medications for opioid use disorder save lives. Washington, DC: The National Academies Press; 2019. Available at: https://www.nap.edu/catalog/25310/medications-for-opioid-use-disorder-save-lives. Accessed February 22, 2021.
44. Substance Abuse and Mental Health Services Administration. Medications for opioid use disorder. In: Treatment improvement protocol (TIP) series 63, full document. HHS Publication No. (SMA) 185063FULLDOC. Rockville, MD: Substance Abuse and Mental Health Services Administration; 2018.
45. Botticelli M. Office of the National Drug Control Policy. Changing the language of addiction. 2017. Available at: https://obamawhitehouse.archives.gov/sites/whitehouse.gov/files/images/Memo%20-%20Changing%20Federal%20Terminology%20Regrading%20Substance%20Use%20and%20Substance%20Use%20Disorders.pdf. Accessed February 22, 2021.
46. Aliferis L. In stylebook, AP directs it reporters: addiction is a 'disease'. California Health Care Foundation; 2017. Available at: https://www.chcf.org/blog/in-stylebook-ap-directs-its-reporters-addiction-is-a-disease. Accessed April 24, 2021.

# Screening for Unhealthy Alcohol and Drug Use in General Medicine Settings

Jennifer McNeely, MD, MS[a,b,*], Leah Hamilton, PhD[a,c]

## KEYWORDS

- Alcohol screening • Drug screening • Primary care • Unhealthy alcohol use
- Unhealthy drug use • Substance use disorders • Implementation

## KEY POINTS

- Guidelines recommend screening adult primary care patients for alcohol and drug use.
- Validated screening tools can quickly and accurately identify unhealthy alcohol and drug use.
- Screening is feasible to incorporate into routine primary care visits, with the thoughtful implementation of strategies that increase the adoption and quality screening in practice
- Patient self-administered screening, integration with electronic health records, and screening during routine primary care visits are recommended.
- Alcohol screening is a quality measure for hospitals, and should consider the higher severity and complexity of substance use among inpatient populations.

## INTRODUCTION

Alcohol and drug use are among the top 10 causes of preventable death in the United States.[1] Alcohol-related deaths have doubled in the past two decades, and now account for more than 72,000 deaths per year.[2] Annual drug overdose deaths have now overtaken alcohol deaths, and are expected to exceed 92,000 in the current year; the highest number ever recorded.[3] The prevalence of substance use and related morbidity has increased with the COVID-19 pandemic, and is likely related to widespread stress, financial problems, social isolation, disruptions to health care and mental health services, and changes in the drug supply.[4–7]

[a] Section on Alcohol, Tobacco, and Drug Use, Department of Population Health, NYU Grossman School of Medicine, 180 Madison Avenue, 17th Floor, New York, NY 10016, USA; [b] Department of Medicine, Division of General Internal Medicine and Clinical Innovation, NYU Grossman School of Medicine, New York, NY 10016, USA; [c] Kaiser Permanente Washington Health Research Institute, 1730 Minor Avenue, Seattle, WA 98101, USA
* Corresponding author.
*E-mail address:* jennifer.mcneely@nyulangone.org

Med Clin N Am 106 (2022) 13–28
https://doi.org/10.1016/j.mcna.2021.08.002
0025-7125/22/© 2021 Elsevier Inc. All rights reserved.

In the general population, alcohol and drug use exist on a spectrum ranging from low-risk use to severe substance use disorders (**Fig. 1**). "Unhealthy substance use" is defined here as any use of alcohol and/or drugs that increases the risk of experiencing adverse health consequences, the severity of which generally increases with the amount and frequency of consumption.[8] Unhealthy substance use includes risky use, problem use, and substance use disorders. An individual with risky use is not experiencing consequences of use, but the quantity or pattern of substance use places them at risk for experiencing negative health effects including traumatic injury, direct health effects of the substances used, poor treatment of other medical conditions, and overdose.[9–11] Those with problem use have at least one active problem related to their substance use, but do not meet criteria for a substance use disorder. Substance use disorders are defined by specific diagnostic criteria, and are classified in the Diagnostic and Statistical Manual, 5th Edition (DSM-5), based on the level of symptoms as mild, moderate, and severe.[12] Individuals with substance use disorders are experiencing 2 or more symptoms (including problems related to use, difficulty controlling use, and physical tolerance or withdrawal) in the past 12 months.

Because tobacco screening and treatment are already integrated into many medical settings, the focus here is on screening for unhealthy use of alcohol and other drugs. For alcohol, although it is now accepted that any level of alcohol use poses some health risk, unhealthy alcohol use refers to consumption that exceeds the daily or weekly guideline-recommended limits. The limit for women and men aged 65 years or older is no more than 3 drinks in a day or 7 drinks per week, whereas for men younger than 65 years, it is no more than 4 drinks in a day or 14 drinks per week.[13] For illicit drugs and cannabis, health risks vary widely depending on the type of drug used, and similar consumption cutoffs have not been established. Presently, any use of illicit drugs or cannabis is classified as unhealthy drug use. Although the actual risk depends on the substance and pattern of use, there is no guideline-recommended "safe" level of drug use, and so for the purposes of screening, any use is considered unhealthy. For prescription medications with potential for misuse, any nonmedical use (ie, use of prescribed medication at increased dose or frequency,

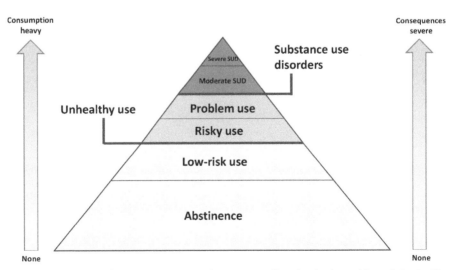

**Fig. 1.** Spectrum of substance use. SUD, substance use disorder. (*Adapted from* Saitz R. Clinical practice. Unhealthy alcohol use. N Engl J Med 2005;352(6):596-607.

or for reasons other than prescribed), or use of medications that were not prescribed, is considered unhealthy because of the risk of health problems and potential for substance use disorders related to over-use.

In the general population, at least 20% of adults have unhealthy alcohol or drug use.[14,15] Among the population with unhealthy use, most individuals have risky or problem use, and not a substance use disorder. In medical populations, the prevalence of unhealthy use tends to be higher, but it varies depending on the clinical setting. In primary care, 20% to 30% of patients can be expected to have risky or problem use of alcohol, whereas approximately 5% to 10% of patients have a substance use disorder.[8,16,17] In the hospital, the severity of use is generally higher, with rates of alcohol use disorder ranging as high as 19% to 50%, and rates of drug use disorders up to 12% to 15%.[18–21]

Most individuals with unhealthy alcohol or drug use, including those with substance use disorders, do not actively seek substance use treatment.[15] Therefore, health care contacts, and primary care visits in particular, may be the only opportunity to identify unhealthy use and provide interventions to prevent worsening substance use–related problems or offer treatment. Yet, most clinicians are not aware of their patients' substance use.[22–24] Screening patients for alcohol and drug use is thus a necessary first step toward transforming health care contacts into opportunities to identify and reduce the negative impact of unhealthy substance use on individuals who use alcohol and drugs.

## DISCUSSION
### Alcohol and Drug Screening Guidelines

The United States Preventive Services Task Force (USPSTF) recommends screening for both alcohol and drug use in adult primary care patients, with a grade B recommendation.[25,26] Alcohol screening has been a guideline-recommended practice for more than two decades, and ranks as the third highest prevention priority for adults in the United States.[27,28] The USPSTF recommends alcohol screening followed by brief counseling in primary care, based on a large evidence base supporting brief interventions for unhealthy alcohol use.[29]

The drug screening recommendation reflects a more recent change (in 2020) by the USPSTF, which had found insufficient evidence in its prior reviews. Because the effectiveness of brief interventions for reducing drug use has not been established, the drug screening recommendation includes the qualifier that "screening should be implemented when services for accurate diagnosis, effective treatment, and appropriate care can be offered or referred."[25,30] Most primary care practices should have the capacity to offer this care, as they do for other complex conditions.[31] Namely, before screening the primary practice should be prepared to assess the severity of use (which can be done with standardized questionnaires), and offer treatment or refer to specialty care for patients who are found to have a substance use disorder or to be at high risk.

### Goals of Screening in Health Care Settings

The goals of screening for substance use as part of medical care can vary depending on the practice setting and resources.

### Informing medical care

For primary care clinicians, perhaps the most important reason for identifying unhealthy alcohol or drug use is to inform a patient's medical care. Substance use can significantly affect disease processes, response to treatment, and exposure to health risks.[2,9–11,32] Identifying unhealthy substance use is necessary for making accurate diagnoses of other medical and psychiatric conditions, and alerts providers to associated health risks (eg, overdose, liver disease) and common comorbid conditions (eg, depression, hypertension). It also has important implications for patient safety, such as alerting providers to medication interactions, or identifying those who could experience acute substance withdrawal symptoms during hospitalization. Knowledge of substance use should also inform priorities for preventive care, which can include screening for viral hepatitis or HIV, depression, pulmonary or liver disease, and other conditions that are more prevalent in individuals with unhealthy alcohol or drug use. Similar to knowing about a patient's past medical history, family history, or social determinants of health, knowing about a patient's substance use helps clinicians formulate effective patient-centered treatment plans.

### Identifying the need for intervention

Another distinct goal is to identify patients who would benefit from interventions to reduce their consumption or are candidates for substance use disorder treatment. Evidence-based interventions can be offered in primary care, and potentially in other health care settings, and include brief motivational counseling interventions for moderate-risk alcohol use and pharmacotherapy for opioid and alcohol use disorders.[14,29,33,34]

### Informing population health

Health care providers and health systems need to understand the prevalence and severity of substance use to better meet the needs of their patient populations. The nature and severity of substance use differ depending on geography and characteristics of the population served, and screening can inform the design of clinical and social services that are most needed.

### Engaging patients and reducing stigma

If done with knowledge and sensitivity, screening can communicate to patients that substance use is a common treatable health condition rather than a moral failing, thus reducing stigma and improving the patient-clinician relationship. Evidence suggests that screening is generally well accepted by patients, and considered by them to be an indicator of higher-quality care.[35,36]

## SCREENING TOOLS FOR MEDICAL SETTINGS

For the purpose of this overview, screening refers to the use of standardized questionnaires to ask individuals about their substance use. Although laboratory tests may detect the presence of substances used very recently (typically hours or $\leq 4$ days after the last use), these tests do not provide the information about quantity, frequency, or problems related to use that is needed to inform medical care. Because screening depends on collecting precise self-reported information from individuals, validated screening questionnaires should be used, and the questions need to be delivered exactly as they were validated. Screening instruments that can be recommended for alcohol and drug screening in medical settings are listed in **Table 1**. Although not an exhaustive list, it includes instruments that are most widely used and are feasible to implement in the context of routine care.[37] All have been validated in adult medical patients, and their performance characteristics are summarized in **Table 2**. The selection of specific instruments should also be informed by the goals of screening, mode of administration, and resources available. Frequently, a 2-step

**Table 1**
**Recommended instruments for use in medical settings to screen for alcohol and drug use in adults**

| Instrument, References | Substances Included | Identifies | No. of Items, Time to Complete (Approximate), Format |
|---|---|---|---|
| Brief screeners for identification of unhealthy use | | | |
| SISQ-Alcohol[38,44] | Alcohol | Unhealthy use | 1 item; 1 min Interviewer or self-administered via electronic app or on paper |
| SISQ-Drug[43,44] | Drugs | Unhealthy use | 1 item; 1 min Interviewer or self-administered via electronic app or on paper |
| SUBS[45] | Tobacco, alcohol, illicit drugs, Rx drugs | Unhealthy use | 4 items; 2 min Interviewer or self-administered via electronic app or on paper |
| Identification of unhealthy use and level of risk | | | |
| AUDIT-C[a,e39,75] | Alcohol | Unhealthy use, level of risk | 3 items; 1–2 min |
| AUDIT[b,e13] | Alcohol | Unhealthy use, level of risk | 10 items; 3 min Interviewer or self-administered |
| TAPS Tool[c,e47] | Tobacco, alcohol, Rx drugs, illicit drugs; identifies specific drug classes | Unhealthy use (TAPS-1); Problem use or SUD (TAPS-2) | 4–25 items; 2–4 min, depending on no. of substances used Interviewer or self-administered on computer/tablet |
| DAST-10[d43] | Drugs | Unhealthy use, level of risk | 10 items; 10 min or less Interviewer or self-administered on paper |

[a] https://cde.drugabuse.gov/sites/nida_cde/files/Audit-C_2014Mar24.pdf.
[b] https://pubs.niaaa.nih.gov/publications/Practitioner/CliniciansGuide2005/guide.pdf.
[c] https://www.drugabuse.gov/taps/
[d] https://cde.drugabuse.gov/sites/nida_cde/files/DrugAbuseScreeningTest_2014Mar24.pdf.
[e] Available in languages other than English.[75,76]

approach is used, with a short screener administered to all patients, and followed by a brief assessment for risk stratification if screening is positive (**Fig. 2**).

### Alcohol Screening Tools

The briefest approach to screening for alcohol use is the validated single-item screening question (*SISQ-Alc*), recommended by the National Institute on Alcohol Abuse and Alcoholism (NIAAA).[38] The SISQ-alcohol can be interviewer- or self-administered and asks about binge drinking in the past year to identify unhealthy alcohol use. Although it is possible for patients to use more alcohol than the guideline-recommended limits even in the absence of binge drinking, validation studies have demonstrated good sensitivity.[38]

**Table 2**
**Performance of alcohol and drug screening instruments in validation studies**

| Instrument | Identification of | Performance (95% Confidence Interval) | Study Population |
|---|---|---|---|
| SISQ-Alcohol | Unhealthy alcohol use | Interviewer-administered[38] Sensitivity: 0.82 (0.73, 0.89) Specificity: 0.79 (0.731, 0.84) Self-administered[44] Sensitivity: 0.73 (0.65, 0.80) Specificity: 0.85 (0.80, 0.89) | Interviewer administered: 286 adult primary care patients Self-administered: 459 adult primary care patients from 2 clinics |
| SISQ-Drug | Unhealthy drug use | Interviewer-administered[43] Sensitivity: 0.94 (0.87, 0.97) Specificity: 0.91 (0.86, 0.95) Self-administered[44] Sensitivity: 0.71 (0.62, 0.79) Specificity: 0.94 (0.91, 0.97) | Interviewer administered: 286 adult primary care patients Self-administered: 459 adult primary care patients from 2 clinics |
| SUBS | Unhealthy tobacco, alcohol, or drug use (illicit or nonmedical prescription drug use) | Tobacco[45] Sensitivity: 0.98 (0.94, 1.0) Specificity: 0.96 (0.92, 0.98) Alcohol Sensitivity: 0.85 (0.79, 0.90) Specificity: 0.77 (0.73, 0.81) Drugs[a] Sensitivity: 0.83 (0.76, 0.88) Specificity: 0.91 (0.88, 0.94) | 586 adult primary care patients from 2 clinics |
| AUDIT-C | Unhealthy alcohol use, high-risk use | Unhealthy use[39] Sensitivity: Men: 0.86 Women: 0.73 Specificity: Men: 0.89 Women: 0.91 Alcohol use disorder Sensitivity: Men: 0.88 Women: 0.87 Specificity: Men: 0.75 Women: 0.85 | 392 male and 927 female adult primary care patients. Results are shown for scores of $\geq 4$ for men and $\geq 3$ for women.[b] |

(continued on next page)

**Table 2**
*(continued)*

| Instrument | Identification of | Performance (95% Confidence Interval) | Study Population |
|---|---|---|---|
| AUDIT | Unhealthy alcohol use, level of risk | Unhealthy use[77]<br>  Sensitivity: 0.64–0.86<br>  Specificity: 0.74–0.94<br>  AUC<br>Alcohol use disorder[77]<br>  Sensitivity: 0.72–0.83<br>  Specificity: 0.67–0.88 | Unhealthy use results from 3 trials conducted in US primary care settings (total N = 2782 adults), using AUDIT cutoffs of ≥3, 4, or 5<br>Alcohol use disorder results from 2 trials conducted in US primary care settings (total N = 1958 adults) using AUDIT cutoff of ≥5 |
| TAPS Tool | Problem use of tobacco, alcohol, and 6 classes of illicit and prescription drugs | Tobacco[47] c<br>  Sensitivity: 0.93 (0.90, 0.95)<br>  Specificity: 0.87 (0.85, 0.89)<br>Alcohol<br>  Sensitivity: 0.74 (0.70, 0.78)<br>  Specificity: 0.79 (0.76, 0.81)<br>Cannabis<br>  Sensitivity: 0.82 (0.76, 0.87)<br>  Specificity: 0.93 (0.91, 0.94)<br>Cocaine, methamphetamine<br>  Sensitivity: 0.68 (0.59, 0.77)<br>  Specificity: 0.99 (0.98, 0.99)<br>Heroin<br>  Sensitivity: 0.78 (0.67, 0.87)<br>  Specificity: 1.00 (0.99, 1.00)<br>Prescription opioids<br>  Sensitivity: 0.71 (0.58, 0.82)<br>  Specificity: 0.99 (0.98, 0.99)<br>Sedatives<br>  Sensitivity: 0.63 (0.47, 0.78)<br>  Specificity: 0.99 (0.98, 0.99) | 2000 adult primary care patients from 5 primary care clinics |

*(continued on next page)*

| Table 2 (continued) | | | |
|---|---|---|---|
| Instrument | Identification of | Performance (95% Confidence Interval) | Study Population |
| DAST-10 | Unhealthy drug use | Unhealthy use[43] Sensitivity: 0.87 (0.79, 0.92) Specificity: 0.93 (0.88, 0.96) | 286 adult primary care patients |

[a] Results shown for any drug use (including illicit and/or prescription drugs). When examined as separate categories, results were as follows: illicit drugs sensitivity 0.81 (95% CI 0.74, 0.87) and specificity 0.97 (0.95, 0.98); prescription drugs sensitivity 0.56 (95% CI 0.41, 0.69) and specificity 0.92 (95% CI 0.89, 0.94).
[b] In another study with 393 female VA patients, the AUDIT-C had a sensitivity and specificity of 0.81 and 0.89, respectively, for unhealthy alcohol use and 0.92 and 0.78, respectively, for alcohol use disorder at a cutoff of $\geq 2$.[42]
[c] Results are for the interviewer-administered version; results were similar for the self-administered TAPS Tool.[47]

To simultaneously screen and assess the level of risk in patients who use alcohol, clinicians can use the 10-item *AUDIT*, developed by the World Health Organization for alcohol use screening in medical settings, or the briefer *AUDIT-C* tool that consists of just the first 3 items of the AUDIT.[29,39,40] The 3-item *AUDIT-C* performs as well as the full 10-item *AUDIT* instrument for identifying unhealthy alcohol use in studies conducted among primary care patients in the United States, and has been implemented throughout the Veterans Health Administration.[39,41,42] However, in settings that have the resources to administer the full *AUDIT*, providers may benefit from the additional information it provides to guide their brief interventions or treatment.

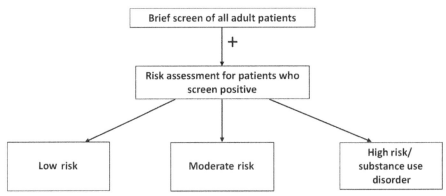

**Fig. 2.** Substance use levels of risk. *Low risk*—Patient is abstinent or uses substances in a way that is not currently associated with negative health consequences or other problems, such as alcohol consumption that does not exceed guideline-recommended levels or occasional cannabis use. *Moderate risk*—Patient is at risk for and may already be experiencing negative health consequences or other problems, such as elevated blood pressure related to alcohol use; atypical chest pain related to cocaine use; or family problems or poor work performance related to opioid use. *High risk*—Patient likely has a substance use disorder, is likely experiencing substance-related health or other types of problems (eg, alcohol use–related cirrhosis or consequences such as separation from family or loss of employment), and is engaging in continued or escalating use despite substance use–related negative consequences. (*Adapted from* [Saitz R. 2005].)

## Drug Screening Tools

Drug screening can also be accomplished with a single-item screening question (*SISQ-Drug*), which can be self-administered and asks about illicit and nonmedical use of prescription drugs.[43,44] A positive response identifies the presence of any unhealthy drug use in the past year, but does not separate illicit drug use from nonmedical use of prescription drugs. An alternative screener, the Substance Use Brief Screen (*SUBS*), elicits information about past-year tobacco, alcohol, illicit drugs, and nonmedical prescription drug use through a single 4-item instrument that is self-administered electronically or on paper.[45]

Assessment of the level of risk for drug use can be accomplished with the 10-item Drug Abuse Screening Test (DAST-10).[43,46] A drawback to the DAST-10 is that it does not identify specific drug classes, which limits its utility in clinical practice. For example, a patient with moderate-risk cannabis use alone could have the same DAST-10 score as a patient with moderate-risk use of opioids and sedatives.

A more optimal approach may be to use a substance-specific screener such as the Tobacco, Alcohol, Prescription Medication, and Other Substance (*TAPS*) tool.[47] The TAPS tool is a screening and assessment instrument that can identify 7 classes of drugs, plus tobacco and alcohol use. It is a 2-part screener, with TAPS-1 identifying any unhealthy use,[48] and TAPS-2 identifying current problem use or substance use disorder.[47] The TAPS is validated in an electronic, patient self-administered format and a more traditional interviewer-administered questionnaire.[47,49] Though originally developed for primary care, the TAPS has also been used in acute care settings such as emergency departments (EDs) and hospital inpatient units.

## Special Considerations for Screening

### Cannabis

Cannabis is the most frequently used drug in the US general population, and among primary care patients.[15] Patients who use cannabis for medical purposes or live in a state where recreational use is legal may perceive cannabis use as being akin to tobacco or alcohol use—that is, carrying some health risks, but not of the same severity as use of other drugs. For these patients, screening instruments that ask about cannabis as a subset of all drug use can seem inappropriate or stigmatizing, and a cannabis-specific screener could facilitate more accurate reporting.[50] One promising single-item screening instrument question is "How often in the past year did you use marijuana?," which was adapted from the SISQ-Drug.[43,51] This screening question, which is undergoing validation, was used in a Washington State primary care study in which 15.8% of patients screened positive for cannabis use.

### Nonmedical use of prescription drugs

Recognition of the potential harms of opioid prescribing has driven interest in screening for nonmedical use of prescription drugs that have misuse potential (opioids, sedatives, and stimulants). Screeners such as the SUBS and TAPS tool include specific questions about nonmedical use, but generally have low sensitivity for identifying it. This may be due in part to confusion on the part of patients about what signifies nonmedical use, and to patients' discomfort with reporting misuse to the prescribing clinician.[52] Other screening tools have been developed specifically for patients who are being prescribed opioids, such as the Opioid Risk Tool (ORT) and the Current Opioid Misuse Measure (COMM), but these are not appropriate for general population screening.

### Screening in specific populations

Instruments available in languages other than English are indicated in **Table 1**. Although the USPSTF guidelines include pregnant women in their recommendation to screen adult primary care patients, screening during pregnancy must take into account the potential legal or social consequences of a positive screening result. The USPSTF currently considers there to be insufficient evidence to support screening of adolescents for alcohol or drug use, but adolescent screening instruments have been developed, and this remains an active area of research.[53]

### Assessment for Substance Use Disorder

For patients who screen positive for alcohol or drug use with a screening score or clinical presentation indicating high-risk or daily use, further assessment for symptoms of substance use disorder is needed to guide clinical care and facilitate treatment. Because primary care clinicians may not have the training or time to conduct a diagnostic interview, symptom checklists have been developed based on the DSM-5 to identify alcohol or drug use disorders.[50,54,55]

### Implementation of Screening in Practice

Despite guidelines from the USPSTF, and federal investments (in the United States) in large-scale "screening, brief intervention, and referral to treatment (SBIRT) programs,"[56] the adoption of screening in practice remains low. In busy primary care practices, the time required for screening, challenges of integrating it into the clinical workflow, poor quality of screening, and lack of clinician knowledge have been identified as the primary barriers.[57,58] Yet, there are examples of successful implementation, including the system-wide adoption of alcohol screening in the US Veterans Health Administration, which screens over 90% of ambulatory care patients for alcohol use,[41] and high screening rates for alcohol and/or drug use that have been achieved in some private health systems.[55,59] Implementation approaches that can facilitate the adoption of screening and enhance its quality are discussed here. Because substance use is stigmatized, it is essential to implement screening thoughtfully, including communicating to patients the reasons for screening, its importance for informing their medical care, lack of judgment or blame, and confidentiality of screening results.[58]

### Self-administered screening

Self-administered screening approaches can increase patient comfort and facilitate more accurate reporting,[59–61] while ensuring fidelity,[50,62,63] and reducing the burden on staff. An implementation feasibility study in 6 primary care clinics found that the one clinic that used a staff-administered screening approach had a screen-positive rate of less than 2% for unhealthy alcohol use, whereas those delivering the same screening instrument with a patient self-administered approach had screen-positive rates of 15% to 37%.[59] Electronic screening tools have the potential to be self-administered online through a patient portal or on a tablet computer or kiosk in the clinic, which can save time in the clinic and facilitate the capture of screening results into the electronic health record (EHR).

### EHR integration

To inform clinical care, substance use information needs to be documented in EHRs, regularly updated, and visible at the point of care.[64] Documenting unhealthy substance use in "social history" fields is inappropriate for a medical condition, and doing so poses barriers to patient care by making the information more difficult to find and less actionable for medical providers. Although the strategy for integrating substance use screening will vary depending on the local EHR and clinical workflows,[65] practices should aim to include it alongside other health maintenance information, or in the patient's problem list.[64]

### Frequency and visit types to target for screening

Evidence is lacking about the optimal frequency of screening, but annual screening is often adopted to balance the need to regularly update substance use information with time and resource constraints.[29,54] Screening once a year was identified as a reasonable frequency in a Veterans Health Administration study, which found that the adjusted probability of converting from a negative to a positive screen 1 year later ranged from 2% to 38%, depending on patient characteristics.[66] In our 6-clinic implementation study, practices that offered screening once per year at any type of primary care visit achieved screening rates of 90% to 95%, whereas those targeting targeted only annual visit types had screening rates of 24% to 72%.[60]

### Screening for alcohol and drug use in the hospital

Screening for substance use might also be considered in the hospital setting, including the ED and on general medical or surgical inpatient units. Although ED and hospital patients are not included in the USPSTF alcohol or drug screening recommendations, screening for alcohol use was adopted in 2006 as a quality care measure by the Joint Commission, which is the major accrediting body for US hospitals,[67] and ED screening is recommended by the American College of Emergency Physicians.[68] Screening in the hospital setting should anticipate that a higher proportion of patients who screen positive will have more severe substance use, as well as complex psychiatric and medical comorbidities, in comparison to primary care.[67] Although prevalence may vary depending on the patient population, in one study, 81% of hospitalized patients with a positive alcohol screen were found to have alcohol use disorder.[21]

The goals of screening in the hospital setting may also differ from those in primary care. At minimum, hospitals should screen to identify inpatients at high risk for acute withdrawal, or for procedural complications related to their substance use. More optimally, screening in the hospital can identify patients with substance use disorders who need medications or linkage to ongoing treatment, as well as those with hazardous or harmful alcohol or drug use who could benefit from counseling and harm reduction interventions. ED and inpatient "screening, brief intervention, and referral to treatment (SBIRT) programs" have been adopted as a strategy for providing this care, but may not be sufficient.[69,70] More robust addiction consult services, which typically involve a team-based approach to managing patients in the hospital and engaging them in postdischarge treatment and harm reduction services, could be better suited to the needs of hospital patients with complex addiction.[71–74]

### SUMMARY

Substance use is a leading cause of morbidity and mortality that frequently goes unidentified and unaddressed in primary care. Guidelines recommend screening adult primary care patients for alcohol and drug use, and routine screening is an important component of high-quality clinical care. Brief screening and assessment tools accurately detect unhealthy alcohol and drug use, and their thoughtful implementation can facilitate the adoption and quality of screening in practice. Bringing well-informed discussions of substance use into the medical visit has the potential to reduce stigma, improve patient care, and increase access to essential treatment.

## CLINICS CARE POINTS

- Screening for alcohol and drug use should be part of routine primary care.
- Brief, validated screening tools should always be used.
- Quality of screening may be enhanced by using patient self-administered screening tools, offered once per year at any routine primary care visit.
- Substance use is stigmatized, and providers should approach screening and counseling with respect for patients and a focus on unhealthy substance use as an important medical problem.

## ACKNOWLEDGMENTS

The authors wish to thank Noa Appleton, MPH, for assistance in preparing the manuscript, and Katharine Bradley, MD, and Gwen Lapham, PhD, for their advice on the content.

## DISCLOSURE

Dr J. McNeely has served as a consultant to the National Committee for Quality Assurance (NCQA). Dr J. McNeely reports intellectual property for a "Substance Use Screening and Intervention Tool" that was developed with funds from the National Institute on Drug Abuse (R34DA040830) and is in the public domain. Drs L. Hamilton and J. McNeely were supported by National Institute on Drug Abuse/National Institutes of Health (NIDA/NIH) cooperative grant awards UG1DA013035 and UG1DA040314.

## REFERENCES

1. Mokdad AH, Marks JS, Stroup DF, et al. Actual causes of death in the United States, 2000. JAMA 2004;291(10):1238–45.
2. White AM, Castle IP, Hingson RW, et al. Using death certificates to explore changes in alcohol-related mortality in the United States, 1999 to 2017. Alcohol Clin Exp Res 2020;44(1):178–87.
3. Ahmad FB, Rossen LM, Sutton P. Provisional drug overdose death counts: National Center for Health Statistics. 2021. Available at: https://www.cdc.gov/nchs/nvss/vsrr/drug-overdose-data.htm. Accessed February 15, 2021.
4. Alexander GC, Stoller KB, Haffajee RL, et al. An epidemic in the midst of a pandemic: opioid use disorder and COVID-19. Ann Intern Med 2020;173(1):57–8.
5. CDC. Increase in Fatal drug overdoses across the United States driven by synthetic opioids before and during the COVID-19 pandemic. 2020. Contract No.: CDCHAN-00438.
6. Czeisler M, Lane RI, Petrosky E, et al. Mental health, substance use, and suicidal ideation during the COVID-19 pandemic - United States, June 24-30, 2020. MMWR Morb Mortal Wkly Rep 2020;69(32):1049–57.
7. Pollard MS, Tucker JS, Green HD Jr. Changes in adult alcohol use and consequences during the COVID-19 pandemic in the US. JAMA Netw Open 2020;3(9):e2022942.
8. Saitz R. Clinical practice. Unhealthy alcohol use. N Engl J Med 2005;352(6):596–607.
9. Mertens JR, Lu YW, Parthasarathy S, et al. Medical and psychiatric conditions of alcohol and drug treatment patients in an HMO: comparison with matched controls. Arch Intern Med 2003;163(20):2511–7.

10. Malta M, Strathdee SA, Magnanini MM, et al. Adherence to antiretroviral therapy for human immunodeficiency virus/acquired immune deficiency syndrome among drug users: a systematic review. Addiction 2008;103(8):1242–57.
11. Danaei G, Ding EL, Mozaffarian D, et al. The preventable causes of death in the United States: comparative risk assessment of dietary, lifestyle, and metabolic risk factors. PLoS Med 2009;6(4):e1000058.
12. American Psychiatric Association. Diagnostic and statistical manual of mental disorders (DSM-5®). Arlington, VA: American Psychiatric Association; 2013.
13. National Institute on Alcohol Abuse and Alcoholism (NIAAA). Helping patients who drink too much: a clinician's guide: National Institute on Alcohol Abuse and Alcoholism (NIAAA) 2005. Available at: http://www.webcitation.org/6YWa6HsYP. Accessed February 15, 2021.
14. Jonas DE, Garbutt JC. Screening and counseling for unhealthy alcohol use in primary care settings. Med Clin North Am 2017;101(4):823–37.
15. Substance Abuse and Mental Health Services Administration. Key substance use and mental health indicators in the United States: results from the 2019 National survey on drug use and health. Rockville, MD: Center for Behavioral Health Statistics and Quality, Substance Abuse and Mental Health Services Administration; 2020. Available at: https://www.samhsa.gov/data/report/2019-nsduh-annual-national-report. Accessed February 15, 2021.
16. Vinson DC, Manning BK, Galliher JM, et al. Alcohol and sleep problems in primary care patients: a report from the AAFP National Research Network. Ann Fam Med 2010;8(6):484–92.
17. Cherpitel CJ, Ye Y. Drug use and problem drinking associated with primary care and emergency room utilization in the US general population: data from the 2005 national alcohol survey. Drug Alcohol Depend 2008;97(3):226–30.
18. Walley AY, Paasche-Orlow M, Lee EC, et al. Acute care hospital utilization among medical inpatients discharged with a substance use disorder diagnosis. J Addict Med 2012;6(1):50–6.
19. Smothers BA, Yahr HT. Alcohol use disorder and illicit drug use in admissions to general hospitals in the United States. Am J Addict 2005;14(3):256–67.
20. Serowik KL, Yonkers KA, Gilstad-Hayden K, et al. Substance use disorder detection rates among providers of general medical inpatients. J Gen Intern Med 2021; 36(3):668–75.
21. Saitz R, Freedner N, Palfai TP, et al. The severity of unhealthy alcohol use in hospitalized medical patients. The spectrum is narrow. J Gen Intern Med 2006;21(4): 381–5.
22. Hallgren KA, Witwer E, West I, et al. Prevalence of documented alcohol and opioid use disorder diagnoses and treatments in a regional primary care practice-based research network. J Subst Abuse Treat 2020;110:18–27.
23. D'Amico EJ, Paddock SM, Burnam A, et al. Identification of and guidance for problem drinking by general medical providers: results from a national survey. Med Care 2005;43(3):229–36.
24. McKnight-Eily LR, Okoro CA, Mejia R, et al. Screening for excessive alcohol use and brief counseling of adults - 17 states and the District of Columbia, 2014. MMWR Morb Mortal Wkly Rep 2017;66(12):313–9.
25. US Preventive Services Task Force. Screening for unhealthy drug use: US preventive services task force recommendation statement. JAMA 2020;323(22): 2301–9.
26. US Preventive Services Task Force. Screening and behavioral counseling interventions to reduce unhealthy alcohol use in adolescents and adults: US

preventive services task force recommendation statement. JAMA 2018;320(18): 1899–909.

27. Solberg LI, Maciosek MV, Edwards NM. Primary care intervention to reduce alcohol misuse ranking its health impact and cost effectiveness. Am J Prev Med 2008;34(2):143–52.

28. Maciosek MV, Coffield AB, Edwards NM, et al. Priorities among effective clinical preventive services: results of a systematic review and analysis. Am J Prev Med 2006;31(1):52–61.

29. O'Connor EA, Perdue LA, Senger CA, et al. Screening and behavioral counseling interventions to reduce unhealthy alcohol use in adolescents and adults: updated evidence report and systematic review for the US Preventive Services Task Force. JAMA 2018;320(18):1910–28.

30. Saitz R. Screening for unhealthy drug use: neither an unreasonable idea nor an evidence-based practice. JAMA 2020;323(22):2263–5.

31. McLellan AT, Starrels JL, Tai B, et al. Can substance use disorders be managed using the chronic care model? Review and recommendations from a NIDA consensus group. Public Health Rev 2014;35(2). Available at: http://www.journalindex.net/visit.php?j=6676.

32. WHO. World Health Organization. The health and social effects of nonmedical cannabis use 2016. Available at: https://www.who.int/substance_abuse/publications/cannabis_report/en/. Accessed February 15, 2021.

33. Mattick RP, Breen C, Kimber J, et al. Buprenorphine maintenance versus placebo or methadone maintenance for opioid dependence. Cochrane Database Syst Rev 2014;(2):Cd002207.

34. Patnode CD, Perdue LA, Rushkin M, et al. Screening for unhealthy drug use: updated evidence report and systematic review for the US Preventive Services Task Force. JAMA 2020;323(22):2310–28.

35. Simonetti JA, Lapham GT, Williams EC. Association Between receipt of brief alcohol intervention and quality of care among veteran outpatients with unhealthy alcohol use. J Gen Intern Med 2015;30(8):1097–104.

36. Miller PM, Thomas SE, Mallin R. Patient attitudes towards self-report and biomarker alcohol screening by primary care physicians. Alcohol Alcohol 2006;41(3):306–10.

37. Harris SK, Csemy L, Sherritt L, et al. Computer-facilitated substance use screening and brief advice for teens in primary care: an international trial. Pediatrics 2012;129(6):1072–82. Available at: http://cde.drugabuse.gov/.

38. Smith PC, Schmidt SM, Allensworth-Davies D, et al. Primary care validation of a single-question alcohol screening test. J Gen Intern Med 2009;24(7):783–8.

39. Bradley KA, DeBenedetti AF, Volk RJ, et al. AUDIT-C as a brief screen for alcohol misuse in primary care. Alcohol Clin Exp Res 2007;31(7):1208–17.

40. Reinert DF, Allen JP. The alcohol use disorders identification test: an update of research findings. Alcohol Clin Exp Res 2007;31(2):185–99.

41. Bradley KA, Williams EC, Achtmeyer CE, et al. Implementation of evidence-based alcohol screening in the Veterans Health Administration. Am J Manag Care 2006;12(10):597–606.

42. Bradley KA, Bush KR, Epler AJ, et al. Two brief alcohol-screening tests from the Alcohol Use Disorders Identification Test (AUDIT): validation in a female Veterans Affairs patient population. Arch Intern Med 2003;163(7):821–9.

43. Smith PC, Schmidt SM, Allensworth-Davies D, et al. A Single-Question Screening Test for Drug Use in Primary Care. Arch Intern Med 2010;170(13):1155–60.

44. McNeely J, Cleland CM, Strauss SM, et al. Validation of self-administered single-item screening questions (SISQs) for unhealthy alcohol and drug use in primary care patients. J Gen Intern Med 2015;30(12):1757–64.

45. McNeely J, Strauss SM, Saitz R, et al. A brief patient self-administered substance use screening tool for primary care: two-site validation study of the substance use brief screen (SUBS). Am J Med 2015;128(7):784, e9–19.

46. Skinner HA. The drug abuse screening test. Addict Behav 1982;7(4):363–71.

47. McNeely J, Wu LT, Subramaniam G, et al. Performance of the tobacco, alcohol, prescription medication, and other substance use (TAPS) tool for substance use screening in primary care patients. Ann Intern Med 2016;165(10):690–9.

48. Gryczynski J, McNeely J, Wu LT, et al. Validation of the TAPS-1: a four-item screening tool to identify unhealthy substance use in primary care. J Gen Intern Med 2017;32(9):990–6.

49. Adam A, Schwartz RP, Wu LT, et al. Electronic self-administered screening for substance use in adult primary care patients: feasibility and acceptability of the tobacco, alcohol, prescription medication, and other substance use (my-TAPS) screening tool. Addict Sci Clin Pract 2019;14(1):39.

50. Bradley KA, Lapham GT, Lee AK. Screening for drug use in primary care: practical implications of the new USPSTF recommendation. JAMA Intern Med 2020; 180(8):1050–1.

51. Lapham GT, Lee AK, Caldeiro RM, et al. Frequency of cannabis use among primary care patients in Washington State. J Am Board Fam Med 2017;30(6):795–805.

52. McNeely J, Halkitis PN, Horton A, et al. How patients understand the term "nonmedical use" of prescription drugs: insights from cognitive interviews. Substance abuse 2014;35(1):12–20.

53. National Institute on Drug Abuse. Screening and assessment tools chart 2021. Available at: https://www.drugabuse.gov/nidamed-medical-health-professionals/screening-tools-resources/chart-screening-tools. Accessed February 15, 2021.

54. SAMHSA. National Council for Behavioral Health. Implementing care for alcohol & other drug use in medical settings: an extension of SBIRT. SBIRT change guide 1.0 2018. Available at: https://integration.samhsa.gov/sbirt/Implementing_Care_for_Alcohol_and_Other_Drug_Use_In_Medical_Settings_-_An_Extension_of_SBIRT.pdf. Accessed February 15, 2021.

55. Sayre M, Lapham GT, Lee AK, et al. Routine assessment of symptoms of substance use disorders in primary care: prevalence and severity of reported symptoms. J Gen Intern Med 2020;35(4):1111–9.

56. Substance Abuse and Mental Health Services Administration (SAMHSA). Screening, brief intervention, and referral to treatment (SBIRT) grantees. Available at: https://www.samhsa.gov/sbirt/grantees. Accessed February 15, 2021.

57. Nilsen P. Brief alcohol intervention–where to from here? Challenges remain for research and practice. Addiction 2010;105(6):954–9.

58. McNeely J, Kumar PC, Rieckmann T, et al. Barriers and facilitators affecting the implementation of substance use screening in primary care clinics: a qualitative study of patients, providers, and staff. Addict Sci Clin Pract 2018;13(1):8.

59. McNeely J, Adam A, Rotrosen J, et al. Comparison of methods for alcohol and drug screening in primary care clinics. JAMA Netw Open 2021;4(5):e2110721.

60. Tourangeau R, Smith TW. Asking sensitive questionsthe impact of data collection mode, question format, and question context. Public Opin Q 1996;60(2):275–304.

61. Spear SE, Shedlin M, Gilberti B, et al. Feasibility and acceptability of an audio computer-assisted self-interview version of the Alcohol, Smoking and Substance

Involvement Screening Test (ASSIST) in primary care patients. Subst Abus 2016; 37(2):299–305.

62. Bradley KA, Lapham GT, Hawkins EJ, et al. Quality concerns with routine alcohol screening in VA clinical settings. J Gen Intern Med 2011;26(3):299–306.

63. Williams EC, Achtmeyer CE, Thomas RM, et al. Factors underlying quality problems with alcohol screening prompted by a clinical reminder in primary care: a multi-site qualitative study. J Gen Intern Med 2015;30(8):1125–32.

64. Tai B, McLellan AT. Integrating information on substance use disorders into electronic health record systems. J Subst Abuse Treat 2012;43(1):12–9.

65. Barclay C, Viswanathan M, Ratner S, et al. Implementing evidence-based screening and counseling for unhealthy alcohol use with epic-based electronic health record tools. Jt Comm J Qual Patient Saf 2019;45(8):566–74.

66. Lapham GT, Rubinsky AD, Heagerty PJ, et al. Probability and predictors of patients converting from negative to positive screens for alcohol misuse. Alcohol Clin Exp Res 2014;38(2):564–71.

67. Makdissi R, Stewart SH. Care for hospitalized patients with unhealthy alcohol use: a narrative review. Addict Sci Clin Pract 2013;8(1):11.

68. Barbosa C, McKnight-Eily LR, Grosse SD, et al. Alcohol screening and brief intervention in emergency departments: review of the impact on healthcare costs and utilization. J Subst Abuse Treat 2020;117:108096.

69. Saitz R. Candidate performance measures for screening for, assessing, and treating unhealthy substance use in hospitals: advocacy or evidence-based practice? Ann Intern Med 2010;153(1):40–3.

70. Hawk K, D'Onofrio G. Emergency department screening and interventions for substance use disorders. Addict Sci Clin Pract 2018;13(1):18.

71. Weinstein ZM, Wakeman SE, Nolan S. Inpatient addiction consult service: expertise for hospitalized patients with complex addiction problems. Med Clin North Am 2018;102(4):587–601.

72. Englander H, Dobbertin K, Lind BK, et al. Inpatient addiction medicine consultation and post-hospital substance use disorder treatment engagement: a propensity-matched analysis. J Gen Intern Med 2019;34(12):2796–803.

73. Englander H, Weimer M, Solotaroff R, et al. Planning and Designing the Improving Addiction Care Team (IMPACT) for hospitalized adults with substance use disorder. J Hosp Med 2017;12(5):339–42.

74. Wakeman SE, Kane M, Powell E, et al. A hospital-wide initiative to redesign substance use disorder care: impact on pharmacotherapy initiation. Subst Abuse 2020;1–8.

75. Sanchez K, Gryczynski J, Carswell SB, et al. Development and feasibility of a spanish language version of the tobacco, alcohol, prescription drug, and illicit substance use (TAPS) tool. J Addict Med 2021;15(1):61–7.

76. World Health Organization. AUDIT: the Alcohol Use Disorders Identification Test : guidelines for use in primary health care. Babor TF, et al. 2nd edition. World Health Organization. Available at: https://apps.who.int/iris/handle/10665/67205.

77. O'Connor EA, Perdue LA, Senger CA, et al. U.S. preventive services task force evidence syntheses, formerly systematic evidence reviews. In: Screening and behavioral counseling interventions to reduce unhealthy alcohol use in adolescents and adults: an updated systematic review for the US preventive services task force. Rockville (MD): Agency for Healthcare Research and Quality (US); 2018.

# Disparities in Addiction Treatment

## Learning from the Past to Forge an Equitable Future

Danielle S. Jackson, MD, MPH[a],*,
Max Jordan Nguemeni Tiako, MD, MS[b,c,1],
Ayana Jordan, MD, PhD[d,1]

### KEYWORDS

- Addiction • Treatment • Disparities • Inequity • Drug policy
- Structural competency • Structural racism

### KEY POINTS

- There is a long history of racialized drug policy in the United States that has determined who is deemed "worthy" of addiction treatment and which racial groups have access to addiction treatment.
- The underlying reasons for disparities in addiction are varied, but many are rooted in structural racism, whereby cultural norms, institutional practices, and policies perpetuate racial group inequity.
- Disparities in addiction treatment continue to widen, despite the development of novel therapeutics in the past 20 years.
- Building community partnerships to effectively address inequities in the social determinants of health is one effective way to improve addiction treatment access, delivery, and outcomes.
- Diversification of the addiction treatment workforce provides a path to mitigating inequities in outcomes among minoritized groups.

[a] Department of Psychiatry, Rutgers- Robert Wood Johnson Medical School, 671 Hoes Lane West, 2nd Floor, Piscataway, NJ 08854, USA; [b] Department of Internal Medicine, Brigham and Women's Hospital, Boston, MA 02115, USA; [c] Harvard Medical School, Boston, MA 02115, USA; [d] Department of Psychiatry, NYU Grossman School of Medicine, New York, NY
[1] Present address: 300 George Street, Suite 901, New Haven, CT 06461, USA
* Corresponding author.
*E-mail address:* danielle.jackson@yale.edu
Twitter: @DrDaniJackson (D.S.J.); @MaxJordan_N (M.J.N.T.); @DrAyanaJordan (A.J.)

Med Clin N Am 106 (2022) 29–41
https://doi.org/10.1016/j.mcna.2021.08.008
0025-7125/22/© 2021 Elsevier Inc. All rights reserved.

## HISTORY OF ADDICTION POLICIES IN THE UNITED STATES
### Early Twentieth Century - the Uncoupling of Addiction from Medical Practice

When discussing disparities in addiction treatment it is important to understand the historical foundation from which these disparities arise. The racialization of drugs and subsequent drug policies date back to the early 1900s.[1,2] Before this, opium was freely imported into the United States (US) and its use unregulated throughout the eighteenth century with little attention from lawmakers or the medical community. The sensationalized propaganda that fueled early drug policy did not begin with opium, however. The racialized association of cocaine use with Black men portrayed as "the negro menace" swiftly ushered in the prohibition of cocaine in the post-Civil War South.[3] Sensational tales in medical journals depicted the Black man as a "cocaine fiend" who when intoxicated developed superhuman strength becoming impenetrable to shock by law enforcement weapons.[4,5] Prohibition of cocaine quickly spread throughout Southern states with most states passing laws making its possession and use punishable by law. The Jim Crow state-enforced segregation laws in Southern states firmly established the roots of racialized drug policy in the US[3]

Until the passage of the Pure Food and Drug Act of 1906, federal regulation of drugs did not exist. The US experienced its first opioid crisis between 1865 and 1913 as a consequence of the unregulated inclusion of opium and its derivatives in patent medications by pharmaceutical companies and the invention of the hypodermic syringe.[6] These patent medications were available by mail, in the local pharmacy, and from physicians without restriction. As medical technology advanced, the formulation and availability of drugs grew, with morphine salts being first derived in 1832 and subsequently heroin in 1897.[6] At that time, addiction was viewed by both the lay public and physicians as a medical condition requiring treatment. Affluent White women were often treated for opioid addiction by their family doctors with the administration of small tinctures of heroin.[7] The Pure Food and Drug Act of 1906, which eliminated opioids and cocaine from patented medication, required medication labeling, and restricted physician prescribing, was the first federal regulation of opioid use.[8] This was swiftly followed by a ban on smoking opium in 1909,[9] with heavy racialized propaganda of opium dens targeting the Chinese immigrant population, despite most widespread use of opium derivatives being of morphine and heroin in pharmaceutical preparations.[4]

The Harrison Narcotics Tax Act of 1914 which called for the taxation and registration of the import of opium and coca derivatives led to the criminalization of substance use (**Fig. 1**).[7,10] This act established opioid use disorder (OUD) "not as a medical condition" and prevented physicians from treating it; many physicians were jailed for treating OUD.[7] Thus, began the era of addiction is viewed as a moral failure, whereby individuals suffering from substance use disorders (SUDs) where seen as menaces to society, with the only acceptable "cure" for addiction being total substance abstinence.

With the temperance movement in full swing, new drug policies swept throughout the country in the first half of the twentieth century.[11] Motivated by racial politics and national anxieties over immigration, early cannabis prohibition first occurred in the Southwestern US targeting immigrants from Mexico.[12,13] As the racist anti-Mexican propaganda grew, it eventually garnered national attention in the 1930s. By this time, the country had repealed the National Prohibition Act of 1920 and a new model of Addiction recovery from alcohol use was established with the foundation of Alcoholics Anonymous in 1935. Anti-Mexican American rhetoric propagated by Harry J. Anslinger, the first commissioner of the newly formed Federal Bureau of Narcotics led to the passage of the Marihuana Tax Act of 1937.[12]

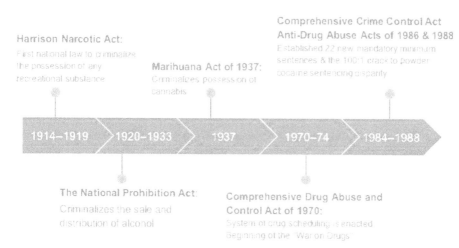

**Fig. 1.** Timeline of drug policy in the United States. ("*from:* [Jordan,A., Mathis,M. Isom, J. Achieving Mental Health Equity: Addictions, Psychiatric Clinics of North America, Volume 43, Issue 3, 2020,Pages 487-500 ]; with permission")

Passage of the Marihuana Tax act of 1937 resulted in heavy taxation on the sale of cannabis which reduced the production of hemp crops in favor of cheaper, synthetic alternatives being developed, and created a negative association between cannabis and individuals from Mexico/South America by renaming *cannabis,* "Marihuana."[13,14] This representation of illicit drug use in the US media at the time played to White American fear. Just as early cocaine bans rose from the racialized association of cocaine use with Black Americans, popular ads, and movies depicting "reefer madness" among Mexican individuals and the "unsuspecting White female victims lured into a life of debauchery" continued the pattern of associating of substance use with non-White ethnic groups.[12]

### Mid-Late Century Criminalization of Substance Use - Policies that Outline the Approach to Drug Use for Over 50 Years

In the decades between 1937 and 1970, there was a relative halt in interest regarding legislation of drugs.[10] Cannabis and psychedelics enjoyed popularity as part of the anti-war "hippie" counterculture in progressive pockets of the country. However, this freedom of drug use changed with the declaration that America's "public enemy number one" was "drug abuse" by Richard Nixon in 1971.[15] During the majority of the period of legislative quiescence, there had not been an increase in the numbers of people using drugs, especially when compared with the peak experienced in the late 1800s during the first opioid crisis.[7]

Racial politics of the time served to capitalize on the need for drug use to be anti-American during a time of rising protests against the Vietnam War and to quell the emergence of Black community leaders and activists for social change in inner cities. Nixon's White House Chief of Staff H.R. Haldeman is quoted as saying "The whole problem is really the Blacks. The key is to devise a system that recognizes this, while not appearing to."[16,17] A national system of systemic and structural racism related to drug use was subsequently reinforced for the next 30-year period.

The 1970 Comprehensive Drug Abuse and Prevention Act, (Title II Controlled Substances Act CSA) placed the control of select plants, drugs, and chemical substances under federal jurisdiction.[18] It prohibited the manufacture, sale, or possession of controlled substances. The CSA classified controlled substances under 5 schedules according to how dangerous they are, potential for misuse and addiction, and legitimacy of medical use, providing the legal framework of the Drug Enforcement Administration authority.[18] Enacted simultaneously with the Racketeer Influenced and Corrupt Organizations Act (RICO), the CSA also allowed for the criminal and civil forfeiture of assets against anyone convicted of violating a drug crime [and later any third party associated with the convicted individual].[10] The broad terminology of the CSA had widespread implications on substance use treatment. It further stigmatized those who used substances as "addicts" and "criminals" and focused on addiction as a moral failing rather than a medical condition causing widespread stigmatization which has largely remained to date.[19–21]

States like New York (NY) doubled down on their focus of portraying addiction as a "criminal enterprise," with the passage of the 1973 eponymous "Rockefeller laws."[22] These laws ushered in the next wave of mass incarceration of predominantly Black and Hispanic men of the late twenty-first century. Although the CSA provided for the establishment of federal treatment centers for OUD with methadone, Black individuals were being disproportionately incarcerated, and left without access to this medical treatment. The Rockefeller laws of 1973 were the first to enact mandatory minimum sentencing based solely on the quantity of drugs possessed, not the nature of the suspected criminal activity. In the period between 1974 and 2002, the NY State prison population increased by 500%, with the proportion of Black and Hispanic individuals comprising 94% of those incarcerated under these drug laws in the year 2000 despite them comprising only 33% of the total state population.[22] Beyond the exclusion of incarcerated Black and Hispanic individuals from methadone treatment programs, methadone treatment was also tightly regulated by the federal government and federal regulation siloed from traditional clinical care setting.[23]

In this same pattern, federal legislation followed state level "tough on crime" drug policies with the passage of the Comprehensive Crime Control Act of 1984, shortly followed by the Anti-Drug Abuse Act of 1986, which established mandatory minimum sentencing for drug-related crimes like the 100:1 sentencing disparity for possession of crystallized "crack" cocaine versus powder cocaine.[24,25] Continuing in the tradition of the racialization of drug use, media outlets portrayed "crack" cocaine use as a problem isolated to the inner-city Black community and those who were "addicted to crack" as more violent than those who used powder cocaine, and lacking in moral fortitude and beyond redemption.[24,26] This served to spread fear and garner popular support among the public limiting the opposition to these draconian laws. The racial hierarchies perpetuated by the War on Drugs resulted in a 6- to 8-fold increase in incarceration for nonviolent drug use between 1985 and 2000.[16,24] The majority of those incarcerated were young Black men.[24]

This overview of US drug policy, racialization of drug use, and support for putative policies toward drug use and addiction over 150 years provides the foundation to understand how many communities of color have been systematically and strategically criminalized for drug use and prevented from accessing addiction treatment.

## STRUCTURAL RACISM LEADING TO DISPARITIES IN ADDICTION

In addition to the lasting effects of racialized drug policy, structural racism is the system in which public policies, institutional practices, cultural representations, and other norms work in various ways to perpetuate racial group inequity.[27] Structural racism influences every sector of addiction treatment from policy to health care delivery and research. In the previous section, we discussed the impact of structural racism through the lens of historical and current drug policies that preferentially advantage the dominant White culture, by disadvantaging minoritized individuals. In this section, we examine how structural racism in health care delivery through access to medication for opioid use disorder (MOUD) and federal regulations (intersection of the carceral system with addiction treatment), leads to inequities in addiction treatment within minoritized communities.

Two out of three US Food and Drug Administration (FDA)-approved treatments for OUD, methadone, and buprenorphine are associated with decreased overdose and mortality risk.[28] However, access to both medications is highly restricted. Since 1972, the federal government has required that methadone be exclusively administered in federally qualified opioid treatment programs (OTPs).[29] In the 1960s and 70s, New York City was home to over 50% of individuals with OUD, and became the epicenter for the creation of methadone treatment clinics[30] The geographic distribution of OTPs became shaped by backlash from mostly upper-class, White residents who feared proximity to individuals with OUD who used heroin.[29] This backlash led to a concentration of OTPs in predominantly Black and Hispanic neighborhoods. To date, methadone treatment remains highly restrictive, despite decades of evidence as a highly effective treatment of OUD.[31] For example, an individual dispensed methadone must wait up to 2 years and have an absence of illicit substance use to obtain 28 days of "take home" (ie, not dispensed daily from the OTP) methadone privileges from an OTP.[32] Recent policy analysis found that 18 out of 30 most common regulations for methadone were inconsistent with best practices recommendations, which may impact access, retention, and success in OUD treatment.[33] An exemption to these regulations now exists due to the COVID-19 pandemic, but the implementation of these exemptions varies greatly depending on geographic location, OTP resources, and OTP medical discretion.[34]

Buprenorphine becomes available as another treatment of OUD in the year 2000 with the passage of the Drug Addiction Treatment Act of 2000 (DATA 2000) and the 2002 FDA approval process. It is well described that its accessibility was heavy marketed to clinicians who accepted commercial insurance in rural and suburban White communities.[35,36] The National Institute of Drug (Ab)use (NIDA) director at the time argued that buprenorphine was better suited as a treatment of suburban, White collar individuals with OUD.[29] The racialization of buprenorphine provides insight into how a less restrictive MOUD was deliberately marketed and advertised to White individuals which resulted in higher utilization among this group, despite tax dollars from diverse populations supporting its development and clinical trial data.[37] It is estimated that 62.3 million dollars in NIH awards supported the development of buprenorphine as a treatment of OUD, but it still remains inaccessible to a large portion of the population.[38] The complex public–private partnership between NIDA and pharmaceutical company Reckitt-Benckiser was so robust that buprenorphine (marketed as Suboxone) was granted FDA approval under the orphan drug designation, a category historically reserved for novel treatments of rare diseases.[29,39]

Today, consequently, studies show that the accessibility of buprenorphine than methadone at the census tract level is significantly associated with racial segregation, with buprenorphine being more available to disproportionately White census tracts and methadone being more available to Black and Hispanic census tracts.[40,41] Additionally, whereas there has been an increase in buprenorphine access over the recent years, most individuals prescribed buprenorphine are White and remain self-pay or have commercial insurance.[37,42] Further, clinicians trained to prescribe buprenorphine are more likely to work in areas with low insurance rates and more likely to decline individuals with Medicaid insurance or require cash payments.[43]

The carceral system provides yet another way through which structural racism shapes existing disparities in SUD treatment, whereby a disproportionate rate of Black and Hispanic individuals remain behind bars due to substance use.[44] A survey showed that court officers favor naltrexone over buprenorphine and methadone to treat OUD,[45] despite the fact that naltrexone is the only one of the 3 treatments not associated with decreased mortality risk.[46] This preference is rooted in substance use stigma, as certain individuals perceive opioid receptor antagonists as "superior" to opioid agonists. It is perplexing and at times deadly to have actors from the carceral system like police involved in the treatment of individuals with SUDs.[47]

Structural racism is a complex web of policies, attitudes, and actions which, in health care, lead to disparities in health outcomes. Addressing these disparities will necessitate deliberate health care policies and accountability at the societal and individual levels to ensure that individuals with SUD receive the best treatment and achieve optimal outcomes. Some solutions that have been proposed include: lifting the regulatory hurdles that limit the workforce of clinicians who prescribe buprenorphine, increase addiction education exposure beginning in all health professions training, and increase educational partnership with nonaddiction clinicians to improve attitudes toward care of individuals with SUD.[48–51] Additionally, evidence shows making methadone more widely available in pharmacies as conducted in Canada, or in primary care clinics would expand access to treatment by decreasing driving distances to OTPs for individuals living in rural areas, and also would help destigmatize OUD treatment.[23,52]

## STRUCTURAL COMPETENCY: A PATIENT-CENTERED APPROACH TO ADDICTION TREATMENT

Structural competency (SC), first introduced into the academic literature in 2014 by Hansen and Metzl, is a tool for health professionals to recognize and respond to health and illness as the downstream effects of broader social, political, and economic structures.[53] SC provides a way forward to address the downstream effects of inequities in addiction as a result of structural racism. Inherent in exercising SC requires a shift of focus from individual clinical interactions toward factors that influence health outcomes outside of the clinical setting. Development of these skills requires clinicians to move the lens beyond the acknowledgment of the social determinants of health (SDOH) of the conditions and environments in which we live that affect our health and health outcomes to understanding and intervening on social conditions that drive health care inequity.[54] There are 5 components to the SC framework which help to change our understanding of the patient and our treatment planning (**Box 1**). They include (1) the recognition of the structures that shape clinical interactions, (2)

---

**Box 1**
**Five components of the structural competency framework**

Recognition of the structures that shape clinical interactions

Recognition of the influence of these structures on health and health outcomes

Responding to structures from within the clinical setting

Learning to respond outside of the clinical setting

Developing structural humility

recognition of the influence of these structures on clinical interactions and health outcomes, (3) responding to structures from within the clinical setting, (4) learning to respond outside of the clinical setting, and (5) developing structural humility.[55] This framework allows clinicians to move away from viewing disease states and health outcomes as an individual issue to a societal condition in need of societal and community-level interventions. Through an understanding and intentional practice of this framework, it is possible to address addiction treatment disparities at multiple levels. Implementation of his framework has successfully been conducted in both undergraduate and graduate medical education programs.[55,56]

Health care models addressing addiction treatment disparities using a structurally competent framework can be immensely useful in the mitigation of health inequity. By incorporating a structural competency framework into clinical practice, clinicians can successfully intervene on SDOH at the individual, institutional, and societal level to improve health outcomes (**Table 1**).[57] In recent years, interventions that overcome structural barriers have been designed and implemented in SUD treatment to increase equitable distribution of access to care and retention in treatment. These interventions include the incorporation of addiction specialists into primary care clinics and federally qualified health clinics (FQHCs), integration of primary care and obstetric care into OTPs, expansion of mobile health units providing harm reduction and health services, establishment of rapid access buprenorphine outpatient clinics connecting patients to care from emergency departments and hospitals, robust hospital-based addiction consultation teams that initiate and facilitate addiction treatment in the hospital setting, and faith-based recovery models embedded in the community.[58–60]

The previous examples demonstrate that disparities in the treatment of SUDs can be addressed successfully both inside and outside the clinical environment by increasing accessibility and barriers to addiction specialists and clinicians' care, implementing harm reduction interventions in acute general medical settings, and engaging in community-based participatory research. Unfortunately, access to such treatment options remains low and has been shown to vary widely based on insurance status, geographic location, and socioeconomic status.[35,37,40,41,61]

## BUILDING DIVERSITY AS A TOOL TO MINIMIZING DISPARITIES IN ADDICTION TREATMENT

A multifaceted approach, including the measures above, is necessary, but not sufficient to eliminate disparities in addiction treatment. The addiction treatment workforce must reflect the diversity of individuals with SUD. This is more salient than ever as rates of drug overdose deaths are increasing more rapidly among Black and Hispanic individuals[62,63] than White individuals and addiction treatment initiation and engagement is highly limited among minoritized populations.[37,64] An addiction treatment workforce, representative of the population most adversely affected by SUDs, is necessary to curb these disproportionate rates of burden.[65,66]

Equity, diversity, inclusion, and belonging in the addiction treatment workforce, enables creative thought resulting in the promotion of new ideas and concepts to address structural racism in addiction treatment.[7] Representation from underrepresented minorities (URM) is essential in the development of policies and addiction treatment paradigms that directly affect communities of color. Given the shared understanding and relevance of what it is to be othered in the US, URM populations are better situated to enact policies that affirm the humanity of minoritized individuals and promote resilience. Further, a diverse addiction treatment workforce minimizes the promotion of racist ideals promulgated in White supremacist culture (the belief

**Table 1**
**Structurally competent versus traditional approaches in clinical practice**

Addressing Addiction Treatment Disparities Using a Structural Competency Framework

| Clinical Scenario | Traditional Approach | Using Structural Competency |
|---|---|---|
| On review of chart notes, a clinician notices elevated rates of Hepatitis C virus (HCV) among persons who inject drugs in the community clinic | The issue may be viewed as an individual problem with no large-scale intervention | The clinician partners with a community organization to provide mobile needle exchange which results in lower HCV rates |
| Patient initiated on buprenorphine in Emergency Department, unable to access continued follow-up due to the lack of transportation, results in the street purchase of heroin for withdrawal symptoms and suffers nonfatal overdose | The clinician attributes follow-up in outpatient care to "lack of compliance" of individual patients. Factors such as distance to clinic and money for transportation are viewed as outside the scope of care | The clinician develops a buprenorphine bridge program in the emergency department, linking patients to buprenorphine treatment at satellite community clinics with underserved neighborhoods |
| Patients with cocaine use disorder experiences nonfatal overdose | The clinician may believe there is no intervention that can be offered, as there is no FDA approved medication therapy for cocaine use disorder | The patient receives counseling based on the principles of harm reduction, a naloxone kit is distributed and referrals are placed to appropriate substance use disorder support groups |

that the dominant narrative, culture, and ideals are superior to others), valuing input, and the promotion of norms from varying perspectives.[27]

Two innovative programs in research and education that are dedicated to increasing the representation of minoritized addiction researchers and clinicians include Learning for Early Careers in Addiction & Diversity (LEAD)[67] and Recognizing and Eliminating disparities in Addiction through Culturally informed Health Care (REACH),[54] respectively. Given the persistent NIH funding gap for minoritized scholars who are more likely to conduct research that affects URM communities, LEAD an NIH-funded initiative, works closely with URM scholars to provide funding and mentoring to develop independent scientists, poised to develop equitable treatment interventions for URM populations with SUD.[68,69] REACH provides an educational immersive experience whereby minoritized scholars interested in pursuing a career in addiction, across disciplines, and medical subspecialties, gain skills specific to taking the best care of minoritized individuals with addiction. Sample topics within REACH include the History & Epidemiology of Addiction, Racism and Health for URM Communities, Advocacy 101, Caring for URMs in the Judicial System, and Structural Competency.[54] The development of a network, solely composed of URM scholars dedicated to taking care of minoritized communities with SUDs, is also another huge benefit of REACH.

An addiction treatment workforce comprised of individuals who know what it feels to be minoritized, are more likely to consciously lead with empathy and compassion, all necessary qualities to work collaboratively with communities who continue to be and have been historically marginalized. Equity, diversity, inclusion, and belonging efforts in addiction treatment leadership must include 3 major areas: (1) promotion of diversity, specifically the inclusion of Black, Hispanic, and Native individuals in key research leadership roles, (2) prioritizing hiring individuals from affected communities into the addiction treatment milieu, and (3) formal inclusion of individuals with community informed expertise (CIE), traditionally known as lived experience, into all aspects of research and clinical care. To achieve compositional diversity, it is necessary that the concepts of inclusion and belonging are integrated into the institutional culture. Inclusion ensures that barriers (seen or unseen) are eliminated so that individuals are willing and able to be fully involved in decision-making. Belonging allows them to be involved as their full authentic self. By following these necessary steps, only then can we set out to eliminate disparities within addiction treatment.[65]

## SUMMARY

Disparities in addiction treatment continue to be perpetuated by a complex interaction of health care delivery and socioeconomic and political barriers built on putative structurally racists policies. The historic backdrop of the racialization of drug use in combination with policies rooted in the utilization of the carceral system to address addiction continues to widen the addiction treatment gap. By approaching addiction treatment using a structurally competent framework, clinicians can begin to address existing disparities, focusing on the extraclinical structures contributing to these outcomes. To be successful, this will require a concerted and deliberate approach of recruiting a diverse addiction treatment workforce that is able to foster close collaboration between policymakers, health care systems, and clinicians. Change requires an investment in training and supporting researchers of color, supporting, and uplifting the voices of minoritized addiction specialists, along with parallel investments in the community, public health infrastructure, and drug policy reform.

## DISCLOSURE

The authors have nothing to disclose.

## REFERENCES

1. Spillane J, McAllister WB. Keeping the lid on: a century of drug regulation and control. Drug Alcohol Depend 2003;70(3):S5–12.
2. Hickman TA. Subjects of desire: race, gender and the personification of addiction. In: The secret leprosy of modern days: narcotic addiction and cultural crisis in the United States, 1870-1920. Amherst: U Mass Press; 2007. p. 59–92.
3. Cohen MM. Jim Crow's drug war: race, coca cola, and the southern origins of drug prohibition. South Cultures 2006;12(3):55–79.
4. Netherland J, Hansen H. White opioids: pharmaceutical race and the war on drugs that wasn't. Biosocieties 2017;12(2):217–38.
5. Hart C. How the myth of the 'negro cocaine fiend' helped shape American Drug Policy. New York, NY: The Nation Company, L.P; 2014.
6. Heimer R, Hawk K, Vermund SH. Prevalent misconceptions about opioid use disorders in the United States produce failed policy and public health responses. Clin Infect Dis 2019;69(3):546–51.
7. Jordan A, Mathis ML, Isom J. Achieving mental health equity: addictions. Psychiatr Clin North Am 2020;43(3):487–500.

8. Murch D. Crack in Los Angeles: crisis, militarization, and black response to the late twentieth-century war on drugs. The J Am Hist 2015;102(1):162–73.

9. Redford A, Powell B. Dynamics of intervention in the war on drugs: the buildup to the Harrison act of 1914. Independent Rev 2016;20:509.

10. Sacco LN. Drug enforcement in the United States: history, policy and trends. Washington, DC: Congressional Research Service; 2014.

11. Musto DF. State and local narcotics control. In: The American disease: origins of narcotic control. 3rd edition. New York: Oxford University Press; 1999. p. 91–120.

12. Krystal H. The Misclassification of medical Marijuana. J Am Acad Psychiatry Law 2018;46(4):472–9.

13. Netherland J, Hansen HB. The war on drugs that wasn't: wasted whiteness, "dirty doctors," and race in media coverage of prescription opioid misuse. Cult Med Psychiatry 2016;40(4):664–86.

14. Whitebread BRI. The marijuana conviction: a history of marijuana conviction in the United States. New York: The Lindesmith Center; 1999.

15. Wood E, Werb D, Marshall BDL, et al. The war on drugs: a devastating public-policy disaster. Lancet 2009;373(9668):989–90.

16. Alexander M. The war on drugs and the new Jim Crow. Race Poverty Environ 2010;17(1):75–7.

17. Baum D. Legalize it all: how to win the war on drugs. New York, NY: Harpers Magazine; 2016.

18. Courtwright DT. The Controlled Substances Act: how a "big tent" reform became a punitive drug law. Drug Alcohol Depend 2004;76(1):9–15.

19. Corrigan P, Schomerus G, Shuman V, et al. Developing a research agenda for understanding the stigma of addictions Part I: lessons from the Mental Health Stigma Literature. Am J Addict 2017;26(1):59–66.

20. Volkow ND, Koob GF, McLellan AT. Neurobiologic advances from the brain disease model of addiction. N Engl J Med 2016;374(4):363–71.

21. Rundle SM, Cunningham JA, Hendershot CS. Implications of addiction diagnosis and addiction beliefs for public stigma: a cross-national experimental study. Drug Alcohol Rev 2021;40(5):842–6.

22. Drucker E. Population impact of mass incarceration under New York's Rockefeller drug laws: an analysis of years of life lost. J Urban Health 2002;79(3):434–5.

23. Joudrey PJ, Edelman EJ, Wang EA. Methadone for opioid use disorder-decades of effectiveness but still miles away in the US. JAMA Psychiatry 2020;77(11):1105–6.

24. Bobo LD, Thompson V. Unfair by design: the war on drugs, race, and the legitimacy of the criminal justice system. Soc Res 2006;73(2):445–72.

25. Vagins D, McCurdy J. Cracks in the system: twenty years of the unjust federal crack cocaine law 2005. Available at: https://www.aclu.org/other/cracks-system-20-years-unjust-federal-crack-cocaine-law. Accessed March 23, 2021.

26. Cobbina JE. Race and class differences in print media portrayals of crack cocaine and methamphetamine. J Criminal Just Pop Cul 2008;15:145–67.

27. 11 terms you should know to better understand structural racism. Racial Equity; 2016. Available at: https://www.aspeninstitute.org/blog-posts/structural-racism-definition.

28. Wakeman SE, Larochelle MR, Ameli O, et al. Comparative effectiveness of different treatment pathways for opioid use disorder. JAMA Netw Open 2020;3(2):e1920622.

29. Hansen H, Roberts SK. Two tiers of biomedicalization: methadone, buprenorphine, and the racial politics of addiction treatment, vol. 14. Bingley: Emerlad Group Publishing; 2012.

30. Joseph H, Stancliff S, Langrod J. Methadone maintenance treatment (MMT): a review of historical and clinical issues. Mt Sinai J Med 2000;67(5–6):347–64.

31. McBournie A, Duncan A, Connolley E, et al. Methadone barriers persist, despite decades of evidence. Health Affairs Blog; 2019. Available at: https://www.healthaffairs.org/do/10.1377/hblog20190920.981503/full/. Accessed April 10,2021.

32. Institute of Medicine (US) Committee on Federal Regulation of Methadone Treatment. In: Rettig RA, Yarmolinsky A, editors. Federal Regulation of Methadone Treatment. Washington, (DC): National Academies Press (US); 1995. p. 120–48. Available at: https://www.ncbi.nlm.nih.gov/books/NBK232108/.

33. Jackson JR, Harle CA, Silverman RD, et al. Characterizing variability in state-level regulations governing opioid treatment programs. J Subst Abuse Treat 2020;115: 108008.

34. Frontz AJ. Opioid treatment programs reported challenges encountered during the COVID-19 pandemic and actions taken to address them. Washington, DC: Substance Abuse and Mental Health Services Administration; 2020. A-09-20-01001.

35. Abraham AJ, Knudsen HK, Rieckmann T, et al. Disparities in access to physicians and medications for the treatment of substance use disorders between publicly and privately funded treatment programs in the United States. J Stud Alcohol Drugs 2013;74(2):258–65.

36. Ducharme LJ, Abraham AJ. State policy influence on the early diffusion of buprenorphine in community treatment programs. Substance Abuse Treat Prev Policy 2008;3(1):17.

37. Lagisetty PA, Ross R, Bohnert A, et al. Buprenorphine treatment divide by race/ethnicity and payment. JAMA Psychiatry 2019;76(9):979–81.

38. Barenie RE, Kesselheim AS. Buprenorphine for opioid use disorder: the role of public funding in its development. Drug Alcohol Depend 2021;219:108491.

39. Campbell ND, Lovell AM. The history of the development of buprenorphine as an addiction therapeutic. Ann N Y Acad Sci 2012;1248:124–39.

40. Goedel WC, Shapiro A, Cerdá M, et al. Association of racial/ethnic segregation with treatment capacity for opioid use disorder in counties in the United States. JAMA Netw Open 2020;3(4):e203711.

41. Hansen HB, Siegel CE, Case BG, et al. Variation in use of buprenorphine and methadone treatment by racial, ethnic, and income characteristics of residential social areas in New York City. J Behav Health Serv Res 2013;40(3):367–77.

42. Olfson M, Zhang V, Schoenbaum M, et al. Trends in Buprenorphine Treatment in the United States, 2009-2018. JAMA 2020;323(3):276–7.

43. Nguemeni Tiako MJ, Culhane J, South E, et al. Prevalence and geographic distribution of obstetrician-gynecologists who treat medicaid enrollees and are trained to prescribe buprenorphine. JAMA Netw Open 2020;3(12):e2029043.

44. Pettit B, Western B. Mass imprisonment and the life course: race and class inequality in U.S. incarceration. Am Soc Rev 2004;69(2):151–69.

45. Andraka-Christou B, Gabriel M, Madeira J, et al. Court personnel attitudes towards medication-assisted treatment: a state-wide survey. J Substance Abuse Treat 2019;104:72–82.

46. Morgan JR, Schackman BR, Weinstein ZM, et al. Overdose following initiation of naltrexone and buprenorphine medication treatment for opioid use disorder in a

United States commercially insured cohort. Drug Alcohol Depend 2019; 200:34–9.

47. Jordan A, Allsop AS, Collins PY. Decriminalising being Black with mental illness. Lancet Psychiatry 2021;8(1):8–9.

48. Marino R, Perrone J, Nelson LS, et al. ACMT position statement: remove the waiver requirement for prescribing buprenorphine for opioid use disorder. J Med Toxicol 2019;15(4):307–9.

49. Fiscella K, Wakeman SE, Beletsky L. Buprenorphine deregulation and mainstreaming treatment for opioid use disorder: X the X Waiver. JAMA Psychiatry 2019;76(3):229–30.

50. Tetrault JM, Petrakis IL. Partnering with psychiatry to close the education gap: an approach to the addiction epidemic. J Gen Intern Med 2017;32(12):1387–9.

51. van Boekel LC, Brouwers EPM, van Weeghel J, et al. Healthcare professionals' regard towards working with patients with substance use disorders: comparison of primary care, general psychiatry and specialist addiction services. Drug Alcohol Depend 2014;134:92–8.

52. Joudrey PJ, Chadi N, Roy P, et al. Pharmacy-based methadone dispensing and drive time to methadone treatment in five states within the United States: a cross-sectional study. Drug Alcohol Depend 2020;211:107968.

53. Metzl JM, Hansen H. Structural competency: theorizing a new medical engagement with stigma and inequality. Soc Sci Med 2014;103:126–33.

54. Apfelbaum JL, Chen C, Mehta SS, et al. Postoperative pain experience: results from a national survey suggest postoperative pain continues to be undermanaged. Anesth analgesia 2003;97(2):534–40, table of contents.

55. Hansen H, Metzl JM. New medicine for the U.S. health care system: training physicians for structural intervention. Acad Med 2017;92(3):279–81.

56. Hansen H, Braslow J, Rohrbaugh R. From cultural to structural competency-training psychiatry residents to act on social determinants of health and institutional racism. JAMA Psychiatry 2018;75:117–8.

57. Marmot M. Social determinants of health inequalities. Lancet 2005;365(9464): 1099–104.

58. Watkins KE, Ober AJ, Lamp K, et al. Collaborative care for opioid and alcohol use disorders in primary care: the SUMMIT randomized clinical trial. JAMA Intern Med 2017;177(10):1480–8.

59. Wakeman SE, Kanter GP, Donelan K. Institutional substance use disorder intervention improves general internist preparedness, attitudes, and clinical practice. J Addict Med 2017;11(4):308–14.

60. Jordan A, Babuscio T, Nich C, et al. A feasibility study providing substance use treatment in the Black church. J Subst Abuse Treat 2021;124:108218.

61. Roberts AW, Saloner B, Dusetzina SB. Buprenorphine use and spending for opioid use disorder treatment: trends from 2003 to 2015. Psychiatr Serv 2018; 69(7):832–5.

62. Hedegaard H, Bastian BA, Trinidad JP, et al. Drugs most frequently involved in drug overdose deaths: United States, 2011 -2016. National Vital Statistics Reports; Hyattsville, MD: National Center for Health Statistics; 2018;67(9).

63. Furr-Holden D, Milam AJ, Wang L, et al. African Americans now outpace whites in opioid-involved overdose deaths: a comparison of temporal trends from 1999 to 2018. Addiction 2021;116(3):677–83.

64. Jordan A, Mathis M, Haeny A, et al. An evaluation of opioid use in black communities: a rapid review of the literature. Harv Rev Psychiatry 2021;29(2):108–30.

65. Jordan A, Jegede O. Building outreach and diversity in the field of addictions. Am J Addict 2020;29(5):413–7.
66. James K, Jordan A. The opioid crisis in black communities. J Law Med Ethics 2018;46(2):404–21.
67. Greenwald MK, Johanson CE, Moody DE, et al. Effects of buprenorphine maintenance dose on mu-opioid receptor availability, plasma concentrations, and antagonist blockade in heroin-dependent volunteers. Neuropsychopharmacology 2003;28(11):2000–9.
68. Ginther D, Schaffer WT, Schnell J, et al. Race, ethnicity, and NIH research awards. Science 2011;333:1015–9.
69. Hoppe TA, Litovitz A, Willis KA, et al. Top choice contributions to the lower rate of NIH awards to African-American/black scientists. Sci Adv 2019;5:eaaw7238.

# The Spectrum of Alcohol Use

## Epidemiology, Diagnosis, and Treatment

Shawn M. Cohen, MD[a],*, Ryan S. Alexander, DO, MPH[a,b,c],
Stephen R. Holt, MD, MS[a]

### KEYWORDS

- Alcohol • Unhealthy alcohol use • Alcohol withdrawal syndrome
- Alcohol use disorder

### KEY POINTS

- Unhealthy alcohol use is common and underrecognized.
- Alcohol withdrawal syndrome can be effectively managed in the clinic and in the hospital; benzodiazepines remain the first line in both settings.
- Complications of alcohol use affect nearly every organ system, and reductions in alcohol use reduce these complications.
- Medications for alcohol use disorder are effective and underutilized.
- Although mutual support such as alcoholic anonymous is the most used behavioral therapy, other therapies such as CBT have more robust evidence.

## DEFINITIONS/EPIDEMIOLOGY

### Introduction

Alcohol is the most commonly used and misused substance in the United States (US) (**Table 1**).[1] More than 50% of the US population report past month alcohol use and more than 85% report lifetime use.[1] The 3 primary types of alcohol available for purchase contain varying concentrations of alcohol: Typically, beer ~5% alcohol by volume (ABV), wine ~12% ABV, and liquor/spirits ~40% ABV. Thus, a standard alcoholic beverage in the US, characterized by approximately 14g of pure alcohol, is defined by different volumes, that is, a 12oz beer, a 5oz glass of wine, or a single 1.5oz "shot" of liquor as illustrated by the National Institute on Alcohol Abuse and Alcoholism (**Fig. 1**).[2] As there are many types, strengths, volumes, and formulations of alcohol that do not clearly fit in these categories, accurately quantifying an individual's level of alcohol use are often challenging.

[a] Program in Addiction Medicine, Section of General Internal Medicine, Yale School of Medicine, 367 Cedar Street, Harkness Hal A, Suite 417A, New Haven, CT 06510, USA; [b] Department of Preventive Medicine, Griffin Hospital, Derby, CT 06418, USA; [c] Department of Internal Medicine, Griffin Hospital, Derby, CT 06418, USA
* Corresponding author.
*E-mail address:* Shawn.cohen@yale.edu

Med Clin N Am 106 (2022) 43–60
https://doi.org/10.1016/j.mcna.2021.08.003
0025-7125/22/© 2021 Elsevier Inc. All rights reserved.

medical.theclinics.com

Not all alcohol use is problematic and not all problematic alcohol use constitutes a disorder. Alcohol use exists across a spectrum (**Fig. 2**) from low-risk drinking to risky and problem drinking followed by alcohol use disorder (AUD).[3] The spectrum is fluid, with individuals transitioning to different risk categories at different times; most individuals who consume alcohol will never develop an AUD.

### Unhealthy Alcohol Use

Unhealthy alcohol use refers to a spectrum of alcohol use that may result in medical/health consequences and includes risky use, problem use, and AUD.

Risky drinking includes binge drinking and/or heavy alcohol use. Binge drinking is defined by the amount of alcohol required to bring the blood alcohol content (BAC) to 0.08 in 2 hours, generally 4 or more standard drinks in a single drinking episode for women or 5 or more for men. Heavy alcohol use is define as more than 3 drinks per day or 7 drinks per week for women and more than 4 drinks per day or 14 drinks per week for men.[3] 65.8 million people met the criteria for binge alcohol use and 16 million met the criteria for heavy alcohol use in the 2019 National Survey on Drug Use and Health (NSDUH).[1]

The presence of an AUD and its severity is determined using criteria outlined in the Diagnostic and Statistical Manual of Mental Disorders, fifth edition (DSM-5).[4] Notably, AUD is the most commonly diagnosed substance use disorder (SUD) in the US, affecting more than 14 million people (**Fig. 3**).[1] Despite this, less than 10% of those with AUD report receiving treatment in the past year[1] and fewer than 20% have ever received treatment.[5]

Screening for unhealthy alcohol use, described in more detail elsewhere in this special issue, start with one of several effective and validated screening tools. Briefly, screening tools for AUD include the single-item screening test for unhealthy alcohol use (**Box 1**), the Alcohol Use Disorders Identification Test (AUDIT) or its abridged version, the AUDIT-C. The CAGE questionnaire is another screening tool but is no longer recommended as it has been supplanted by the AUDIT-C which has a higher sensitivity for identifying risky use.

AUD is a serious medical problem associated with significant morbidity and mortality. New data from the CDC reveal that, on average, more than 95,000 individuals die each year from alcohol-related causes[6] and it is estimated that alcohol use is the third greatest modifiable risk factor leading to death in the US.[7] By comparison, estimates of the considerable morbidity and mortality related to illicit drug use remain less than that associated with unhealthy alcohol use, despite the current epidemic of opioid overdose deaths.[8]

### Prevalence in the clinical setting

Unhealthy alcohol use is underrecognized in the outpatient and inpatient setting and is a leading cause of hospitalization. Despite high rates of unhealthy alcohol use and AUD in the primary care setting, screening and diagnosis are often missed. Some advocate for a shift in addressing alcohol use in the clinic to an approach similar to addressing other chronic illnesses.[9] In the hospital setting, positive screening results for moderate-high risk alcohol use are as high as 11%–18%[10,11] and in one study over three-quarters of screen-positive patients met criteria for AUD.[11] Alcohol withdrawal alone accounted for 5% of all admissions in a national VA sample in 2013.[12] Alcohol was the 20th most expensive inpatient condition contributing to Medicaid expenditures in 2017.[13] The overall impact of alcohol on the health care system is likely underrecognized.

# What Is a Standard Drink?

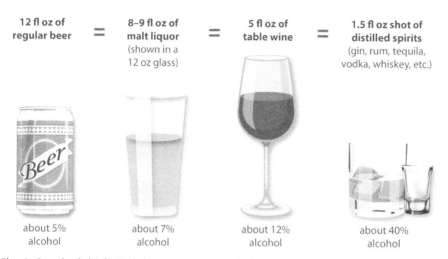

<table>
<tr><td>**12 fl oz of regular beer**</td><td>=</td><td>**8–9 fl oz of malt liquor** (shown in a 12 oz glass)</td><td>=</td><td>**5 fl oz of table wine**</td><td>=</td><td>**1.5 fl oz shot of distilled spirits** (gin, rum, tequila, vodka, whiskey, etc.)</td></tr>
<tr><td>about 5% alcohol</td><td></td><td>about 7% alcohol</td><td></td><td>about 12% alcohol</td><td></td><td>about 40% alcohol</td></tr>
</table>

**Fig. 1.** Standard drink. Each beverage portrayed above represents one standard drink (or one alcohol drink equivalent), defined in the United States as any beverage containing .6 fL oz or 14 g of pure alcohol, expressed here as alcohol by volume (alc/vol). Although the standard drink amounts are helpful for following health guidelines, they may not reflect customary serving sizes. (Figure from National Institute of Alcohol Abuse and Alcoholism (NIAAA)[2])

## NEUROBIOLOGY

Physiologically, alcohol acts primarily as a central nervous system (CNS) depressant. The acute effects of alcohol are transient and positively correlate with blood alcohol

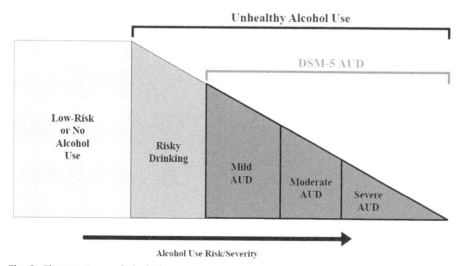

**Fig. 2.** The spectrum of alcohol use.

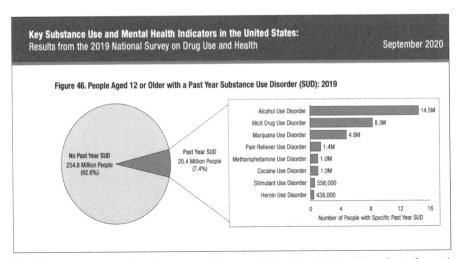

**Fig. 3.** Past year rates of substance use disorders. Note: The estimated number of people with substance use disorders is not mutually exclusive because people could have use disorders for more than 1 substance. (Figure from National Survey on Drug Use and Health 2019, SAMHSA[1])

concentration (BAC). At lower BAC levels, alcohol is an anxiolytic producing relaxation and social disinhibition. As BAC increases, one begins to experience ataxia, impaired judgment, and delayed reaction time. BAC levels exceeding 300 to 400 mg/dL may lead to significant sedation, reduced respiratory drive, coma, or death.[14]

Molecularly, alcohol's primary effect as a CNS depressant is the result of both activation of inhibitory ion channels, primarily GABA, and the downregulation of excitatory ion channels, primarily glutamate, in the brain (**Fig. 4**).[15] In addition to GABA/glutamate effects, acute intoxication produces a dopamine surge and moderate opioid agonism that positively reinforces drinking behavior.

Long-standing alcohol use leads to neural adaptations that seek to restore homeostasis between excitatory and inhibitory neural signaling.[16] In response to the persistent excess of GABA and deficiency of glutamate, the brain reduces the amount of intrinsic GABA (and other inhibitory neurotransmitters), and enhances the intrinsic excitatory signaling.[17,18] This physiologic adaptation to prolonged alcohol exposure predisposes the system to a relative GABA deficiency when the exogenous GABAergic signal (alcohol) is removed in the setting of alcohol cessation. This compensatory maladaptation is the source of alcohol withdrawal syndrome (AWS).

In addition, as alcohol is intrinsically neurotoxic, prolonged, heavy alcohol use can contribute to global cerebral neuron loss, permanently altering brain function.[19] Neurotoxicity is proposed to occur through various mechanisms including excitotoxicity from unbalanced upregulation of glutamate during alcohol withdrawal (as outlined above) as well as inflammatory damage (oxidative stress), metabolic derangement (hyperammonemia), and nutritional deficiencies (thiamine, folate). In addition to CNS

---

**Box 1**
**Single item screen for alcohol positive screen is any response greater than 0**

How many times in the past year have you had X or more drinks in a single day?

X = 5 for men, 4 for women

damage, prolonged alcohol use causes peripheral nervous system (PNS) damage which can result in a debilitating alcohol-related polyneuropathy.

## ALCOHOL BIOMARKERS

Lab testing, often referred to as biomarkers, can be used to help identify acute and chronic alcohol use. Direct measurement of blood alcohol level (BAL) is useful in detecting intoxication and acute use of alcohol.

Biomarkers of chronic alcohol use are more varied. Nonspecific testing can include measurements of aspartate aminotransferase (AST) assessing hepatic inflammation, gamma-glutamyl transferase (GGT), which is more specific for alcohol-related hepato-toxicity, and mean corpuscular volume (MCV) for macrocytosis. More specific tests include urine ethyl glucuronide (EtG) which can be detected 5 days after use and serum carbohydrate deficient-transferrin (CDT) which can be used to detect heavy alcohol use from the prior 2 weeks. Both tests can be limited by false positives particularly in the setting of liver disease.[20] Phosphatidylethanol (PEth) has shown utility in patients with liver disease but the optimal cutoff point is unclear.[21]

These laboratory tests are not a replacement for thorough patient history and should only be interpreted in the appropriate clinical context.

## ALCOHOL WITHDRAWAL MANAGEMENT
### Course

The symptoms of AWS can begin as little as 6 hours after last alcohol use and peak around 72 hours after last use.[22,23] Notably, symptoms can begin before the BAC reaches zero. Mild and moderate symptoms often predominate early and include anxiety, tremors, difficulty sleeping, decreased appetite, diaphoresis, headache, and nausea. Hallucinations, which may be auditory, tactile, or visual, are also relatively common, affecting up to 2% of all individuals who experience AWS.[24] This syndrome, known as alcohol hallucinosis, is distinct from alcohol withdrawal delirium such that disorientation and autonomic hyperactivity are absent.

### Severe or complicated alcohol withdrawal

Severe AWS includes the presence of seizures and/or delirium, that is, delirium tremens (DTs).[25] Seizures, typically grand mal seizures, occur in less than 3% of patients and can occur as early as 8 hours after the cessation of alcohol with peak occurrence

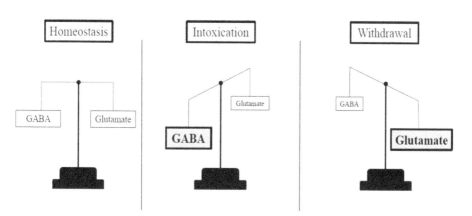

**Fig. 4.** Simplified neurobiology of alcohol intoxication and withdrawal.

at 24 hours.[4,22] DTs is potentially lethal and the most severe complication of AWS. It is characterized by disorientation and autonomic hyperactivity, including tachycardia, hypertension, fever, and psychomotor agitation. Symptoms of DTs typically begin 3 days after the start of AWS and can last between 1 and 8 days.[23] Mortality rates due to DTs have declined to nearly 1% and are most often attributable to arrhythmia, seizures, concurrent illness, and hyperthermia.[23,26]

Given its potential mortality, early identification of patients at highest risk of severe withdrawal is of paramount importance. Prior episodes of DTs and AWS have consistently been associated with future incidence whereas other findings including historical features (age >65, concurrent acute illness) and laboratory results (BAL>200, hypokalemia, thrombocytopenia) have been less consistent.[27–30] Scoring systems such as the PAWSS have been developed to aid in prediction but have not been widely validated.[31]

### Ambulatory Treatment

Although the treatment of AWS often requires hospital-based management, ambulatory management can be considered in willing patients with mild/moderate symptoms, no risk factors for severe AWS, and reliable community support.[25] In appropriately selected patients, ambulatory management has been associated with dramatic reductions in treatment duration and cost.[32] This approach requires a willing support person who can help facilitate near-daily follow-up visits, monitor the individual's alcohol withdrawal symptoms, manage medications, and assess for clinical deterioration that might warrant hospitalization.

Benzodiazepines are first-line therapy for treating AWS in the outpatient setting due to the wealth of studies showing a reduction in significant outcomes including seizures, DTs, and symptom scores.[33–35] Long-acting benzodiazepines such as chlordiazepoxide or diazepam are preferred over shorter-acting medications but should be avoided in the setting of advanced hepatic disease; in this case, lorazepam would be preferred. Gabapentin, an anticonvulsant, has been shown as an effective alternative to benzodiazepines for outpatient AWS treatment and has the benefit of being an effective treatment for AUD as well (**Table 1**).[36] Although neither benzodiazepines nor gabapentin has been shown to reduce seizures or DTs in the outpatient setting, the wealth of data using benzodiazepines in the inpatient setting makes these agents the first-line choice for outpatients as well.

### Hospital-Based Treatment

Standardized hospital protocols for the treatment of AWS are an important framework for providing high-quality treatment in the inpatient setting. These often include approved medications, symptom-based scoring, and preselected adjunctive treatments. Using such protocols has been shown to reduce the length of stay, ICU length of stay, intubation, and improve adherence to evidence-based care.[37–39] Workup of a hospitalized patient with AWS should also involve laboratory testing including complete blood count, complete metabolic panel including magnesium and phosphate levels, blood alcohol level, and urine drug screen. Hospitalization can also be an opportunity to engage in preventative care including HIV testing, HCV testing, and indicated vaccinations such as the pneumococcal vaccine.

As in the ambulatory setting, benzodiazepines remain first-line therapy in the hospital setting (see **Table 1**). Diazepam, due to its rapid onset, long half-life, and multiple routes of administration (oral, IV, IM), is often preferred except in the case of advanced liver disease due to active hepatic metabolites; in such cases, lorazepam is preferred. Symptom-triggered therapy (STT), giving medication based on a validated symptom

**Table 1**
**Example regimens for the treatment of alcohol withdrawal syndrome**

| Outpatient | | |
|---|---|---|
| | Benzodiazepine fixed dose | Day 1- diazepam 10 mg four times daily |
| | | Day 2 - diazepam 10 mg three times daily |
| | | Day 3 - diazepam 10 mg two times daily |
| | | Day 4 - diazepam 10 mg one time daily |
| | | Additional PRN doses provided as well |
| | Gabapentin fixed dose | Day 1 - gabapentin 300 mg every 6 h |
| | | Day 2 - gabapentin 300 mg every 8 h[a] |
| | | Day 3 - gabapentin 300 mg every 12 h |
| | | Day 4 - gabapentin 300 mg daily |
| | | Additional PRN dose available as well |
| Inpatient | Benzodiazepine symptom triggered | Diazepam 10 mg q2-4 hours PRN CIWA >10 |
| | | • if the history of complicated withdrawal add diazepam 10 mg q6 hours until using minimal PRNs then decrease to 5 mg q6hrs then stop |
| | Phenobarbital front loading | 10 mg/kg[b] ideal body weight IV/IM followed by up to 5–7 d oral taper (example taper 65 mg BID x2d then 32 mg BID x2d) |
| | | • can get additional doses of 130–260 mg IV/IM PRN for continued symptoms |

[a] If interested in gabapentin as MAUD can continue at gabapentin 300 mg q6hrs and increase to 600 TID after 2 to 3 d.
[b] Often given in 3 divided IM doses 3 h apart.

score, is the preferred method of treatment due to evidence it reduces the length of stay and total benzodiazepine use when compared with a prolonged benzodiazepine fixed-dose approach.[40,41] Using an additional brief, fixed-dose taper or a front-loading treatment is appropriate for those at highest risk for severe withdrawal.

The most commonly used, validated scoring system is the Clinical Institute Withdrawal Assessment for Alcohol -revised (CIWA-Ar), a 10-item symptom scale. Importantly, the CIWA-Ar requires some training to administer and also requires an alert, oriented, and reasonably cooperative patient to reliably generate a score.[22] In the setting of significant delirium or obtundation, alternatives such as the Minnesota Detoxification Scale (MINDS) score or Richmond Agitation Sedation Scale (RASS) can be used to guide therapy.[25,38]

Phenobarbital, a barbiturate, with its rapid onset and long-acting effects, is increasingly viewed as an alternative to benzodiazepines in the treatment of AWS, particularly for use as initial treatment to rapidly control symptoms or as rescue therapy in those not responding to benzodiazepines.[37,42,43] Despite concerns about the increased risk of respiratory depression with barbiturates, large observational studies have shown no increased rates of adverse events compared with benzodiazepines.[42,44] Due to their different mechanism of action at the GABA receptor, barbiturates can provide additional benefits compared to benzodiazepines, potentially mediating cross-tolerance with alcohol and providing inhibition at the NMDA receptor which plays an important role in the symptoms of AWS.[18] Nonetheless, as data for benzodiazepines are more robust, they remain first-line treatment with barbiturates a reasonable alternative.

Other anticonvulsants such as carbamazepine and gabapentin have been shown to be effective at treating the symptoms of AWS; however, their use should be limited to mild to moderate alcohol withdrawal or as adjuncts given lack of data on the prevention of manifestations of severe alcohol withdrawal.[25]

### Additional Therapies

Alcohol withdrawal seizures should prompt a full neurologic examination. In patients with recurrent seizures, focal findings on examination, or with a change in seizure type/pattern further workup including neuroimaging, EEG, and neurology consultation may be required. Intravenous administration of benzodiazepines is first-line treatment for withdrawal seizures and has also been shown to prevent recurrent seizures.[45] Phenobarbital is considered an effective second-line agent.[43]

Vitamin deficiencies and electrolyte abnormalities are commonly encountered in AWS. Thiamine is routinely administered to prevent and treat Wernicke–Korsakoff syndrome (WKS), further reviewed below. Electrolytes including magnesium and phosphate should be measured and repleted.

Lastly, as a fulminant manifestation of an underlying chronic, relapsing disease, the inpatient management of AWS must include addressing AUD itself, with referrals to outpatient treatment, behavioral therapy, and initiation of pharmacotherapy before discharge, if within the patient's goals.

## MEDICAL AND PSYCHIATRIC COMPLICATIONS

As a small molecule that easily diffuses into all tissues in the body, alcohol can lead to pathologic conditions in multiple organ systems (**Table 2**). Below is an overview of selected complications of unhealthy alcohol use.

### Alcohol-Related Cardiomyopathy

Alcohol-related cardiomyopathy, a diagnosis of exclusion, is a dilated cardiomyopathy diagnosed by dilation and dysfunction of both ventricles in the setting of chronic heavy alcohol use.[46] Manifestations and treatment are similar to other forms of heart failure with reduced ejection fraction, including guideline-directed medical therapy.

| Table 2 Medical and psychiatric complications of alcohol use | |
|---|---|
| **Organ System** | **Effect of Alcohol** |
| Cardiovascular | *Acute:* Atrial Fibrillation (ie, Holiday Heart Syndrome) <br> *Chronic:* Cardiomyopathy, coronary artery disease, hypertension |
| Hepatic | *Acute:* Alcoholic hepatitis <br> *Chronic:* Steatohepatitis, Cirrhosis |
| Gastrointestinal | *Acute:* Pancreatitis, gastritis <br> *Chronic:* Chronic pancreatitis with pancreatic insufficiency, esophageal cancer |
| Neuropsychiatric | *Acute:* Wernicke encephalopathy, seizure[a], delirium[a], hallucinosis[a] <br> *Chronic:* Korsakoff Syndrome, peripheral neuropathy, stroke, dementia |
| Pulmonary | *Acute:* Aspiration pneumonitis or pneumonia |
| Rheumatologic/MSK | *Acute:* Rhabdomyolysis, trauma <br> *Chronic:* Gout |
| Renal/Metabolic | *Acute:* Ketoacidosis, refeeding syndrome, Hypomagnesemia |
| Hematologic | *Chronic:* Macrocytic anemia, thrombocytopenia |

[a] In the setting of alcohol withdrawal syndrome.

Additionally, focusing on reduction in alcohol use is an essential component of treatment as several studies have shown marked improvement in cardiac function following a significant reduction in alcohol consumption.[47]

### Alcohol-Associated Liver Disease

Alcohol remains one of the most common causes of liver disease in the US.[48] Alcohol-related hepatitis is an acute manifestation of the toxic effect of alcohol on the liver. It can present with rapid onset of jaundice, right upper quadrant pain, development of ascites, and fever, and can occur during binge drinking episodes or even after several weeks of abstinence. Diagnosis is generally clinical, with accompanying elevations in bilirubin and transaminases; however, in the setting of confounding factors, a biopsy may be required.[49] Mild to moderate disease (as defined by Maddrey Discriminant Function score < 32) has a low risk of death, requiring only supportive care, whereas severe disease has a mortality ranging from 14% to 50%[48] and is typically treated with prednisilone.[50]

Cirrhosis secondary to alcohol use is the leading indication for liver transplantation in the US.[51] Management is identical to cirrhosis from other causes, including avoidance of alcohol. While alcohol cessation has been shown to improve survival, recent recommendations do not require fixed intervals of cessation as a prerequisite for transplantation.[48] It is notable that posttransplant survival in patients with cirrhosis secondary to alcohol is similar to those with other indications for transplantation.[52]

### Wernicke–Korsakoff Syndrome

WKS is a potentially fatal neuropsychiatric disease caused by Vitamin B1 (thiamine) deficiency and is more common among individuals with AUD.[53] Early manifestations of Wernicke encephalopathy are altered mental status, oculomotor abnormalities (nystagmus and gaze palsies), and gait ataxia, which are reversible with thiamine replacement. Without treatment, the syndrome progresses to the irreversible Korsakoff's syndrome (KS) defined by an impairment in working memory causing anterograde amnesia. The syndrome is underrecognized and thus often goes untreated.[54]

Treatment for WKS is IV or IM thiamine replacement given that oral thiamine is poorly absorbed and intravenous and intramuscular thiamine is well tolerated.[55,56] A typical treatment dose is 500 mg IV every 8 hours for 3 days although data comparing the efficacy of different regimens are generally lacking.[57] In addition, WKS prophylaxis with routine IV/IM thiamine administration at a dose of 100 mg once per day is generally recommended for hospitalized individuals with current heavy alcohol use.[25,55]

## MEDICATIONS FOR ALCOHOL USE DISORDER

Treatment of AUD begins with a conversation regarding the goals of treatment. Although abstinence is a stated goal for some individuals, others may find that committing to a reduction of alcohol is more feasible than complete abstinence. Reduction of heavy alcohol use has been shown to improve physical and mental health, enhance the quality of life, and decrease mortality.[58–60]

As reviewed below, MAUD is effective at reducing alcohol use and increasing rates of abstinence (**Table 3**). Despite the evidence in support of MAUD, they remain underutilized in all treatment settings.[61–63] If medications are used and the patient is amenable, partnership with family or close friends to assist with medication management, a treatment modality known as network therapy,[64] has been shown to be effective particularly with disulfiram.[65]

**Table 3**
Medications for alcohol use disorder

| Medication | Naltrexone | Acamprosate | Disulfiram | Gabapentin | Topiramate |
|---|---|---|---|---|---|
| Dose | 50 mg PO daily or 380 mg IM monthly | 666 mg three times daily | 250 mg daily[b] | 600 mg three times daily[a] | 100 mg two times daily[a] |
| Contraindication | Currently on opioids Decompensated liver disease | Renal Failure | Avoid in unstable cardiac disease | | |
| Who to use in | First-line goal of abstinence or reduction in drinking | Goal of abstinence | Goal of abstinence | Withdrawal symptoms If other indications | If other meds ineffective |
| Tips | No recommendation for LFTs before starting if going to delay care | Abstinent to start | Better in directly observed therapy or with partner; Avoid alcohol-containing products; Can cause idiosyncratic hepatitis | Can also use to treat mild/moderate withdrawal; Not FDA approved Dose adjustment based on renal function | Some data in cocaine use disorder; Not FDA approved Dose adjustment based on renal function |

[a] Gabapentin and topiramate should be titrated up to an effective dose.
[b] Can increase to 500 mg if no reaction to 250 mg.

### Food and Drug Administration (FDA) Approved Medications

Naltrexone is a mu opioid receptor antagonist; its effectiveness in treating AUD is thought to be mediated by a decrease in alcohol cravings and pleasurable effects associated with alcohol use.[66] Available as a 50 mg pill taken once daily or a 380 mg intramuscular injection given monthly, numerous studies support naltrexone's efficacy in improving alcohol-related outcomes.[67–69] Alternative oral dosing strategies such as needed dosing in the setting of anticipated triggers have also been shown effective.[70] Naltrexone is contraindicated in patients taking opioids, and whereas hepatitis is listed as an adverse effect, recent studies have shown it to be safe in most stages of liver dysfunction leading SAMHSA to recommend that naltrexone can be started before obtaining liver function tests.[71,72] Advanced liver disease (Child–Pugh Class C) should prompt a discussion of risks and benefits.

Acamprosate is a GABA and glutamate neuromodulator, available in 333 mg pills dosed as 2 pills 3 times daily. Several large meta-analyses have shown it to be effective at a reduction in return to drinking, reduction in any drinking, and increased cumulative abstinence.[68,69,73] Acamprosate is renally excreted and dose should be adjusted for renal impairment and it is contraindicated at CrCl less than 30. Diarrhea is the most common side effect.

Disulfiram is an inhibitor of aldehyde dehydrogenase with the ingestion of alcohol, blood aldehyde levels increase leading to an aversive reaction. This "disulfiram reaction" is often characterized by flushing, tachycardia, diaphoresis, nausea, vomiting, and headache.[74] It is typically dosed as 250 mg daily and is only appropriate in patients whose goal is abstinence. Although a large metanalysis of randomized controlled trials showed no difference in outcomes with disulfiram, a metanalysis of open-label trials, believed to be the more appropriate study design for a deterrent medication, showed it to be effective, particularly for patients with a partner who can help improve adherence.[65,69,75] Disulfiram should be avoided in patients with advanced liver disease given the risk of acute hepatitis and in those with significant cardiac disease given the hemodynamic changes that may accompany the disulfiram reaction.

### Non–FDA-Approved Medications

Of the non–FDA-approved medications with trials assessing their use in AUD, topiramate, and gabapentin have the most robust data. Topiramate, an anticonvulsant, has had several RCTs showing efficacy to reduce heavy alcohol use, improving abstinence, and increasing safe drinking at doses up to 300 mg.[76,77] Side effects were more common with topiramate including paresthesias, dizziness, weight loss, anorexia, and difficulty concentrating; however, serious adverse events were not more common than placebo. A slow uptitration starting at a dose of 25 mg in the evening, increasing by 25 to 50 mg every 5 to 7 days, to a target dose of 100 mg twice daily is essential to minimizing side effects.

Gabapentin, another anticonvulsant and a GABA agonist, also has several RCTs evaluating its efficacy for the reduction of alcohol use. Two studies have shown an increase in abstinence and decrease in heavy drinking; the first yielded a dose–response relationship up to 1800 mg per day and the second showed benefits specifically in patients with symptoms of early alcohol withdrawal.[78,79] Gabapentin is typically started at a dose of 300 mg TID and increased over several weeks to a target dose of 600 to 900 mg TID, as tolerated.

## BEHAVIORAL TREATMENT

The recommended treatment for AUD involves both pharmacotherapy and behavioral therapy, though behavioral treatments are often overemphasized at the expense of pharmacotherapy. Behavioral treatments seek to achieve the following goals: to gain an improved understanding of one's addiction, to enhance motivation to change harmful behaviors, teach healthy coping skills, and to provide social and psychological support to optimize recovery.[80]

### Screening and Brief Intervention

Brief interventions (BIs) aim to address harmful alcohol use among patients in primary care settings who have at-risk alcohol use. BI is often used in conjunction with screening, as discussed above, and the 2 together are referred to as SBI. BI is typically minutes in duration and is conducted by primary care or emergency department providers. One simple approach, initially developed for tobacco cessation, is "the 5 A's" (Ask, Advise, Assess, Assist, Arrange): Ask about alcohol use, advise about unhealthy alcohol use, and concern about harms, assess the severity of alcohol misuse, assist the patient in developing a plan, and finally arrange for follow-up or referral to specialty care. SBI has been shown to be effective in reducing unhealthy alcohol use among individuals who report at-risk drinking behaviors.[81] The US Preventive Services Task Force (USPSTF) recommends routine SBI for adults in the primary care setting with a grade B recommendation.[82]

### Mutual Support And 12-Step Facilitation

Among individuals with AUD who received any treatment in 2019, the most common type of treatment reported (>50%) was mutual support programs such as alcoholics anonymous (AA).[1] AA is the prototypical 12-step facilitation program, though numerous others have emerged in recent years (eg, SMART recovery, Refuge recovery). Despite often being thought synonymous with treatment, few data exist evaluating the effect of mutual support groups on treatment outcomes in AUD. Nonetheless, numerous advantages, including the accessibility, the highly structured process, the low-cost, and the potential for sustained relapse prevention among engaged members, make mutual support groups an attractive adjunct to treatment.[83]

TSF is a manualized program that leads a participant through a standardized, stepwise, treatment algorithm that facilitates their participation and progression through treatment steps. Despite conflicting evidence regarding the efficacy of TSF for the treatment of AUD, TSF is likely as effective as other behavioral therapies in improving alcohol-related outcomes.[84]

### Cognitive-Behavioral Therapy

CBT is a commonly used and widely studied treatment for AUD, with small to moderate effect sizes, similar to other behavioral modalities.[85] The approach is a therapist-driven, structured intervention that aims to help patients better understand the thoughts, feelings, and behaviors that lead to alcohol use, and then to develop skills to address and cope with the underlying psychopathology. A plan is developed to prepare for future triggers or urges to drink alcohol and to create a relapse prevention strategy using psychotherapeutic techniques. Despite its benefits, access is limited to CBT. Computer-based CBT may be one mechanism to increase access to CBT and studies has been shown to be effective for AUD.[86]

### Other Behavioral Interventions

In addition to the common interventions mentioned above, some other approaches should be mentioned. Motivational interviewing (MI) or motivational enhancement therapy (MET) is an important, nonjudgmental, collaborative approach to interviewing that helps patients realize the harms of their alcohol use. This approach can be used in any setting and should be used when other behavioral treatments have not been successful. It can be viewed as a philosophic approach to interviewing that intends to promote self-actualization rather than serving as a stand-alone treatment.

## NEW ADVANCES IN TREATMENT

Research continues into both new avenues for medication treatment and behavioral treatment of AUD. The effectiveness of off-label medications, such as prazosin and varenicline, has continued to be assessed as the search for new medications and targets for treatment continues.[87] There are also numerous emerging technology-based interventions that use apps and internet resources to promote recovery from AUD that are being studied.[88]

Perhaps most impactful may be continued advocacy by the alcohol clinical trials initiative (ACTIVE) toward MAUD clinical trial endpoints focusing on WHO drinking level reduction rather than the current endpoints of abstinence and no heavy drinking. Given the clear benefit of reduction of drinking level,[58–60] this could lead to approval of more effective medications and reframing of the definition of treatment success to be more inclusive and person-centered.

## SUMMARY

As the most commonly used and misused substance in the US, alcohol exacts a considerable toll on morbidity and mortality. Decades of research have highlighted the precise neurobiological mechanisms by which alcohol acts in the brain, including its reinforcing effects via dopaminergic transmission. Management of alcohol intoxication includes supportive care, whereas benzodiazepines remain the mainstay of treatment for alcohol withdrawal. Several pharmacologic and behavioral approaches have demonstrable evidence in the long-term management of AUD. Ongoing research may identify novel therapeutic targets that may aid in treatment.

## CLINICS CARE POINTS

- Benzodiazepines remain first line treatment of alcohol withdrawal in the inpatient and outpatient setting. They are most often used with a standardized symptom scale with the addition of a standing taper or front loading in high risk patients.
- Medications for alcohol use disorder are effective and underused in both the clinic and the hospital.
- Behavioral treatment, while also effective, is often overemphasized at the expense of medication.
- Treatment of alcohol use disorder should be person-centered; both abstinence and reduction of alcohol use goals may be appropriate as both goals are evidence-based and beneficial.

## DISCLOSURE

The authors have nothing to disclose.

## REFERENCES

1. Substance Abuse and Mental Health Services Administration. Key substance use and mental health indicators in the United States: results from the 2019 National Survey on Drug Use and Health (HHS Publication No. PEP20-07-01-001, NSDUH series H-55). Rockville, MD: Center for Behavioral Health Statistics and Quality, Substance Abuse and Mental Health Services Administration; 2020. Available at: https://www.samhsa.gov/data/.

2. National Institute on Alcohol Abuse and Alcoholism. What is a standard drink?. Available at: https://www.niaaa.nih.gov/alcohols-effects-health/overview-alcohol-consumption/what-standard-drink. Accessed July 2, 2021.

3. National Institute on Alcohol Abuse and Alcoholism. Alcohol facts and statistics 2020. Available at: https://www.niaaa.nih.gov/publications/brochures-and-fact-sheets/alcohol-facts-and-statistics.

4. American Psychiatric Association. Diagnostic and statistical manual of mental disorders: DSM-5. 5th edition. Arlington, VA: American Psychiatric Association; 2013.

5. Grant BF, Goldstein RB, Saha TD, et al. Epidemiology of DSM-5 alcohol use disorder: results from the National Epidemiologic Survey on Alcohol and Related Conditions III. JAMA Psychiatry 2015;72(8):757–66.

6. Esser MB, Sherk A, Liu Y, et al. Deaths and years of potential life lost from excessive alcohol use - United States, 2011-2015. MMWR Morb Mortal Wkly Rep 2020; 69(30):981–7.

7. Mokdad AH, Marks JS, Stroup DF, et al. Correction: actual causes of death in the United States, 2000. JAMA 2005;293(3):293–4.

8. Miller TR, Nygaard P, Gaidus A, et al. Heterogeneous costs of alcohol and drug problems across cities and counties in California. Alcohol Clin Exp Res 2017; 41(4):758–68.

9. Rehm J, Anderson P, Manthey J, et al. Alcohol use disorders in primary health care: what do we know and where do we go? Alcohol Alcohol 2016;51(4):422–7.

10. Wakeman SE, Herman G, Wilens TE, et al. The prevalence of unhealthy alcohol and drug use among inpatients in a general hospital. Subst Abus 2020;41(3): 331–9.

11. Saitz R, Freedner N, Palfai TP, et al. The severity of unhealthy alcohol use in hospitalized medical patients. The spectrum is narrow. J Gen Intern Med 2006;21(4): 381–5.

12. Steel TL, Malte CA, Bradley KA, et al. Prevalence and variation of clinically recognized inpatient alcohol withdrawal syndrome in the Veterans Health Administration. J Addict Med 2020;14(4):300–4.

13. Liang L, Moore B, Soni A. National inpatient hospital costs: the most expensive conditions by payer, 2017. HCUP Statistical Brief #261. Month 2020. Agency for Healthcare Research and Quality, Rockville, MD. www.hcup-us.ahrq.gov/reports/statbriefs/sb261-Most-Expensive-Hospital-Conditions-2017.pdf.

14. Heatley MK, Crane J. The blood alcohol concentration at post-mortem in 175 fatal cases of alcohol intoxication. Med Sci Law 1990;30(2):101–5.

15. Woodward JJ. The pharmacology of alcohol. In: Miller SC, Fiellin DA, Rosenthal RN, et al, editors. The ASAM principles of addiction medicine. 6th edition. Philadelphia: Wolters Kluwer; 2019. p. 107–24.

16. Koob GF, Bloom FE. Cellular and molecular mechanisms of drug dependence. Science 1988;242(4879):715–23.

17. Clapp P, Bhave SV, Hoffman PL. How adaptation of the brain to alcohol leads to dependence: a pharmacological perspective. Alcohol Res Health 2008;31(4): 310–39.

18. Littleton J. Neurochemical mechanisms underlying alcohol withdrawal. Alcohol Health Res World 1998;22(1):13–24.

19. Most D, Ferguson L, Harris RA. Molecular basis of alcoholism. Handb Clin Neurol 2014;125:89–111.

20. Merlin JS, Warner EA, Starrels JL. Laboratory assessment. In: Miller SC, Fiellin DA, Rosenthal RN, et al, editors. The ASAM principles of addiction medicine. 6th edition. Philadelphia: Wolters Kluwer; 2019. p. 348–58.

21. Stewart SH, Koch DG, Willner IR, et al. Validation of blood phosphatidylethanol as an alcohol consumption biomarker in patients with chronic liver disease. Alcohol Clin Exp Res 2014;38(6):1706–11.

22. Wartenberg AA. Management of alcohol intoxication and withdrawal. In: Miller SC, Fiellin DA, Rosenthal RN, et al, editors. The ASAM principles of addiction medicine. 6th edition. Philadelphia: Wolters Kluwer; 2019. p. 704–22.

23. Schuckit MA. Recognition and management of withdrawal delirium (delirium tremens). N Engl J Med 2014;371(22):2109–13.

24. Stephane M, Arnaout B, Yoon G. Alcohol withdrawal hallucinations in the general population, an epidemiological study. Psychiatry Res 2018;262:129–34.

25. The ASAM clinical practice guideline on alcohol withdrawal management. J Addict Med 2020;14(3S):1–72.

26. Naranjo CA, Sellers EM. Clinical assessment and pharmacotherapy of the alcohol withdrawal syndrome. Recent Dev Alcohol 1986;4:265–81.

27. Ferguson JA, Suelzer CJ, Eckert GJ, et al. Risk factors for delirium tremens development. J Gen Intern Med 1996;11(7):410–4.

28. Goodson CM, Clark BJ, Douglas IS. Predictors of severe alcohol withdrawal syndrome: a systematic review and meta-analysis. Alcohol Clin Exp Res 2014; 38(10):2664–77.

29. Salottolo K, McGuire E, Mains CW, et al. Occurrence, predictors, and prognosis of alcohol withdrawal syndrome and delirium tremens following traumatic injury. Crit Care Med 2017;45(5):867–74.

30. Wood E, Albarqouni L, Tkachuk S, et al. Will this hospitalized patient develop severe alcohol withdrawal syndrome?: the rational clinical examination systematic review. JAMA 2018;320(8):825–33.

31. Maldonado JR, Sher Y, Das S, et al. Prospective validation study of the Prediction of Alcohol Withdrawal Severity Scale (PAWSS) in medically Ill inpatients: a new scale for the prediction of complicated alcohol withdrawal syndrome. Alcohol Alcohol 2015;50(5):509–18.

32. Hayashida M, Alterman AI, McLellan AT, et al. Comparative effectiveness and costs of inpatient and outpatient detoxification of patients with mild-to-moderate alcohol withdrawal syndrome. N Engl J Med 1989;320(6):358–65.

33. Amato L, Minozzi S, Vecchi S, et al. Benzodiazepines for alcohol withdrawal. Cochrane Database Syst Rev 2010;(3):CD005063.

34. Holbrook AM, Crowther R, Lotter A, et al. Meta-analysis of benzodiazepine use in the treatment of acute alcohol withdrawal. CMAJ 1999;160(5):649–55.

35. Mayo-Smith MF. Pharmacological management of alcohol withdrawal. A meta-analysis and evidence-based practice guideline. American Society of Addiction Medicine Working Group on pharmacological management of alcohol withdrawal. JAMA 1997;278(2):144–51.

36. Leung JG, Hall-Flavin D, Nelson S, et al. The role of gabapentin in the management of alcohol withdrawal and dependence. Ann Pharmacother 2015;49(8): 897–906.

37. Duby JJ, Berry AJ, Ghayyem P, et al. Alcohol withdrawal syndrome in critically ill patients: protocolized versus nonprotocolized management. J Trauma Acute Care Surg 2014;77(6):938–43.

38. Heavner JJ, Akgun KM, Heavner MS, et al. Implementation of an ICU-specific alcohol withdrawal syndrome management protocol reduces the need for mechanical ventilation. Pharmacotherapy 2018;38(7):701–13.

39. Melkonian A, Patel R, Magh A, et al. Assessment of a hospital-wide CIWA-Ar protocol for management of alcohol withdrawal syndrome. Mayo Clin Proc Innov Qual Outcomes 2019;3(3):344–9.

40. Saitz R, Mayo-Smith MF, Roberts MS, et al. Individualized treatment for alcohol withdrawal. A randomized double-blind controlled trial. JAMA 1994;272(7): 519–23.

41. Daeppen JB, Gache P, Landry U, et al. Symptom-triggered vs fixed-schedule doses of benzodiazepine for alcohol withdrawal: a randomized treatment trial. Arch Intern Med 2002;162(10):1117–21.

42. Nisavic M, Nejad SH, Isenberg BM, et al. Use of phenobarbital in alcohol withdrawal management - A retrospective comparison study of phenobarbital and benzodiazepines for acute alcohol withdrawal management in general medical patients. Psychosomatics 2019;60(5):458–67.

43. Young GP, Rores C, Murphy C, et al. Intravenous phenobarbital for alcohol withdrawal and convulsions. Ann Emerg Med 1987;16(8):847–50.

44. Askgaard G, Hallas J, Fink-Jensen A, et al. Phenobarbital compared to benzodiazepines in alcohol withdrawal treatment: a register-based cohort study of subsequent benzodiazepine use, alcohol recidivism and mortality. Drug Alcohol Depend 2016;161:258–64.

45. D'Onofrio G, Rathlev NK, Ulrich AS, et al. Lorazepam for the prevention of recurrent seizures related to alcohol. N Engl J Med 1999;340(12):915–9.

46. Bozkurt B, Colvin M, Cook J, et al. Current diagnostic and treatment strategies for specific dilated cardiomyopathies: a scientific statement from the American Heart Association. Circulation 2016;134(23):e579–646.

47. Nicolas JM, Fernandez-Sola J, Estruch R, et al. The effect of controlled drinking in alcoholic cardiomyopathy. Ann Intern Med 2002;136(3):192–200.

48. Crabb DW, Im GY, Szabo G, et al. Diagnosis and treatment of alcohol-associated liver diseases: 2019 practice guidance from the American Association for the Study of Liver Diseases. Hepatology 2020;71(1):306–33.

49. Crabb DW, Bataller R, Chalasani NP, et al. Standard definitions and common data elements for clinical trials in patients with alcoholic hepatitis: recommendation from the NIAAA alcoholic hepatitis consortia. Gastroenterology 2016;150(4): 785–90.

50. Louvet A, Thursz MR, Kim DJ, et al. Corticosteroids Reduce risk of death within 28 days for patients with severe alcoholic hepatitis, compared with pentoxifylline or placebo-a meta-analysis of individual data from controlled trials. Gastroenterology 2018;155(2):458–468 e458.

51. Cholankeril G, Ahmed A. Alcoholic liver disease replaces hepatitis C virus infection as the leading indication for liver transplantation in the United States. Clin Gastroenterol Hepatol 2018;16(8):1356–8.

52. Lucey MR, Schaubel DE, Guidinger MK, et al. Effect of alcoholic liver disease and hepatitis C infection on waiting list and posttransplant mortality and transplant survival benefit. Hepatology 2009;50(2):400–6.
53. Sechi G, Serra A. Wernicke's encephalopathy: new clinical settings and recent advances in diagnosis and management. Lancet Neurol 2007;6(5):442–55.
54. Caine D, Halliday GM, Kril JJ, et al. Operational criteria for the classification of chronic alcoholics: identification of Wernicke's encephalopathy. J Neurol Neurosurg Psychiatry 1997;62(1):51–60.
55. Pruckner N, Baumgartner J, Hinterbuchinger B, et al. Thiamine substitution in alcohol use disorder: a narrative review of medical guidelines. Eur Addict Res 2019;25(3):103–10.
56. Wrenn KD, Slovis CM. Is intravenous thiamine safe? Am J Emerg Med 1992; 10(2):165.
57. Day E, Bentham PW, Callaghan R, et al. Thiamine for prevention and treatment of Wernicke-Korsakoff Syndrome in people who abuse alcohol. Cochrane Database Syst Rev 2013;(7):CD004033.
58. Laramee P, Leonard S, Buchanan-Hughes A, et al. Risk of all-cause mortality in alcohol-dependent individuals: a systematic literature review and meta-analysis. EBioMedicine 2015;2(10):1394–404.
59. Witkiewitz K, Kranzler HR, Hallgren KA, et al. Drinking risk level reductions associated with improvements in physical health and quality of life among individuals with alcohol use disorder. Alcohol Clin Exp Res 2018;42(12):2453–65.
60. Roerecke M, Gual A, Rehm J. Reduction of alcohol consumption and subsequent mortality in alcohol use disorders: systematic review and meta-analyses. J Clin Psychiatry 2013;74(12):e1181–9.
61. Harris AH, Oliva E, Bowe T, et al. Pharmacotherapy of alcohol use disorders by the Veterans Health Administration: patterns of receipt and persistence. Psychiatr Serv 2012;63(7):679–85.
62. Joudrey PJ, Kladney M, Cunningham CO, et al. Primary care engagement is associated with increased pharmacotherapy prescribing for alcohol use disorder (AUD). Addict Sci Clin Pract 2019;14(1):19.
63. Mark TL, Kranzler HR, Song X. Understanding US addiction physicians' low rate of naltrexone prescription. Drug Alcohol Depend 2003;71(3):219–28.
64. Galanter M. Network therapy for addiction: a model for office practice. Am J Psychiatry 1993;150(1):28–36.
65. Skinner MD, Lahmek P, Pham H, et al. Disulfiram efficacy in the treatment of alcohol dependence: a meta-analysis. PLoS One 2014;9(2):e87366.
66. O'Malley SS, Jaffe AJ, Rode S, et al. Experience of a "slip" among alcoholics treated with naltrexone or placebo. Am J Psychiatry 1996;153(2):281–3.
67. Garbutt JC, Kranzler HR, O'Malley SS, et al. Efficacy and tolerability of long-acting injectable naltrexone for alcohol dependence: a randomized controlled trial. JAMA 2005;293(13):1617–25.
68. Bouza C, Angeles M, Munoz A, et al. Efficacy and safety of naltrexone and acamprosate in the treatment of alcohol dependence: a systematic review. Addiction 2004;99(7):811–28.
69. Jonas DE, Amick HR, Feltner C, et al. Pharmacotherapy for adults with alcohol use disorders in outpatient settings: a systematic review and meta-analysis. JAMA 2014;311(18):1889–900.
70. Kranzler HR, Tennen H, Armeli S, et al. Targeted naltrexone for problem drinkers. J Clin Psychopharmacol 2009;29(4):350–7.

71. Springer SA. Monitoring of liver function tests in patients receiving naltrexone or extended-release naltrexone. In: PCSS providers' clinical support system: MAT training. 2014. Available at: http://pcssmat.org/wp-content/uploads/2014/2010/PCSS-MAT-NTX-Liver-Safety-Guideline2011.pdf.

72. SAMHSA. Clinical advances in non-agonist therapies. Rockville, MD: US Department of Health and Human Services; 2016.

73. Rosner S, Hackl-Herrwerth A, Leucht S, et al. Acamprosate for alcohol dependence. Cochrane Database Syst Rev 2010;(9):CD004332.

74. Reus VI, Fochtmann LJ, Bukstein O, et al. The American Psychiatric Association practice guideline for the pharmacological treatment of patients with alcohol use disorder. Am J Psychiatry 2018;175(1):86–90.

75. Azrin NH, Sisson RW, Meyers R, et al. Alcoholism treatment by disulfiram and community reinforcement therapy. J Behav Ther Exp Psychiatry 1982;13(2):105–12.

76. Ma JZ, Ait-Daoud N, Johnson BA. Topiramate reduces the harm of excessive drinking: implications for public health and primary care. Addiction 2006; 101(11):1561–8.

77. Blodgett JC, Del Re AC, Maisel NC, et al. A meta-analysis of topiramate's effects for individuals with alcohol use disorders. Alcohol Clin Exp Res 2014;38(6):1481–8.

78. Mason BJ, Quello S, Goodell V, et al. Gabapentin treatment for alcohol dependence: a randomized clinical trial. JAMA Intern Med 2014;174(1):70–7.

79. Anton RF, Latham P, Voronin K, et al. Efficacy of gabapentin for the treatment of alcohol use disorder in patients with alcohol withdrawal symptoms: a randomized clinical trial. JAMA Intern Med 2020;180(5):728–36.

80. Flanagan JC, Jones JL, Jarnecke AM, et al. Behavioral treatments for alcohol use disorder and post-traumatic stress disorder. Alcohol Res 2018;39(2):181–92.

81. Kaner EF, Beyer FR, Muirhead C, et al. Effectiveness of brief alcohol interventions in primary care populations. Cochrane Database Syst Rev 2018;2:CD004148.

82. O'Connor EA, Perdue LA, Senger CA, et al. Screening and behavioral Counseling interventions to reduce unhealthy alcohol use in adolescents and adults: an updated systematic review for the U.S. Preventive Services Task Force. Rockville (MD): Agency for Healthcare Research and Quality (US); 2018 (Evidence Synthesis, No. 171.). Available at: https://www.ncbi.nlm.nih.gov/books/NBK534916/.

83. Kelly JF, Magill M, Stout RL. How do people recover from alcohol dependence? A systematic review of the research on mechanisms of behavior change in Alcoholics Anonymous. Addict Res Theor 2009;17(3):236–59.

84. McKellar J, Stewart E, Humphreys K. Alcoholics anonymous involvement and positive alcohol-related outcomes: cause, consequence, or just a correlate? A prospective 2-year study of 2,319 alcohol-dependent men. J Consult Clin Psychol 2003;71(2):302–8.

85. Magill M, Ray L, Kiluk B, et al. A meta-analysis of cognitive-behavioral therapy for alcohol or other drug use disorders: treatment efficacy by contrast condition. J Consult Clin Psychol 2019;87(12):1093–105.

86. Kiluk BD, Devore KA, Buck MB, et al. Randomized trial of computerized cognitive behavioral therapy for alcohol use disorders: efficacy as a virtual stand-alone and treatment add-on compared with standard outpatient treatment. Alcohol Clin Exp Res 2016;40(9):1991–2000.

87. Witkiewitz K, Litten RZ, Leggio L. Advances in the science and treatment of alcohol use disorder. Sci Adv 2019;5(9):eaax4043.

88. Fowler LA, Holt SL, Joshi D. Mobile technology-based interventions for adult users of alcohol: a systematic review of the literature. Addict Behav 2016;62: 25–34.

# Current Best Practices for Acute and Chronic Management of Patients with Opioid Use Disorder

Alyssa Peterkin, MD[a],*, Jordana Laks, MD, MPH[b],
Zoe M. Weinstein, MD, MS[c]

## KEYWORDS

- Opioids • Buprenorphine • Methadone • Naltrexone • Fentanyl • Harm reduction
- Overdose • Epidemic

## KEY POINTS

- Racist drug policy and enforcement sets the backdrop for the modern-era opioid use epidemic, characterized by increasing rates of opioid use disorder, steep growth in overdose deaths, and increased use of high-potency synthetic opioids such as fentanyl.
- Medications for opioid use disorder remain underutilized despite well-known benefits in reducing morbidity and mortality.
- People with opioid use disorders have a high prevalence of comorbid medical and psychiatric disorders.

## EPIDEMIOLOGY

The current opioid use epidemic originates in a long history of opium use, trade, and criminalization dating back to ancient civilizations.[1] In the United States, opium consumption increased dramatically in the nineteenth century with rising morphine use in medical settings.[2] Criminalization of recreational opium use in the 1900s targeted Chinese-American immigrants, beginning a pattern of US drug laws rooted in racism.[3] The War on Drugs and Rockefeller Laws created draconian sentencing laws, including

[a] Grayken Center for Addiction Medicine, Section of General Internal Medicine, Department of Medicine, Boston University School of Medicine, Boston Medical Center, 801 Massachusetts Avenue, Room 2070, Boston, MA 02118, USA; [b] Grayken Center for Addiction Medicine, Section of General Internal Medicine, Department of Medicine, Boston University School of Medicine, Boston Medical Center, 801 Massachusetts Avenue, Room 2103B, Boston, MA 02118, USA; [c] Grayken Center for Addiction Medicine, Section of General Internal Medicine, Department of Medicine, Boston University School of Medicine, Boston Medical Center, 801 Massachusetts Avenue, Room 2039, Boston, MA 02118, USA
* Corresponding author.
*E-mail address:* Alyssa.peterkin@bmc.org

Med Clin N Am 106 (2022) 61–80
https://doi.org/10.1016/j.mcna.2021.08.009
0025-7125/22/© 2021 Elsevier Inc. All rights reserved.

mandatory life sentences for selling or possessing drugs, with black and Hispanic individuals accounting for the majority incarcerated for drug offenses.[4] Despite similar rates of drug use across racial and ethnic groups, from the 1960s to the 1990s, media portrayals centered on urban, black, and Hispanic communities.[4]

Punitive and racist drug policy set the backdrop for the current epidemic of problematic opioid use and opioid use disorder (OUD). OUD is defined by 11-point criteria outlined in the *Diagnostic and Statistical Manual of Mental Disorders* (Fifth Edition), which include cravings, withdrawal, tolerance, loss of control, and use despite harms within the past 12 months.[5] Meeting 2 to 3 of those criteria indicates mild severity; 4 to 5, moderate; and 6 or more, severe OUD.[5] Worldwide, approximately 26.8 million people meet criteria for OUD with disproportionately high prevalence seen in the United States and Canada. In the United States nearly 500,000 people died of an opioid-involved overdose between 1999 and 2019.[6]

### Timeline of the Opioid Overdose Epidemic

The modern epidemic of opioid overdose deaths is categorized into 3 waves (**Fig. 1**).[6] The first wave started in the late 1990s with an increase in prescription opioid overdoses. Driven by pharmaceutical companies' false assurances that prescription opioids could not cause addiction, as well as increased public attention to pain management, sales of opioid analgesics quadrupled between 1999 and 2010.[7] Concurrently, rates of overdose deaths and substance use treatment admissions increased 4-fold.[7]

The second wave started in 2010 with an increase in heroin-involved overdose deaths that surpassed the rate of prescription opioid-involved overdose deaths by 2015 (see **Fig. 1**). Many people initiated opioid use with prescription pills and later transitioned to heroin because of its lower cost and increased availability.[8,9] Increasing heroin use and overdose deaths were disproportionately concentrated in the Northeast and Midwest among younger individuals aged 20 to 34 years.[9] Contrasting with the first wave's more geographically homogeneous increase in prescription opioid, overdoses peaked in 50- to 64-year-olds.[9]

Illicitly manufactured fentanyl and other high-potency synthetic opioids (HPSOs) account for the third wave in opioid overdose deaths. In 2011, increasing production and distribution of these substances led to widespread adulteration of the drug supply and

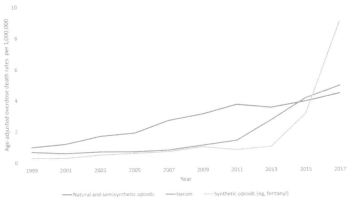

**Fig. 1.** Opioid overdose deaths by opioid category, 1999 to 2017. *Data from* NCHS National Vital Statistics System.[18]

substitution of "heroin" with HPSOs, predominantly in the Northeast and Midwest where they could be sold as a white powder.[8,10] Fentanyl is approximately 30 to 50 times more potent than diacetylmorphine (heroin), carrying a substantially elevated overdose risk.[10] HPSO-related overdose deaths increased 11-fold from 2011 to 2017 (see **Fig. 1**). In Canada, HPSOs accounted for 74% of opioid-related deaths in 2017.[11]

The most recent data during the coronavirus disease 2019 pandemic demonstrate a significant acceleration in opioid overdose mortality driven by HPSOs coupled with psychostimulants.[12] Approximately 81,230 drug overdose deaths occurred in the United States in the 12 months ending in May 2020, the largest number ever recorded in a 1-year period.[12] Emerging data point to disproportionate overdose increases in non-Hispanic black and Hispanic populations.[13]

### Risk Factors for Opioid Use Disorder and Opioid Overdose

Risk factors for developing OUD include younger age, male sex, unemployment, and lower income.[14,15] Although women are more likely to misuse prescription opioids, heroin use is more common in men.[14] From 1999 to 2017, opioid overdose deaths increased in both sexes, but rates were higher for men than for women each year.[16]

Although the media has featured non-Hispanic white rural and suburban communities as the face of the opioid overdose crisis, rates of opioid misuse and OUD are similar among non-Hispanic white, black, and Hispanic people.[15,16] Between 2015 and 2017, disproportionately high increases in HPSO-involved deaths were seen in large metropolitan areas; black individuals had the steepest increase in overall opioid overdose mortality.[17]

### Pharmacology

The term "opiates" refers to naturally occurring alkaloids derived from the opium poppy, including morphine and codeine. Opioids are a broader category referring to all chemical compounds, including synthetic and semisynthetic opioids, which function at opioid receptors.

Opioids are classified by their effect on the $\mu$-opioid receptor (MOR) and their synthetic process (**Table 1**).[19] Full agonists bind to and activate the MOR. Partial agonists and mixed agonists stimulate the MOR to a lower degree and exhibit a "ceiling effect" in which analgesia and respiratory depression plateau with increasing doses. Antagonists bind but do not activate the MOR, blocking agonists from binding.

Differences in opioid activity are attributed to their relative activation and affinity for opioid receptors.[19] Opioids with a high affinity bind tightly and competitively to the MOR.[20] For example, buprenorphine, a partial agonist with high affinity for the MOR, can displace full agonists with a lower affinity leading to precipitated withdrawal.[21] Precipitated withdrawal occurs when full agonists are rapidly displaced from opioid receptors.

Metabolism of opioids occurs mainly in the liver by cytochrome P450 enzymes with renal excretion.[19] Genetic polymorphisms in CYP3A and CYP2D6 influence individuals' opioid metabolism, toxicity levels, and efficacy.[21] Medications inhibiting or inducing CYP450 enzymes can increase or decrease serum opioid levels, particularly methadone (**Table 2**).[19]

### Neurobiology

#### Opioid receptors

Endogenous peptides naturally stimulate opioid receptors located both within the central nervous system and peripheral tissues (**Table 3**). MOR activation is responsible for

**Table 1**
Commonly used opioids classified by their activity at the opioid receptor, synthetic process, and specific pharmacodynamic properties[19,21]

| Receptor Activity | Opioid Name | Natural or Synthetic | Pharmacologic Properties |
|---|---|---|---|
| **Agonists** | Morphine | Natural | Multiple active metabolites; avoid in renal failure due to accumulation of metabolites |
| | Codeine | Natural | Converted to morphine by CYP2D6 |
| | Diacetylmorphine (heroin) | Semisynthetic | When injected, acetyl groups facilitate rapid blood-brain barrier crossing → metabolized into morphine, its active metabolite |
| | Oxycodone | Synthetic | Inhibits release of vasopressin, somatostatin, insulin, and glucagon |
| | Hydrocodone | Semisynthetic | Converted to hydromorphone by CYP2D6 |
| | Hydromorphone | Semisynthetic | About 2–8 times more potent than morphine with shorter half-life |
| | Meperidine | Synthetic | Metabolite, normeperidine, is highly toxic with a long half-life, accumulates in patients with renal dysfunction, and is not reversible by naloxone |
| | Methadone | Synthetic | Long and variable half-life (7–59 h), highest risk of accumulation during titration. Can cause QTc prolongation |
| | Fentanyl | Synthetic | Highly lipophilic. Approximately 100 times more potent than morphine |
| | Tramadol | Synthetic | Multiple mechanisms of action: MOR agonist and norepinephrine and serotonin reuptake inhibitor. Active metabolite has a long half-life. Naloxone reverses respiratory depression but not other components of tramadol overdose |
| **Partial agonists** | Buprenorphine | Synthetic | Partial agonist with ceiling effect on respiratory depression and analgesia; high affinity to the MOR; poor oral bioavailability |
| | Butorphanol | Synthetic | Mixed agonist/antagonist with ceiling effect on analgesia; formulated parenterally and as a nasal spray to treat migraines |
| **Antagonist** | Naloxone | Semisynthetic | High affinity for the MOR, prevents or reverses the effects of opioid agonists for 30–60 min |
| | Naltrexone | Synthetic | Longer-acting and more potent than naloxone; blocks opioid agonist effects at the CNS μ-, kappa-, and gamma-opioid receptors |

*Abbreviation:* CNS, central nervous system.

**Table 2**
**Common medication interactions with methadone[22]**

| Medication | Methadone Serum Level | |
|---|---|---|
| | Increase | Decrease |
| | Amiodarone | Rifampicin |
| | Ketoconazole | Carbamazepine |
| | Fluconazole | Phenytoin |
| | Ciprofloxacin | Phenobarbital |
| | Azithromycin | Efavirenz |

the primary effects of opioid agonists: analgesia, euphoria, respiratory depression, sedation, bradycardia, miosis, and reduced gastric motility, as well as physical dependence (ie, tolerance and withdrawal).[23]

## Reward System Activation

Opioids activate the mesolimbic reward system leading to dopamine release in the nucleus accumbens, producing euphoria.[24] Neurobiological studies suggest that people with OUD develop changes in the amygdala, basal ganglia, and prefrontal cortex that alter the brain reward system and memory formation, driving compulsive drug use and cravings.[23,24]

## Opioid Tolerance and Withdrawal

Physical opioid dependence is a potent driver of developing OUD. Repeated exposure to exogenous opioids induces opioid receptor neuroadaptations that cause opioid receptor desensitization, that is, tolerance. Higher doses of opioids are needed to activate the mesolimbic system and produce comparable amounts of dopamine release. Desensitization of this neuronal pathway prevents individuals from deriving pleasure from normally rewarding activities, such as eating.[23,24]

Opioid activation of MORs in the locus coeruleus inhibits norepinephrine release causing sedation and respiratory depression. Repeated opioid exposure heightens the activity of locus coeruleus neurons, causing people to feel normal with exogenous opioid use. Cessation of opioid use then results in excessive norepinephrine activity, which causes the autonomic hyperactivity symptoms of opioid withdrawal (**Fig. 2**). Opioids are thus needed to avoid the intolerable opioid withdrawal syndrome.

**Table 3**
**Opioid receptor subtypes, locations, and primary effects[20]**

| Opioid Receptor | Locations | Primary Effects |
|---|---|---|
| Mu (μ) | Cerebral cortex, medial thalamus, amygdala, spinal cord | Mu1: supraspinal analgesia, respiratory depression, euphoria, sedation, decreased gastrointestinal motility, physical dependence<br>Mu2: respiratory depression, sedation, pruritus, prolactin release |
| Kappa (κ) | Brain stem, spinal cord, peripheral tissues | Spinal analgesia, sedation, miosis, respiratory depression, dysphoria, diuresis |
| Delta (δ) | Cortex and basal ganglia | Spinal analgesia, inhibition of dopamine release |

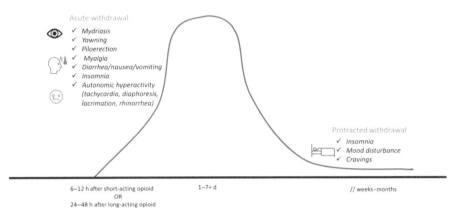

**Fig. 2.** Opioid withdrawal signs and symptoms.[27]

## WITHDRAWAL MANAGEMENT
### Opioid Withdrawal Signs and Symptoms

Opioid withdrawal includes autonomic hyperactivity (tachycardia, hypertension, hyperthermia, lacrimation, and rhinorrhea), gastrointestinal symptoms, piloerection, mydriasis, myalgias, anxiety, and insomnia (see **Fig. 2**). The Clinical Opiate Withdrawal Scale (COWS) is used to quantify withdrawal severity and monitor for improvement with treatment. The COWS assesses 11 signs and symptoms on a scale from 0 to 47, with 5 to 12 representing mild, 13 to 24 moderate, and greater than 24 moderately severe and then severe symptoms.[25]

### Opioid Withdrawal Timeline

People with physiologic dependence to opioids may begin to experience opioid withdrawal within 6 hours of cessation of short-acting opioids such as oxycodone, fentanyl, or heroin. Withdrawal symptoms may not appear for more than 24 hours after the last dose of long-acting opioids such as methadone. Without treatment, symptoms worsen over a period of days and wane within a few weeks.[26] Some individuals experience protracted withdrawal, including mood dysregulation, insomnia, and cravings for months after last use.[27]

### Medical management of withdrawal

Methadone and buprenorphine are the first-line treatments for opioid withdrawal. Adjuvant medications may help control symptoms but are considered second line and should only be used without an opioid agonist with the patient's explicit request and consent. Adjuvant medications include nonopioid analgesics, $\alpha_2$-adrenergic agonists for anxiety or restlessness, and medications to relieve mood, sleep, and gastrointestinal symptoms. If opioid agonist treatment is initiated, adjuvant medications should be used sparingly for the first 72 hours to avoid masking withdrawal symptoms that could be better managed by aggressive titration of opioid agonists (**Table 4**).

Opioid agonists may be started once the patient exhibits mild opioid withdrawal symptoms (COWS >5). Given buprenorphine's high MOR affinity and partial agonist properties, there is some risk of precipitated withdrawal when initiating buprenorphine. Dosing of buprenorphine should be delayed at least 12 hours after last short-acting opioid use and up to 48 hours after a long-acting opioid. Clinicians may also choose to defer buprenorphine initiation until patients exhibit more significant

**Table 4**
**Opioid withdrawal treatment medications[22,26]**

| Medication | Initial Dose | Additional Doses | Taper[a] |
|---|---|---|---|
| **Opioid agonist** | | | |
| Methadone | 20 mg po | 10 mg po q 2–4 h PRN, up to 40 mg/first day of treatment | Decrease by 5–10 mg po per day |
| Buprenorphine | 2–8 mg SL | 2–4 mg SL q 2–4 h PRN, up to 16 mg SL per day | Decrease by 2–4 mg SL per day |
| **Adjunctive agents** | | | |
| **$\alpha_2$-adrenergic agonist** | | | |
| Clonidine | 0.1 mg po | 0.1–0.2 mg po qid PRN anxiety | |
| Lofexidine | 0.54 mg po | 0.54 mg po qid PRN anxiety | |
| **Gastrointestinal medications** | | | |
| Loperamide | 4 mg po | 2 mg po qid PRN diarrhea | |
| Dicyclomine | 20 mg po | 20 mg po qid PRN abdominal cramping | |
| **Analgesics** | | | |
| Ibuprofen | 600 mg po | 600 mg po tid PRN body aches | |
| Acetaminophen | 650 mg po | 650 mg po qid PRN body aches | |
| Ketorolac | 15–30 mg IV/IM | 15–30 mg IV/IM qid PRN body aches | |
| **Sleep and mood medications** | | | |
| Hydroxyzine | 25 mg po | 25 mg po qid PRN anxiety | |
| Trazodone | 25–50 mg po QHS PRN insomnia | | |

*Abbreviations:* IM, intramuscular; IV, intravenous; po, by mouth; PRN, as needed; QHS, at bedtime; qid, four times daily; SL, sublingual; tid, three times daily.

[a] Ideal treatment plan involves stabilization on opioid agonist and not tapering these medications.

withdrawal with a COWS score of 8 to 12.[28] When there is particular concern about precipitated withdrawal (eg, history of precipitated withdrawal, recent long-acting opioid use), starting at lower doses of buprenorphine can help avoid precipitated withdrawal (see Lose-dose buprenorphine induction).

Withdrawal management with detoxification alone is not recommended for people with OUD. Detoxification is highly associated with opioid use recurrence, overdose, and death.[28–31] People should be offered induction and stabilization on opioid agonist medications. However, this is not feasible in all clinical circumstances, and some patients may not desire long-term opioid agonist treatment.

In outpatient and inpatient settings, opioid withdrawal can be managed similarly; however, there are legal restrictions on outpatient use of opioid agonists. In the United States, only Drug Enforcement Administration (DEA)-X-waivered prescribers can prescribe buprenorphine outpatient, and methadone for OUD can only be dispensed at DEA-licensed opioid treatment programs (OTPs). Inpatient clinicians may dispense dose medications per their clinical judgment.[32]

### Medications for opioid use disorder

Medications for opioid use disorder (MOUD) are the gold-standard treatment of OUD. MOUD alleviate opioid withdrawal and cravings and normalize brain changes. At present, in the United States there are 3 Food and Drug Administration-approved MOUD: methadone, buprenorphine, and naltrexone. In Canada, slow-release oral morphine (SROM) is an alternative treatment of patients for whom first-line treatments were unsuccessful.[33,34] Although not widely available, injectable hydromorphone and diacetylmorphine are considered treatment options for patients with OUD who have not fully benefited from first-line agents in Canada.[35,36] Injectable hydromorphone and diacetylmorphine have identical efficacy, which includes high rates of treatment retention and reduction in nonprescribed opioid use.[36]

In the United States in 2019, less than 20% of people with OUD received MOUD.[37] Disparities in treatment exist. White individuals with OUD are 35 times more likely than black individuals to receive buprenorphine, and black and Hispanic pregnant people with OUD are less likely to receive any MOUD.[38,39]

**Methadone.** As the oldest treatment of OUD, methadone has substantial evidence supporting its efficacy and safety, including in pregnant people (**Box 1**).[22,40] In the United States, methadone can only be accessed through OTPs, highly regulated clinics in which patients must present for observed methadone dosing. In Canada, however, methadone for OUD can be prescribed and dispensed daily at a pharmacy.[41]

**Buprenorphine.** Buprenorphine was first approved for OUD in the United States through the Drug Addiction and Treatment Act in 2000. Similar to methadone, buprenorphine demonstrates efficacy in mortality reduction, treatment retention, and abstinence and improved occupational stability and psychosocial outcomes and may also be used during pregnancy.[42,43] Buprenorphine interacts with few drugs and has not been associated with clinically significant QTc prolongation.[44]

Buprenorphine is available as a monoproduct or in combination with naloxone. Naloxone, an MOR antagonist, has poor oral bioavailability and will not precipitate withdrawal when taken sublingually. The combination of naloxone with buprenorphine serves as a deterrent to intravenous use, which will precipitate withdrawal. As a monoproduct, buprenorphine can be administered as a buccal film, injection, implant, or transdermal patch, although only the injection and implant formulations are indicated for treatment of OUD.[22]

---

**Box 1**
**Methadone efficacy[22,40]**

Methadone is associated with
  Increased treatment retention
  Increased employment
  Improved birth outcomes
  Decreased substance use
  Decreased mortality
  Decreased criminal activity
  Decreased human immunodeficiency virus and hepatitis seroconversion

**Naltrexone.** Naltrexone, an MOR antagonist, is available as a tablet and a monthly extended-release intramuscular (IM) injection.[22,26] Naltrexone is a treatment option for patients who prefer nonopioid agonist treatment and/or patients with co-occurring alcohol use disorder and OUD.

Oral naltrexone is only effective in certain highly monitored settings in which treatment is mandated and therefore should not be considered a first-line treatment of OUD. Treatment retention with IM naltrexone decreases with each subsequent dose of IM naltrexone. Homelessness, injection drug use (IDU), and mental illness are risk factors for premature treatment discontinuation.[45] Owing to loss of opioid tolerance with IM naltrexone, there is a higher risk of opioid overdose after drug recurrence when compared with buprenorphine and methadone.[26] In addition, naltrexone has not shown the same morbidity and mortality benefits as opioid agonists and therefore should be considered second line.[40]

**Slow-release oral morphine.** SROM, a long-acting MOR agonist, is an alternative treatment option for people with OUD refractory to methadone and buprenorphine, based on Canadian national guidelines.[33] SROM should be prescribed after consultation with an addiction specialist and is dispensed daily under direct observation by a pharmacist. Similar to methadone, SROM is associated with treatment retention and reduced opioid cravings (**Fig. 3**).[46]

### Dosing and induction methods

**Methadone.** The general guideline for methadone dose titration is "start low and go slow," meaning methadone is initiated at a low dose such as 10 to 20 mg by mouth and increased gradually with daily monitoring over days to weeks. The legal limit on initial methadone dosing in OTPs is a maximum of 30 mg by mouth per day with only one clinical assessment or 40 mg by mouth if there is a second clinical assessment.[47] Peak effects of methadone occur 2 to 4 hours after the dose. Following a dose adjustment, it generally takes 5 days, the equivalent of 4 to 5 half-lives, for plasma levels to achieve a steady state. Doses are typically increased by increments

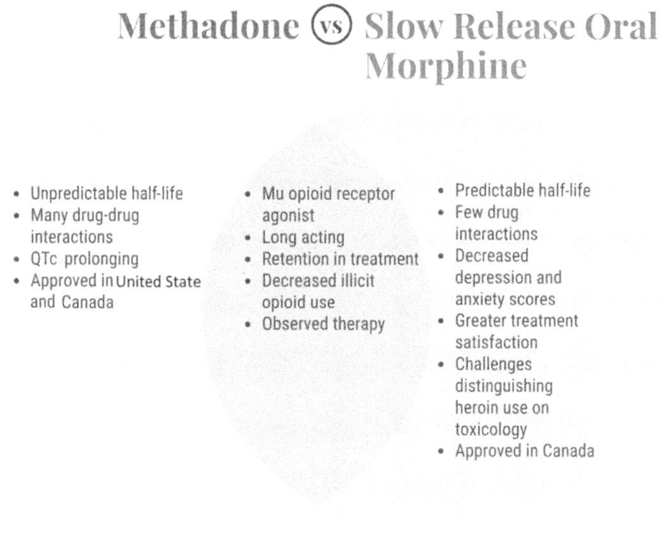

## Methadone (vs) Slow Release Oral Morphine

- Unpredictable half-life
- Many drug-drug interactions
- QTc prolonging
- Approved in United State and Canada

- Mu opioid receptor agonist
- Long acting
- Retention in treatment
- Decreased illicit opioid use
- Observed therapy

- Predictable half-life
- Few drug interactions
- Decreased depression and anxiety scores
- Greater treatment satisfaction
- Challenges distinguishing heroin use on toxicology
- Approved in Canada

**Fig. 3.** Comparing long-acting opioid agonists: methadone and slow-release oral morphine.[46]

of 5 to 10 mg by mouth of methadone every 3 to 5 days taking into account opioid withdrawal, cravings, and risk of oversedation.[22] Slower dose titration should be considered for individuals with recent loss of tolerance, severe respiratory disease, or severe hepatic dysfunction.

Lower doses of methadone such as 20 to 40 mg by mouth daily are adequate for withdrawal management; however, higher doses are typically needed to suppress cravings and block effects of other opioid agonists (**Fig. 4**).[48] Overdose risk is the highest during the initial weeks of methadone treatment owing to ongoing cravings leading to additional opioid use.[49] Higher doses of methadone (>100 mg) are associated with treatment retention and decreased heroin use. Treatment should be flexible and individualized. For example, some people are able to abstain from nonprescribed opioid use with methadone 60 mg by mouth, whereas others will require higher doses such as 120 mg by mouth to achieve adequate reduction of cravings and effective opioid blockade.[50]

**Buprenorphine.** Buprenorphine can be initiated through traditional induction or low- or high-dose methods. In a traditional induction, a period of opioid abstinence ranging from 8 to 48 hours and opioid withdrawal are required before starting buprenorphine to decrease the chances of precipitating withdrawal.[22,53] Traditional inductions start with 2 to 4 mg buprenorphine administered sublingually (SL) as an initial dose and titrating up to 8 to 16 mg SL on the first day until opioid withdrawal symptoms and cravings abate. On the second and third days, patients may receive additional 4 mg SL doses if needed for ongoing cravings or withdrawal to increase the daily dose to a maximum of 24 mg SL by day 3.

**Low-dose buprenorphine induction** Low-dose induction, also known as the Bernese method, is a novel approach to buprenorphine inductions that starts at very low doses of buprenorphine followed by incremental dose increases while patients continue taking full opioid agonists.[54] Low-dose inductions address 2 major concerns. First, undergoing the opioid-free period required for traditional buprenorphine initiation can be very challenging. Second, as HPSOs further dominate the drug supply, traditional buprenorphine inductions are increasingly leading to precipitated withdrawal.[50] This precipitated withdrawal may be due in part to HPSO's lipophilic properties causing increased volume distribution and slower clearance from the body when compared with heroin.[55]

Data, mostly through case reports, demonstrate several effective dosing strategies (**Table 5**).[53,54,56,57] Many low-dose induction strategies present logistical challenges. For example, some strategies use buprenorphine formulations approved for pain (ie, transdermal patches) that must be prescribed off-label to treat OUD. Low-dose induction with buprenorphine films or tablets requires cutting the films or tablets into quarters or eighths, which may be prohibited by pharmacy policies.[56]

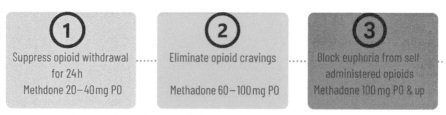

**Fig. 4.** Methadone dosing milestones.[51,52] Note: The doses in this figure are ranges; actual dosing will vary by individual.

**Table 5**
Sample low-dose buprenorphine induction strategies[53,54,56-58]

| | Inpatient | | Outpatient | |
| --- | --- | --- | --- | --- |
| | **Buprenorphine Formulation** | | | |
| | Transdermal Patch + Sublingual Film | Buccal Film + Sublingual Film | Sublingual Film/Tablet | |
| **Outline of protocol** | | | | |
| Day 1 | 20mcg/hr for buprenorphine patch[a][b] | 225 μg po daily[c] | 0.5 mg SL daily | 0.5 mg SL bid[d] |
| Day 2 | Continue patch + start buprenorphine SL 2–4 mg every 2–4 h as needed[a] (limit to 8 mg buprenorphine SL) | 225 μg po bid | 0.5 mg SL bid | 1 mg SL bid[d] |
| Day 3 | Administer previous day's buprenorphine dose + 2–4 mg as needed[a] (limit to 16 mg buprenorphine SL) | 450 μg po bid | 1 mg SL bid | 1mg SL tid[d] |
| Day 4 | [e] | 2 mg SL bid | 2 mg SL bid | 2 mg SL tid[d] |
| Day 5 | | 4 mg SL bid | 3 mg SL bid | 4 mg SL tid[d][e] |
| Day 6 | | 4 mg SL tid[e] | 4 mg SL bid | |
| Day 7 | | 4 mg SL tid; 8 mg SL bid | 12 mg SL daily[e] | |

*Abbreviations:* CR, controlled-release; bid, twice daily; po, by mouth; tid, three times daily.
[a] Full opioid agonists are tapered at the provider's discretion.
[b] 20mcg/hr for buprenorphine patch delivers approximately 0.48 mg buprenorphine per day.
[c] 225μg po buprenorphine is equivalent to approximately 0.5 mg sublingual buprenorphine.
[d] Oxycodone CR 80 mg tid used on days 1 to 3 and switched to oxycodone CR 80 mg bid on day 4.
[e] All other opioids should be stopped.

**High-dose buprenorphine induction** High-dose buprenorphine inductions have been useful in emergency departments (EDs) to rapidly manage opioid withdrawal and to facilitate early linkage to MOUD treatment. One single-site ED study found that high-dose (>12 mg) buprenorphine inductions were safe and well tolerated.[59] The protocol initiates 4 to 8 mg buprenorphine SL for COWS greater than 8 and then reassesses within 1 hour for improvement of withdrawal symptoms or precipitated withdrawal. If opioid withdrawal has improved but persists, an additional buprenorphine 8 to 24 mg SL is administered.[59]

**Naltrexone.** Naltrexone is an opioid antagonist with high receptor affinity; thus, guidelines recommend waiting 7 to 10 days since the last opioid use before initiating naltrexone to prevent precipitating withdrawal. The 380-mg extended-release depot naltrexone is administered every 28 days.

**Slow-response oral morphine.** SROM is available as an extended-release capsule and has been approved for a maximum daily dose of 400 mg/d as treatment of OUD in Canada. The typical starting dose of SROM is 30 to 60 mg by mouth, which is subsequently increased every 48 hours.[34] Compared with methadone, SROM has fewer drug-drug interactions, less cardiotoxicity, and a more predictable half-life (see **Fig. 3**).[46]

## MEDICAL AND PSYCHIATRIC COMPLICATIONS OF OPIOID USE
### Medical Complications

In addition to the increased risk of overdose and addiction, long-term opioid use is associated with numerous medical complications (**Table 6**).[60–62] Long-term opioid use suppresses the immune system, leading to higher risk of invasive pneumococcal infections.[63] Hypogonadism related to decreased hypothalamic-pituitary axis function may decrease testosterone levels and cause sexual dysfunction.[60] Decreased estradiol and progesterone can manifest as irregular menses and amenorrhea.[64]

### Infections
Unsafe injection practices including reusing and sharing needles and injection equipment have fostered the spread of hepatitis C and human immunodeficiency

**Table 6**
**Opioid-related medical complications[2]**

| System | Complications |
| --- | --- |
| Cardiovascular | Endocarditis, septic emboli, valvular heart disease, arrhythmias, mycotic aneurysms, hypotension |
| Central nervous system | Brain abscess, meningitis, central sleep apnea, stroke, seizure, overdose, neuropathy |
| Endocrine | Sexual dysfunction, osteoporosis, hypogonadism |
| Gastrointestinal | Liver failure, hepatitis, constipation |
| Integumentary | Abscess, cellulitis, necrotizing soft tissue infection, septic thrombophlebitis, hyperpigmentation, venous insufficiency |
| Musculoskeletal | Osteomyelitis, epidural abscess, septic arthritis, tetanus, pyomyositis, tenosynovitis, fractures, rhabdomyolysis |
| Pulmonary | Pneumonia (aspiration and community acquired), pneumothorax, tuberculosis, septic pulmonary embolism, noncardiogenic pulmonary edema, foreign body deposition, granulomatosis |
| Renal | Nephropathy, amyloidosis |

virus (HIV). During the current opioid epidemic, IDU has led to doubling of serious bacterial infections increasing morbidity and mortality while reducing life expectancy.[65,66] People injecting HPSOs inject more frequently increasing the risk of injection-related complications.[67] In North America, 16% of infective endocarditis is associated with IDU.[68]

### Psychiatric Complications

Opioid use, withdrawal, and OUD can cause psychiatric symptoms and exacerbate underlying disorders. Psychiatric conditions that precede opioid use or persist following a period of abstinence are consistent with a chronic condition, whereas substance-induced psychiatric disorders typically manifest within 30 days of intoxication or withdrawal.[5] Insomnia is common, because opioid use and withdrawal disrupt rapid eye movement sleep causing decreased sleep time and increased sleep latency.[69] Sleep disturbances often persist for months even after a period of abstinence and may increase risk of drug use recurrence. In addition, opioid withdrawal symptoms can mimic depression and anxiety disorders.[70]

### Co-occurring disorders

In the United States, 1 in 4 adults with OUD have a serious mental illness often requiring a complex treatment course.[37,71] Co-occurring mental illness has been linked to higher risk of overdose.[71]

History of a mood disorder, anxiety disorder, or another substance use disorder (SUD) dramatically increases the risk of OUD.[72] Nicotine, alcohol, and cannabis use disorders are the most common co-occurring SUDs in people with OUD.[71] People with OUD, particularly women, also report disproportionately high rates of childhood physical, emotional, and sexual abuse.[73] The prevalence of posttraumatic stress disorder is high; veterans are particularly susceptible to OUD because of physical and emotional trauma and high rates of chronic prescribed opioids.[74] Prescription opioid misuse and OUD substantially increases the risk of suicidal ideation; people with OUD have 14 times higher risk of completed suicide after an attempt.[75,76] A comprehensive approach treating both OUD and co-occurring disorders is paramount to improving outcomes.

### Behavioral Treatments

Evidence supports the use of psychosocial interventions both independently and in conjunction with MOUD, with particular benefits shown when combining psychosocial and pharmacologic treatments (**Table 7**).[75]

When compared with treatment as usual, the addition of contingency management (CM) or counseling to methadone treatment is associated with greater treatment attendance and lower dropout.[75] Buprenorphine therapy combined with community reinforcement and family training is associated with reduced opioid and other substance use.[75] The addition of cognitive behavioral therapy to primary care-based buprenorphine treatment increased abstinence in people with prescription opioid-related OUD, although no differences were seen in treatment retention or abstinence in people using heroin.[77,78] CM coupled with naltrexone leads to higher rates of treatment retention and medication adherence.[75]

Mutual support groups are often used, although more rigorous research is needed to understand their relative benefits and risks.[40] Narcotics Anonymous and Alcoholics Anonymous are based on fellowship, spirituality, and motivation for abstinence. In contrast, Self-Management and Recovery Training support groups focus on self-empowerment and evidence-based interventions.

**Table 7**
**Psychosocial interventions for opioid use disorder[76]**

| Psychosocial Intervention | Key Concept | Example |
|---|---|---|
| Contingency management | Using tangible incentives and other reinforcements to increase a target behavior such as abstinence | Patient has the opportunity to pick from a grab bag after urine drug screen results are negative for fentanyl |
| Motivational interviewing | Exploring ambivalence and eliciting internal motivation to change | Provider assesses patient with newly diagnosed OUD for readiness and motivation to stop using opioids |
| Cognitive behavioral therapy | Understanding that thoughts and emotions can impact behavior | Patient who avoids a main road due to fear of being offered heroin is asked to take a closer look at his negative thoughts, ie, What are the chances.... |
| Community reinforcement and family training | Using strategies for family and friends can use to assist loved one make change | A mother calmly tells her son she will no longer call his manager when he is hungover to cancel work but instead offers to help him get ready for work |

*Data from Herron*, Abigail, Timothy Koehler Brennan. The ASAM Essentials of Addiction Medicine. 2nd ed. Wolters Kluwer; 2015.

## *Harm Reduction for Opioid Use Disorder*

Harm reduction is an essential component of care for people with OUD (**Table 8**). To reduce overdose morbidity and mortality, clinicians should prescribe naloxone to people using opioids and counsel patients and their loved ones on ways to prevent and respond to overdose (see **Table 8**). People who inject opioid drugs should also undergo frequent HIV screening, and clinicians should recommend preexposure prophylaxis and/or postexposure prophylaxis when indicated.

**Fig. 5** summarizes harm reduction interventions that are essential components of comprehensive care for people with OUD.

**Table 8**
**Counseling tips for opioid overdose prevention and response**

| Overdose Prevention | Overdose Response Plan |
|---|---|
| • Avoid mixing drugs, particularly sedatives like opioids, benzodiazepines, and alcohol<br>• "Start low and go slow" = Test a small amount of drug first and go slow<br>• Use less after a period of abstinence<br>• Test the drug strength and purity (eg, fentanyl testing) | • Do not use alone<br>• Keep the door unlocked or ajar<br>• Ask a friend to check on you<br>• Make sure you and others around you have naloxone<br>• Provide rescue breathing |

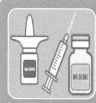

## Opioid overdose prevention and response

- Start low and go slow
- Drug testing for potency and purity
- Avoid mixing drugs
- Avoid using alone
- Keep naloxone available and accessible
- Overdose response training for self and family/friends

## Safer injecting practices

- Use sterile syringes and equipment
- Wash or sterilize hands before and after injecting
- Avoid licking needles
- Avoid high-risk injection sites (arms and hands are lowest risk sites
- Use each needle only once ("One shot, one syringe and works")
- Refer to sterile syringe programs

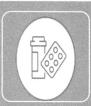

## Screening and prevention of HIV, viral hepatitis, and STIs

- Frequent HIV and HCV screening and linkage to treatment
- Prescribe HIV PrEP and PEP when indicated
- Vaccinate against HBV
- Screen for and treat STIs and offer condoms

**Fig. 5.** Harm reduction counseling and interventions for people with OUD. HCV, hepatitis C virus; HIV, human immunodeficiency virus; PEP, postexposure prophylaxis; PrEP, preexposure prophylaxis; STIs, sexually transmitted infections.

## CONCLUSIONS

Opioid use dates back to centuries, but the recent surge in prescription and illicit opioid use has contributed to an unprecedented increase in overdose deaths and morbidity due to infectious complications. Genetics, psychosocial risk factors, alterations in brain reward pathways, and physiologic opioid dependence drive the development of OUD. Preventing associated harms, ensuring equitable access to MOUD, and addressing co-occurring disorders and social needs are crucial in curbing opioid-related morbidity and mortality.

## CLINICS CARE POINTS

- Prescription opioids, heroin, and HPSOs, respectively, have contributed to the first, second, and third waves of opioid overdose deaths.
- Black people have experienced the steepest increase in overall opioid overdose mortality and experience significant barriers to treatment access.
- Opioid detoxification alone is not recommended and is associated with high rates of opioid recurrence, overdose, and death due to loss of opioid tolerance.
- Methadone and buprenorphine are associated with increased treatment retention, improved psychosocial outcomes, and reduced mortality.

## DISCLOSURE STATEMENT

The authors have nothing to disclose.

## REFERENCES

1. Brook K, Bennett J, Desai SP. The Chemical History of Morphine: An 8000-year Journey, from Resin to de-novo Synthesis. J Anesth Hist 2017;3(2):50–5.
2. Courtwright DT. Preventing and Treating Narcotic Addiction — A Century of Federal Drug Control. N Engl J Med 2015;373(22):2095–7.
3. McCaffrey P. How American opium Politics led to the Establishment of International Narcotics. 2019. Available at: http://nrs.harvard.edu/urn-3:HUL.InstRepos: 42004195. [Accessed 24 March 2021].
4. James K, Jordan A. The Opioid Crisis in Black Communities. J Law Med Ethics 2018;46(2):404–21.
5. American Psychiatric Association. Diagnostic and Statistical manual of mental disorders. Fifth Edition. Arlington, VA: American Psychiatric Association; 2013.
6. Centers for Disease Control and Prevention. Understanding the Epidemic. 2021. Available at: https://www.cdc.gov/drugoverdose/epidemic/index.html. [Accessed 28 March 2021].
7. Vital Signs: Overdoses of Prescription Opioid Pain Relievers — United States, 1999–2008. Available at: http://www.cdc.gov/mmwr/preview/mmwrhtml/ mm6043a4.htm. [Accessed 28 February 2021].
8. Ciccarone D. The Triple Wave Epidemic: Supply and Demand Drivers of the US Opioid Overdose Crisis. Int J Drug Policy 2019;71:183–8.
9. Unick G, Ciccarone D. US Regional and Demographic Differences in Prescription Opioid and Heroin-Related Overdose Hospitalizations. Int J Drug Policy 2017;46: 112–9.
10. Ciccarone D. Editorial for "US Heroin in Transition: Supply Changes, Fentanyl Adulteration and Consequences" IJDP Special Section. Int J Drug Policy 2017; 46:107–11.
11. Special Advisory Committee on the Epidemic of Opioid Overdoses. National Report: Apparent Opioid-Related Deaths in Canada (January 2016 to June 2017). 2017. Available at: https://www.canada.ca/en/public-health/services/ publications/healthy-living/apparent-opioid-related-deaths-report-2016-2017- december.html. [Accessed 25 March 2021].
12. Centers for Disease Control and Prevention. Increase in Fatal Drug Overdoses Across the United States Driven by Synthetic Opioids Before and During the COVID-19 Pandemic. Emergency Preparedness and Response. 2020. Available at: https://emergency.cdc.gov/han/2020/han00438.asp. [Accessed 4 March 2021].
13. Khatri UG, Pizzicato LN, Viner K, et al. Racial/Ethnic Disparities in Unintentional Fatal and Nonfatal Emergency Medical Services–Attended Opioid Overdoses During the COVID-19 Pandemic in Philadelphia. JAMA Netw Open 2021;4(1): e2034878.
14. Han B, Compton WM, Blanco C, et al. Prescription Opioid Use, Misuse, and Use Disorders in U.S. Adults: 2015 National Survey on Drug Use and Health. Ann Intern Med 2017;167(5):293–301.
15. Jones CM. The paradox of decreasing nonmedical opioid analgesic use and increasing abuse or dependence — An assessment of demographic and substance use trends, United States, 2003–2014. Addict Behav 2017;65:229–35.

16. Hedegaard H, Arialdi M, Miniño MW. Drug overdose deaths in the United States, 1999–2017. 2018. Available at: https://www.cdc.gov/nchs/data/databriefs/db329-h.pdf. [Accessed 30 March 2021].

17. Lippold KM. Racial/Ethnic and Age Group Differences in Opioid and Synthetic Opioid–Involved Overdose Deaths Among Adults Aged ≥18 Years in Metropolitan Areas — United States, 2015–2017. MMWR Morb Mortal Wkly Rep 2019; 68:967–73.

18. Centers for Disease Control and Prevention. Drug Overdose Deaths in the United States, 1999–2017. Available at: https://www.cdc.gov/nchs/data/databriefs/db329_tables-508.pdf#page=4. [Accessed 25 March 2021].

19. Trescot AM, Datta S, Lee M, et al. Opioid pharmacology. Pain Physician 2008; 11(2 Suppl):S133–53.

20. Opioid Agonists, Partial Agonists, Antagonists: Oh My! Pharmacy Times. Available at: https://www.pharmacytimes.com/contributor/jeffrey-fudin/2018/01/opioid-agonists-partial-agonists-antagonists-oh-my. [Accessed 1 March 2021].

21. Nafziger AN, Barkin RL. Opioid Therapy in Acute and Chronic Pain. J Clin Pharmacol 2018;58(9):1111–22.

22. Substance Abuse and Mental Health Services Administration. Medications for Opioid Use Disorder. Treatment improvement protocol (TIP) Series 63. HHS Publication No. (SMA) 18-5063. Rockville, MD: Substance Abuse and Mental Health Services Administration; 2018.

23. Kosten TR, George TP. The Neurobiology of Opioid Dependence: Implications for Treatment. Sci Pract Perspect 2002;1(1):13–20.

24. Koob GF, Volkow ND. Neurobiology of addiction: a neurocircuitry analysis. Lancet Psychiatry 2016;3(8):760–73.

25. Wesson DR, Ling W. The Clinical Opiate Withdrawal Scale (COWS). J Psychoactive Drugs 2003;35(2):253–9.

26. Schuckit MA. Treatment of Opioid-Use Disorders. N Engl J Med 2016;375(4): 357–68.

27. Center for Substance Abuse Treatment. Protracted Withdrawal. 2010. Available at: https://store.samhsa.gov/sites/default/files/d7/priv/sma10-4554.pdf. [Accessed 16 February 2021].

28. Gowing L, Ali R, White JM, et al. Buprenorphine for managing opioid withdrawal. Cochrane Database Syst Rev 2017;(2):1–83.

29. Amato L, Davoli M, Minozzi S, et al. Methadone at tapered doses for the management of opioid withdrawal. Cochrane Database Syst Rev 2005;3:1–58.

30. Bentzley BS, Barth KS, Back SE, et al. Discontinuation of buprenorphine maintenance therapy: perspectives and outcomes. J Subst Abuse Treat 2015;52:48–57.

31. American Society of Addiction Medicine.The ASAM National Practice Guideline for the Treatment of Opioid Use Disorder: 2020 Focused Update. J Addict Med 2020;14(2S):1–91.

32. Noska A, Mohan A, Wakeman S, et al. Managing Opioid Use Disorder During and After Acute Hospitalization: A Case-Based Review Clarifying Methadone Regulation for Acute Care Settings. J Addict Behav Ther Rehabil 2015;4(2):1–11.

33. Bruneau J, Ahamad K, Goyer M-È, et al. Management of opioid use disorders: a national clinical practice guideline. CMAJ 2018;190(9):E247–57.

34. British Columbia Centre on Substance use and B.C. Ministry of Health. A Guideline for the Clinical Management of Opioid Use Disorder. 2017. Available at: https://www.bccsu.ca/wp-content/uploads/2017/06/BC-OUD-Guidelines_June2017.pdf. [Accessed 25 March 2021].

35. Fairbairn N, Ross J, Trew M, et al. Injectable opioid agonist treatment for opioid use disorder: a national clinical guideline. CMAJ 2019;191(38):E1049–56.

36. Oviedo-Joekes E, Guh D, Brissette S, et al. Hydromorphone Compared With Diacetylmorphine for Long-term Opioid Dependence: A Randomized Clinical Trial. JAMA Psychiatry 2016;73(5):447.

37. Substance Abuse and Mental Health Services Administration. Key Substance Use and Mental Health Indicators in the United States: Results from the 2019 National Survey on Drug Use and Health. Center for Behavioral Health Statistics and Quality, Substance Abuse and Mental Health Services Administration. Center for Behavioral Health Statistics and Quality, Rockville, MD: Substance Abuse and Mental Health Services Administration; 2020.

38. Lagisetty PA, Ross R, Bohnert A, et al. Buprenorphine Treatment Divide by Race/Ethnicity and Payment. JAMA Psychiatry 2019;76(9):979.

39. Schiff DM, Nielsen T, Hoeppner BB, et al. Assessment of Racial and Ethnic Disparities in the Use of Medication to Treat Opioid Use Disorder Among Pregnant Women in Massachusetts. JAMA Netw Open 2020;3(5):e205734.

40. Strang J, Volkow ND, Degenhardt L, et al. Opioid use disorder. Nat Rev Dis Primer 2020;6(1):1–28.

41. Calcaterra SL, Bach P, Chadi A, et al. Methadone Matters: What the United States Can Learn from the Global Effort to Treat Opioid Addiction. J Gen Intern Med 2019;34(6):1039–42.

42. Fudala PJ, Bridge TP, Herbert S, et al. Office-based treatment of opiate addiction with a sublingual-tablet formulation of buprenorphine and naloxone. N Engl J Med 2003;349(10):949–58.

43. Sordo L, Barrio G, Bravo MJ, et al. Mortality risk during and after opioid substitution treatment: systematic review and meta-analysis of cohort studies. BMJ 2017; 357:j1550.

44. Krantz MJ, Garcia JA, Mehler PS. Effects of Buprenorphine on Cardiac Repolarization in a Patient with Methadone-Related Torsade de Pointes. Pharmacother J Hum Pharmacol Drug Ther 2005;25(4):611–4.

45. Cousins SJ, Radfar SR, Crèvecoeur-MacPhail D, et al. Predictors of Continued Use of Extended-Released Naltrexone (XR-NTX) for Opioid-Dependence: An Analysis of Heroin and Non-Heroin Opioid Users in Los Angeles County. J Subst Abuse Treat 2016;63:66–71.

46. Kimmel S, Bach P, Walley AY. Comparison of Treatment Options for Refractory Opioid Use Disorder in the United States and Canada: a Narrative Review. J Gen Intern Med 2020;35(8):2418–26.

47. Substance Abuse and Mental Health Services Administration. Statutes, Regulations, and Guidelines. 2020. Available at: https://www.samhsa.gov/medication-assisted-treatment/statutes-regulations-guidelines. [Accessed 28 March 2021].

48. Strain EC, Bigelow GE, Liebson IA, et al. Moderate- vs High-Dose Methadone in the Treatment of Opioid Dependence: A Randomized Trial. J Am Med Assoc 1999;281(11):1000.

49. Baxter LES, Campbell A, DeShields M, et al. Safe Methadone Induction and Stabilization: Report of an Expert Panel. J Addict Med 2013;7(6):377–86.

50. Bisaga A. What should clinicians do as fentanyl replaces heroin? Addiction 2019; 114(5):782–3.

51. Donny E, Walsh S, Bigelow G, et al. High-dose methadone produces superior opioid blockade and comparable withdrawal suppression to lower doses in opioid-dependent humans. Psychopharmacology (Berl) 2002;161(2):202–12.

52. Donny EC, Brasser SM, Bigelow GE, et al. Methadone doses of 100 mg or greater are more effective than lower doses at suppressing heroin self-administration in opioid-dependent volunteers. Addiction 2005;100(10):1496–509.

53. Raheemullah A, Lembke A. Initiating Opioid Agonist Treatment for Opioid Use Disorder in the Inpatient Setting: A Teachable Moment. JAMA Intern Med 2019; 179(3):427–8.

54. Randhawa PA, Brar R, Nolan S. Buprenorphine–naloxone "microdosing": an alternative induction approach for the treatment of opioid use disorder in the wake of North America's increasingly potent illicit drug market. CMAJ 2020;192(3):E73.

55. Huhn AS, Hobelmann JG, Oyler GA, et al. Protracted renal clearance of fentanyl in persons with opioid use disorder. Drug Alcohol Depend 2020;214:108147.

56. Weimer MB, Guerra M, Morrow G, et al. Hospital-based Buprenorphine Microdose Initiation. J Addict Med 2021;15(3):255–7.

57. Becker WC, Frank JW, Edens EL. Switching From High-Dose, Long-Term Opioids to Buprenorphine: A Case Series. Ann Intern Med 2020;173(1):70–1.

58. Ghosh SM, Klaire S, Tanguay R, et al. A Review of Novel Methods To Support The Transition From Methadone and Other Full Agonist Opioids To Buprenorphine/Naloxone Sublingual In Both Community and Acute Care Settings. Can J Addict 2019;10(4):41–50.

59. Herring AA, Vosooghi AA, Luftig J, et al. High-Dose Buprenorphine Induction in the Emergency Department for Treatment of Opioid Use Disorder. JAMA Netw Open 2021;4(7):e2117128.

60. Baldini A, Von Korff M, Lin EHB. A Review of Potential Adverse Effects of Long-Term Opioid Therapy: A Practitioner's Guide. Prim Care Companion CNS Disord 2012;14(3):1–12.

61. Visconti AJ, Sell J, Greenblatt AD. Primary Care for Persons Who Inject Drugs. Am Fam Physician 2019;99(2):109–16.

62. Li A, Rosenthal ES, Rapoport AB, et al. Opioid use disorder and infectious complications in persons who inject drugs. Int Anesthesiol Clin 2020;58(2):4–11.

63. Wiese AD, Griffin MR, Schaffner W, et al. Opioid Analgesic Use and Risk for Invasive Pneumococcal Diseases. Ann Intern Med 2018;168(6):396–404.

64. Katz N, Mazer NA. The Impact of Opioids on the Endocrine System. Clin J Pain 2009;25(2):170–5.

65. Murphy SL, Xu J, Kochanek KD, et al. Mortality in the United States, 2017 2018.

66. Ronan MV, Herzig SJ. Hospitalizations Related To Opioid Abuse/Dependence And Associated Serious Infections Increased Sharply, 2002–12. Health Aff (Millwood) 2016;35(5):832–7.

67. Stein MD, Anderson B. Injection frequency mediates health service use among persons with a history of drug injection. Drug Alcohol Depend 2003;70(2):159–68.

68. Murdoch DR. Clinical Presentation, Etiology, and Outcome of Infective Endocarditis in the 21st Century: The International Collaboration on Endocarditis–Prospective Cohort Study. Arch Intern Med 2009;169(5):463.

69. Angarita GA, Emadi N, Hodges S, et al. Sleep abnormalities associated with alcohol, cannabis, cocaine, and opiate use: a comprehensive review. Addict Sci Clin Pract 2016;11(1):9.

70. Renner JA. Managing Common Psychiatric Conditions in Patients with Substance Use Disorders. Presented at the: Provider Clinical Support System; July 2019. Available at: https://cf8b2643ab1d3c05e8f6-d3dc0d8f838e182b6b722cea42bb6a35.ssl.cf2.rackcdn.com/aaap_7bb681c846586f06c60ece6a6c18277e.pdf. [Accessed 24 February 2021].

71. Jones CM, McCance-Katz EF. Co-occurring substance use and mental disorders among adults with opioid use disorder. Drug Alcohol Depend 2019;197:78–82.

72. Blanco C, Alderson D, Ogburn E, et al. Changes in the prevalence of non-medical prescription drug use and drug use disorders in the United States: 1991–1992 and 2001–2002. Drug Alcohol Depend 2007;90(2):252–60.

73. Santo T, Campbell G, Gisev N, et al. Prevalence of childhood maltreatment among people with opioid use disorder: A systematic review and meta-analysis. Drug Alcohol Depend 2021;219:108459.

74. Mills KL, Teesson M, Ross J, et al. The impact of post-traumatic stress disorder on treatment outcomes for heroin dependence. Addict Abingdon Engl 2007;102(3):447–54.

75. Dugosh K, Abraham A, Seymour B, et al. A Systematic Review on the Use of Psychosocial Interventions in Conjunction With Medications for the Treatment of Opioid Addiction. J Addict Med 2016;10(2):91–101.

76. Herron A, Brennan TK. The ASAM essentials of addiction medicine. 2nd ed. Philadelphia, PA: Wolters Kluwer; 2015.

77. Fiellin DA, Barry DT, Sullivan LE, et al. A Randomized Trial of Cognitive Behavioral Therapy in Primary Care-based Buprenorphine. Am J Med 2013;126(1):74.e11–7.

78. Moore BA, Fiellin DA, Cutter CJ, et al. Cognitive behavioral therapy improves treatment outcomes for prescription opioid users in primary-care based buprenorphine treatment. J Subst Abuse Treat 2016;71:54–7.

# Understanding Stimulant Use and Use Disorders in a New Era

Daniel Ciccarone, MD, MPH[a],*, Steve Shoptaw, PhD[b]

## KEYWORDS

- Cocaine • Methamphetamine • Fentanyl • Epidemiology • Pharmacology
- Neurobiology • Medication treatments • Behavioral treatments

## KEY POINTS

- Rising mortality related to stimulants, eg cocaine and methamphetamine, represent a fourth wave of the US overdose crisis.
- Methamphetamine supply, purity and potency have increased to historically high levels following shifts in chemical production.
- Substance use involving mixing of stimulants with opioid use is now common in the US.
- The medical complications of stimulant use occur in many organ systems; the most serious of which involve the CV and CNS systems.
- Chronic methamphetamine use can lead to neurodegeneration, cognitive impairment, and psychiatric and psychomotor syndromes.
- Evidence for pharmacotherapies for stimulant use disorders is mounting, eg agonists for cocaine use disorder and mirtazapine (single therapy) as well as naltrexone-XL plus high-dose bupropion (combination therapy) for methamphetamine use disorder.
- Contingency management is the behavioral therapy with the greatest efficacy for producing sustained abstinence from cocaine and methamphetamine use.

## EPIDEMIOLOGY

The United States is in an era of unprecedented levels of drug-related mortality, evidenced by an exponential increase in deaths over a recent 38-year period.[1] The recent drivers of overdose deaths are illicit opioids, mortality from which has been described as a triple wave phenomenon.[2–4] Most recently, illicit stimulant use (including

[a] Justine Miner Professor of Addiction Medicine, Department of Family and Community Medicine, University of California, San Francisco, MU3-E, Box 900, 500 Parnassus Avenue, San Francisco, CA 94143-0900, USA; [b] Professor and Vice Chair for Research, Department of Family Medicine, University of California, Los Angeles, 10880 Wilshire Boulevard, Suite 1800, Los Angeles, CA 90024, USA
* Corresponding author.
*E-mail address:* daniel.ciccarone@ucsf.edu

Med Clin N Am 106 (2022) 81–97
https://doi.org/10.1016/j.mcna.2021.08.010
0025-7125/22/© 2021 Elsevier Inc. All rights reserved.

psychostimulants, predominantly methamphetamine, as well as cocaine) and medical consequences, including overdose, are increasing. This article provides a review of the published literature on stimulants including the epidemiology, pharmacology, neurobiology, medical and psychiatric consequences, withdrawal management, and medical and behavioral treatments.

National surveys reveal increased methamphetamine use prevalence 2016 to 2019,[5] but with considerable regional and demographic variation.[6] The national prevalence of past-year cocaine use in 2019 is estimated at 5.5 million, increasing since 2011.[5] Illicit supplies are growing as well as shifting. Seizures of methamphetamine, a proxy for supply, have increased in all US census regions including those in which supply was historically low.[7] Correspondingly, for example, methamphetamine use is increasing in Massachusetts, a state where its use was uncommon in the past.[8] According to US Drug Enforcement Agency data, cocaine production estimates and US border seizures are at 10-year high levels as of 2019.[9]

Extending from the triple wave epidemic of opioid-related overdose deaths, a fourth wave of high mortality involving methamphetamine and cocaine use has been gathering force.[10] From 2012 to 2018 psychostimulant-related mortality has increased 5-fold (from 0.8 to 3.9/100,000) and cocaine-related mortality 3-fold (from 1.4 to 4.5/100,000 pop.).[11] Rates for methamphetamine-involved deaths are higher among men and non-Hispanic American Indian or Alaska Native and non-Hispanic White individuals.[12]

The current increase in stimulant-related deaths, although poorly understood, seem to be entwined with the ongoing opioid epidemic.[6,13–16] Polydrug use, for example, the co-use of stimulants and opioids, may partially explain the increase in stimulant-related deaths; this finding is increasingly common.[6] For example, the 3-fold increase nationally, 2015 to 2017, in methamphetamine use among those reporting past-month heroin use.[17] Nationally, in 2019, 76% of cocaine-related overdose deaths also involved an opioid; for psychostimulant-related deaths, 54% also involved an opioid, with co-involvement increasing over time.[16] The co-use of stimulants with high-potency synthetic opioids, for example, fentanyl and fentanyl analogs, is particularly concerning. In 2016, synthetic opioids were involved in deaths attributable to psychostimulants (14%) and cocaine (40%).[14] The reasons for co-use of stimulants, particularly methamphetamine, with synthetic opioids requires exploration.

In addition to the illicit stimulants discussed elsewhere in this article, there are increasing numbers of novel psychoactive substances (NPS), including novel stimulants such as substituted cathinones. Eutylone and N-ethylpentylone are among the 2 most common NPS stimulants according to recent US Drug Enforcement Agency seizure data,[9] toxicologic surveillance,[18] and wastewater analyses.[19]

The prevalence of use data are scarce, and a recent estimate using multiple sources indicated that fewer than 3% of US adults have used any NPS in the past 12 months; estimates for younger persons were higher.[20] An estimated 5.8% of young adults aged 18 to 25 years reported past year misuse of prescription stimulants in 2019, decreasing from 7.3% in 2015.[5]

## PHARMACOLOGY

Methamphetamine supply, purity, and potency have increased nationally to historically high levels after shifts in source and chemical production.[9] Methamphetamine purity and potency now exceed 90% after several changes: a decrease in US domestic production and an increase in Mexico-based production[21]; a historic shift from ephedrine-based to several variants of phenyl-2-propanone–based chemical production[22]; and increases in the D-isomer to L-isomer ratio (ie, the potency is defined by the proportion of D-isomer).[22] Methamphetamine typically exists in a racemic mixture of these 2 stereo-isomers, which have some known physiologic differences: L-methamphetamine has strong peripheral $\alpha$-adrenergic activity, whereas D-methamphetamine has 3 to 5 times the central nervous system activity (eg, increased euphoria as well as mental health problems and addiction liability).[23] The broad clinical implications of increasing availability and use of potent D-methamphetamine need explication.

Illicit or street methamphetamine comes in liquid (rarely used on the street), powder, crystalline, and pill (sometimes prescription mimics) forms.[9] Powder methamphetamine (eg, Meth, Speed, or Crank) is the HCL salt of racemic methamphetamine; crystal methamphetamine (eg, Crystal, Ice, or Tina) tends to be a purer form of D-methamphetamine and is more smokable as such.[23,24] Intake can be through oral ingestion, nasal insufflation (ie, snorting), vapor inhalation (ie, smoking, including "hot railing"), insertion per rectum (ie, "booty bumping"), and injecting (intravenously [IV]) (ie, "slamming").[25] The plasma half-life after intake is 9 to 11 hours, depending on the route of administration. IV and intranasal routes lead to peak effects within 15 minutes, whereas the smoking and oral routes take longer. Bioavailability is 100% for IV and 60% to 80% for other routes. After use, approximately 70% of a dose is excreted in the urine within 24 hours.[26]

Cocaine (benzoylmethylecgonine) is a naturally occurring alkaloid extracted from the leaves of the *Erthroxylon coca* plant, indigenous to the Andean region of South America. The powder form of cocaine (eg, Coke, Blow, or Snow) is the hydrochloride salt, which is water soluble and consumable by nasal insufflation and IV routes. The basic or bicarbonate form is well-known as 'crack' and is typically smoked or inhaled unless converted by acidification to a more soluble, and thus injectable, form. Cocaine HCL is typically not smoked because its vaporization temp is too high.[23] Inhaled (smoked) cocaine has the fastest onset of action (3–5 seconds) followed by IV (1–3 minutes) and nasal insufflation (>10 minutes). Inhaled cocaine leads to rapid cycling of use given its immediate effect and short duration of action. Its half-life is 0.7 to 1.5 hours with rapid metabolism by the liver and excretion in the urine.[27,28]

Cocaine is often consumed along with heroin, a combination known as a "speedball."[23] The expected effects are to boost the euphoria from heroin; this practice is more common once physical dependence to heroin sets in. The combination of methamphetamine and strong opioids, for example, heroin or fentanyl, is known as a "goofball." This combination was historically less common than the cocaine and heroin speedball, but seems to be getting more common.[6,29] The combinations of stimulants and synthetic opioids seems to be driving the recent mortality wave.[16]

Synthetic cathinones are a class of NPS structurally similar to cathinone, a naturally occurring chemical derived from the khat plant (*Catha edulis*), which is native to East Africa and the Arabian Peninsula. Cathinones are the chemical analogues of amphetamine and were once marketed as "bath salts" or "legal highs" to avoid regulation, and often sold as counterfeit MDMA (aka, Ecstasy). Synthetic cathinones are usually consumed in pill or capsule form, but smoking and insufflation, and more rarely injection, routes are options. There is a range of dosing (1–300 mg), onset of action (2–120 minutes), and duration of effect (0.25–6.00 hours), depending on the substance; many have unknown pharmacokinetics. Regulation, beginning in 2011 in the United States, led to a decrease in some of the initial products; however, a diversity of cathinones has sprung up since.[30]

### Neurobiology

The neurobiology of methamphetamine has been well-described in several excellent reviews.[31,32] In brief, methamphetamine is a potent indirect agonist at the noradrenaline, dopamine, and serotonin receptors and thus stimulates releases of these monoamines in the central and peripheral nervous system. Mechanisms that combine to enhance neurotransmitter release include redistribution from neuron synapse storage vesicles to the cytosol; increased (reversed) transport from cytosol to synapse; blockade as well as decreased expression of membrane transporters; inhibition of monoamine oxidase (metabolism); and increasing the activity of tyrosine hydroxylase (increasing dopamine production).[33] Methamphetamine is twice as potent at releasing noradrenaline than dopamine and 60-fold more effective at releasing serotonin.[26]

Methamphetamine acts on the major central nervous system (CNS) dopaminergic, noradrenergic, and serotonergic pathways.[34] Dopaminergic circuits, mediating reward and reinforcement processes, include mesolimbic, mesocortical circuit, and nigrostriatal pathways. Noradrenergic regions include the prefrontal cortex (cognitive processes), hippocampus (memory consolidation), and medial basal forebrain (arousal). The serotonergic system is diffuse and includes regulation of diverse functions, for example, those involving pain perception, reward, satiety, and impulsivity, among others. The opioidergic pathways are also affected, with intertwined effects on drug reinforcement and craving.[34]

The CNS effects of acute methamphetamine use include arousal, euphoria, positive mood, and improvements in cognitive function, as well as anxiety. Use over time leads to the downregulation of receptors and depletion of monoamine stores. It is increasingly evident that chronic methamphetamine use is involved in neuroinflammation and degeneration processes. Three molecular cascades are being investigated: oxidative stress, neurotoxic, and neuroinflammation. These neurobiological cascades are associated with altered brain metabolism and parallels in chronic dysfunction similar to other degenerative CNS diseases.[33]

Cocaine also boosts postsynaptic monoamine levels, not through the mechanisms outlined elsewhere in this article for methamphetamine leading to greater release of neurotransmitters, but through presynaptic reuptake blockade.[27] In addition to boosting the dopaminergic reward pathways, repeated cocaine exposure leads to significant neuroadaptations in the excitatory neurotransmitter glutamate,[35] as well as brain pathways that respond to stress. Cocaine use disorders frequently co-occur with stress-related disorders and stress can contribute to the recurrence of use.[36]

Similar to methamphetamine and cocaine, synthetic cathinones are psychomotor stimulants that exert their effects by impairing monoamine transporter function. Ring-substituted cathinones, for example, mephedrone, promote neurotransmitter release (like methamphetamine), whereas pyrrolidine-containing cathinones (eg, 3,4-methylenedioxypyrovalerone) act through reuptake blockage (like cocaine).[30]

### Medical and Psychiatric Complications

The medical complications of stimulant use are diverse and occur in many organ systems (**Table 1**). The major mechanisms of organ injury include ischemia, excess central and peripheral nervous system stimulation, and direct toxicity.[23] The etiology of methamphetamine-related mortality is multifaceted and includes, for example, the cardiovascular (common), pulmonary, CNS, and renal systems; in addition, intentional and unintentional fatal injuries stemming from use are common.[26]

The most serious medical complications, leading to the most mortality, are cardiovascular and cerebrovascular.[33] Psychostimulants cause harm in these systems through excessive sympathetic nervous system stimulation; cocaine has an additional prothrombotic effect.[37] In the acute setting, chest pain is a more common presentation from cocaine than methamphetamine use. Chest pain is the most common complaint of persons using cocaine presenting to the emergency department[38]; however, only a minority of patients have evidence of ischemia (10%) or acute myocardial infarction (6%).[39] Acute coronary syndrome is more likely due to vasospasm over plaque rupture.[40,41] Myocardial

**Table 1**
**Medical complications of stimulant use**

| Organ system | Acute | Chronic |
|---|---|---|
| Nervous system | | |
| Agitation | | Psychotic symptoms, mood disorders / Cerebrovascular disease/ stroke / Cognitive impairment |
| | Hallucinations, especially tactile / Dyskinesia / Seizures | Movement disorders for example, dystonic reactions, akathisia, choreoathetosis, tardive dyskinesia |
| Cardiovascular system | | |
| Tachycardia | | |
| | Hypertension / Coronary artery vasospasm / Myocardial infarction / Arrhythmias / Thoracic aortic dissection | Malignant hypertension / Myocarditis / Cardiomyopathy / Pulmonary hypertension / Accelerated atherosclerosis |
| Pulmonary | Cough, shortness of breath / Reactive airways disease / Pulmonary edema, hemorrhage / Pneumothorax | Acute coronary syndrome / Interstitial pneumonitis / Bronchiolitis obliterans / Pulmonary hypertension |
| Renal | Acute renal failure | |
| | Renal ischemia / Glomerulonephritis / Chronic renal failure | |
| Gastrointestinal | | Gastric ulceration and perforation |
| Reduced gastric motility | | Intestinal infarction |
| | GI bleeding | Ischemic colitis |
| Liver | | |
| Viral hepatitis and HIV | | |
| Endocrine | Reduced prolactin | Increased, normal, or decreased prolactin / Normal testosterone, cortisol, LH, thyroid hormones |
| Increased epinephrine, CRH, ACTH, cortisol and LH | Musculoskeletal | Movement disorders (see CNS) |
| Rhabdomyolysis | Head and neck | Rhinitis |
| Rhinitis, sinusitis | Corneal ulcers | Relieve drug-related symptoms (craving) |
| Improve mood, cognition, motivation | | Perforated nasal septum / Nasal and gingival ulceration / Dental decay and |

(continued on next page)

| Organ system | Acute | Chronic |
|---|---|---|
| **Table 1**<br>**(continued)** | | |
| | | periodontal disease<br>Xerostomia |
| Immune system | | |
| Vasculitis syndromes | | |
| Sexual function | | |
| Erectile dysfunction | | |
| Irregular menses | | |
| Reproductive | Vaginal bleeding | FDA category C<br>Placenta previa<br>Low birth weight |
| | Abruption placenta<br>Premature rupture of<br>membranes | |
| Dermatologic | | |
| Skin and soft tissue<br>infections | | |
| General/other | | |
| Dehydration | | Weight loss |
| | Hyperthermia | Nutritional deficits |

References:[23,27,32,37,45,103]

*Abbreviations:* ACTH, adrenocorticotropic hormone; CRH, corticotropin-releasing hormone; FDA, US Food and Drug Administration; LH, luteinizing hormone.

infarction owing to plaque rupture is seen in a minority of cases and more likely stemming from cocaine use owing to its prothrombic effect. Hypertension can be acute or chronic.[37] Cardiac arrythmias can develop in persons using high dose psychostimulants. Long-term use leads to chronic hypertension, cardiomegaly, congestive heart failure, and myocardial ischemia. Myocarditis is considered a precursor to the development of dilated cardiomyopathy, a significant clinical problem among persons using psychostimulants.[42,43] Hypertensive, or hypertrophic, cardiomyopathy is less common; this entity results from profound chronic hypertension.[37] Injury to the cerebrovascular system also occurs owing to persistent hypertension. Stoke, particularly hemorrhagic stroke, is found at higher rates among psychostimulant users.[44,45]

There is mounting evidence that chronic methamphetamine use leads to neurodegeneration, cognitive impairment, and psychiatric and psychomotor syndromes.[33] Cognitive impairment stemming from methamphetamine use is across multiple domains, including executive function, memory, learning and processing speed, and motor and language skills.[46] Cocaine use is associated with milder or more transient deficits.[45]

Premorbid impairments may account for some of these findings. Psychotic symptoms are common stemming from occasional use and become more frequent with regular, high-dose, or high-potency (eg, D-methamphetamine) use. Psychotic symptom expression among persons who use methamphetamine may indicate an underlying vulnerability to schizophrenia,[45] although there are important differences: persons with methamphetamine-induced psychotic symptoms have fewer negative symptoms (ie, blunted affect, disorganization, social withdrawal) and similar levels of positive symptoms (ie, grandiosity, hallucinations, paranoia) compared with individuals with schizophrenia.[32] Comorbid mood disorders are also common among those meeting the criteria for methamphetamine use disorder.[47] Abnormal psychomotor symptoms include tremors, dyskinesia, and akathisia, as well as repetitive and compulsive behaviors, for example, tweaking (owing to tactile hallucinations; ie, formication).[23] Neurodegeneration of dopaminergic CNS pathways, secondary to chronic methamphetamine use, may lead to premature development of Parkinson's disease and parkinsonism.[45] It is important to recognize that premorbid conditions, for example, genetics, family history, and childhood trauma or isolation, can lead to both substance use disorders and psychiatric syndromes.[33,45]

Nationwide, HIV diagnoses are edging up among persons who inject drugs; this increase is more profound among White persons who inject drugs.[48,49] Recent outbreaks of HIV discovered among persons who inject drugs in several US states accentuate this trend, along with increasing viral hepatitis infection rates.[50–53] Injection stimulant use, both of cocaine and methamphetamine, has been associated with HIV seroconversion, whether through injection practices or high-risk sexual behavior, often in patterns of polydrug use.[6,54–56] Methamphetamine also incurs an increased physiologic risk of HIV acquisition[57] and is associated with lower rates of viral suppression among people living with HIV and therefore an enhanced risk of transmission.[58]

The long-term use of stimulants is frequently preformed in cycles of bingeing and abstinence.[23] Cohort studies estimate that, after the initiation of cocaine use, 7% of persons meet the criteria for cocaine use disorder at 1 year, with a 15% cumulative probability of cocaine use disorder after 10 years.[59] Stimulant use disorder is a chronic relapsing condition. The criteria for meeting the diagnosis come from the *Diagnostic and Statistical Manual*, Fifth Edition, published by the American Psychiatric Association.[60] Eleven criteria are detailed including, for example, craving; a failure to satisfy important school, home, or work obligations; a consistent desire to control use; and continued use despite psychological or physical difficulties. Three levels of severity of illness are diagnosed based on number of criteria met within a 12-month period: mild disorder (2–3 criteria), moderate disorder (4–5 criteria), or severe disorder (6 or more). The development of stimulant use disorder is strongly influenced by early childhood adversity. A recent national study found a statistically significant relationship between the number of self-reported adverse childhood experiences and stimulant use and use disorders among adult respondents.[61]

### Management of Stimulant Withdrawal Symptoms

Abstinence after prolonged use can produce withdrawal symptoms defined by the *Diagnostic and Statistical Manual*, Fifth Edition, which include trouble sleeping, trouble concentrating, tiredness, fatigue, irritability, agitation, anxiety, sadness, depression, and an inability to perform normal activities.[60]

In the inpatient and emergency department settings, patients with stimulant-related agitation are usually managed with antipsychotics,[62] although these medications show no efficacy for sustaining abstinence after discharge. In outpatient settings, withdrawal symptoms are usually mild-to-moderate in severity; most are short lived[63] and mostly absent after 5 weeks. In contrast, the craving for stimulants diminishes slowly, contributing to continued use or recurrence of use in the first weeks and months of abstinence.[63] Longer term abstinence from stimulants leads some to attribute decreases in cognitive abilities, especially in settings of continued episodic use, as protracted withdrawal.[64] Because no medications show consistent effects in treating stimulant withdrawal,[65] treatments are largely behavioral (eg, cognitive–behavioral therapies, behavioral activation, 12-step facilitation and contingency management)—all of which require patients to allot cognitive resources to sustain abstinence—resources that may be diminished from the direct effects of the stimulants themselves and from the effects of stimulant withdrawal symptoms. In addition, patients who experience repeated use and recurrence of use as a consequence of failures of treatments to successfully resolve withdrawal can lose motivation to remain in treatment. There are some innovations, however. One new approach that enhances cognitive reserve is repetitive transcranial magnetic stimulation. A pilot study showed superiority in decreasing methamphetamine withdrawal symptoms compared with a sham condition in a small study of men acutely abstinent from methamphetamine use disorder.[66]

### Medication Treatments for Stimulant Use Disorder

Evidence-based treatments, whether pharmacologic or behavioral, can be considered for use to the extent they show superiority over placebo or other comparisons along defined targets (**Table 2**). Although there are no medications approved by the US Food and Drug Administration for cocaine or methamphetamine use disorders, clinical research shows that some medications show statistically significant and clinically relevant outcomes over placebo. A small number of medications have data in placebo-controlled trials showing measurable decreases in stimulant use. The point worth remembering is that this benefit is due to a medication or medications, a benefit to patients that occurs directly related to the medication, and a benefit that accrues to the patient without needing to allot psychological energy or motivational resources regarding their stimulant use (or nonuse).

One rule to evaluate the strength of findings reported by studies on stimulant pharmacotherapy outcomes involves whether positive outcomes are observed from 2 or more trials of a medication and/or whether there is a single, well-powered study. With this in mind, there are 4 medications or classes of medications that show consistent signals of efficacy for improving cocaine use outcomes. Dopamine agonists show the most consistent findings for efficacy.[67] Significant cocaine abstinence outcomes are seen for D-amphetamine over placebo at doses between 30 and 60 mg with a flexible dosing plan and 60 mg as a fixed dose in patients with cocaine dependence.[68,69] A finding also seen for cocaine abstinence outcomes at 60 mg for people with cocaine and opioid use disorders.[70] Showing cocaine abstinence outcomes are improved at higher agonist doses, 1 trial evaluated extended release mixed amphetamine salts and showed dose-dependent effects (60 mg, 80 mg) over placebo for decreasing cocaine use among participants with both cocaine use disorder and attention deficit hyperactivity disorder.[71]

A second medication involves repeated trials showing significant improvements in cocaine abstinence outcomes for topiramate over placebo,[72,73] with cocaine use outcomes also decreased for 1 trial in a subset of participants with cocaine and alcohol use disorder.[74] Despite this consistency, a frequent side effect for topiramate involves cognitive dysfunction that can interfere with daily functioning. This side effect can be minimized by titrating the dose to a steady state in weekly increases, with abstinence

| Table 2 | |
|---|---|
| **What would effective medication and behavioral treatments for stimulant use disorder do?[a]** | |
| **Pharmacologic Targets** | **Behavioral Targets** |
| Full agonist | Achieve remission |
| Block stimulant effect (antagonists) | Prevention of recurrence of use |
| Relieve drug-related symptoms (cravings) | Improve mood, cognition, and motivation |
| Alter biological mechanisms of stimulant use disorder | Decrease cravings |

[a] Addiction is a chronic, relapsing disorder. Multiple treatments are usually required before remission is achieved.

outcomes observed at steady state. A combination pharmacotherapy that combines extended release mixed amphetamine salts and topiramate produced 2 trials showing strong replication findings in decreasing cocaine use, especially among participants who had a greater frequency of cocaine use at baseline.[75,76] An honorable mention in the list of medications for cocaine use disorder is disulfiram. Multiple trials have been conducted on the medication. Two systematic reviews that evaluated the complex set of trial findings regarding use of disulfiram for cocaine use disorder concluded, however, that if there is a signal for disulfiram,[77] it is not replicable and there is a signal that disulfiram actually decreases retention in trials compared with placebo.[78]

These findings underscore the importance of replicating findings from single trials, especially when trials are small and/or have conflicting findings. There does seem, however, to be sufficient evidence to consider an agonist approach, or the combination topiramate and extended release mixed amphetamine salts strategy, when developing a treatment plan for patients with cocaine use disorder. It is worth restating that none of these medications have been evaluated for use as a treatment for cocaine use disorder by the US Food and Drug Administration.

Using the same metric for considering medications to improve drug use outcomes for methamphetamine use disorder, 1 medication and 1 combination pharmacotherapy deserve consideration. The single pharmacotherapy involves mirtazapine (30 mg/d). In a small, 12-week randomized, placebo-controlled trial[79] and a larger, 36-week replication study,[80] nearly identical superior signals in methamphetamine use over placebo were observed for mirtazapine for decreasing methamphetamine use. It is worth noting that both trials were conducted in San Francisco and both trials were conducted among men who have sex with men and transgender women. It is also worth noting that the majority of methamphetamine decreases occurred in the first 12 weeks, with the mirtazapine group maintaining their abstinence gains to the end of the study. A recent multisite, fully powered, 12-week trial of combination pharmacotherapy of extended release naltrexone and oral daily bupropion (450 mg) showed significant decrease in methamphetamine use.[81] The trial was the largest methamphetamine clinical trial ever (n-403). It is worth noting that the extended release naltrexone was administered every 3 weeks with the high-dose bupropion condition to address the tendency of pharmacotherapy trials to evaluate suboptimal study doses. The number needed to treat using the combination is 9, which compares favorably with other medications used for substance use disorder. It remains unclear if the combination pharmacotherapy can be used with patients with methamphetamine use disorder who have moderate or severe opioid use disorder. Still, the consistency of the findings from these 2 studies with clear signals of efficacy provide a rationale for considering their use in clinical settings.

### Behavioral Treatments for Stimulant Use Disorder

There is a mature evidence base describing outcomes for behavioral treatments for cocaine and methamphetamine use disorders. Behavioral treatments with efficacy for cocaine also show efficacy for methamphetamine. Taking advantage of the number of completed trials, systematic reviews and meta-analyses describe signals of efficacy for behavioral treatments of cocaine and stimulant use disorders. It is worth noting that the ability to respond to behavioral therapies for stimulant use disorders is linked to the availability of dopamine D2 and D3 receptors[82,83] and the cognitive ability to avoid making decisions of risk in the setting of recent loss.[84,85] Because all behavior reflects brain activity, it is encouraging to note that behavioral therapies have neural and cognitive correlates that predict treatment outcome and signal key neurocognitive mechanisms in recovery from stimulant use disorder.

### Contingency management

Contingency management is the behavioral therapy with greatest efficacy for producing sustained abstinence from cocaine and methamphetamine use. The therapy works by providing incentives of increasing value for successive biomarkers documenting stimulant abstinence. It is based on the principles of operant behavior.[86] The operant principles of contingency management were first applied to determining who qualified for take home medications in methadone treatment clinics.[87] The principles were adapted for use in treating cocaine use disorder in the 1990s.[88] The original method of providing vouchers in exchange for urine samples documenting stimulant abstinence was adapted further by using a fish bowl method that provided increasing numbers of draws for prizes from the fish bowl with consecutive samples documenting stimulant abstinence.[89] Four meta-analyses of clinical trials measuring the signal for contingency management report an effect size ("d") between 0.4 and 0.6.[90–93] The size of this signal is such that, if contingency management were a medication, it would be the standard of care. A frequent complaint about contingency management is that the therapy works by paying people to make healthy choices that they should make without incentives. However, there are limits to the contingency management paradigm: it works only when participants have some intention to change their stimulant use behaviors.[94] Another concern expressed notes that, until recently, contingency management was only available in research clinics and a limited number of public health treatment settings. Notably the Veterans Administration Healthcare System now provides contingency management treatment of cocaine use disorder.[95] Scale-up of contingency management and addressing sticky issues in providing resources for the contingency management schedules in insurance markets, both privately and publicly funded, is currently underway.

### Cognitive–behavioral therapy

Cognitive–behavioral therapy involves teaching a set of common principles to patients to facilitate remission, to return to abstinence after use and recurrence of use, and to prevent recurrence of use. Cognitive–behavioral therapies are didactic and taught over a series of weeks in individual or group formats. Manuals are available online to deliver cognitive behavioral therapy[96,97] and the therapy is now available to engage on-line (www.CBT4CBT.com). Cognitive–behavioral therapies show weaker and less consistent signals of efficacy compared with contingency management.[98,99] The effects noted elsewhere in this article on direct stimulant effects and withdrawal symptoms in eroding cognitive capacity can interfere with some patients being able to engage the learning process in the short term. However, there are data showing that, even with the relatively weaker signal for cognitive–behavioral therapy over contingency management during early recovery, data do show significant improvements in abstinence outcomes at distal follow-up evaluations. One explanation for this observation is that some investigators believe that the skills for recurrence of use prevention are best learned in real time by applying the skills to return to abstinence during recurrence of use of stimulants. In individual trials, there is a consistent sleeper effect for cognitive–behavioral therapy, where abstinence outcomes improve over time as patients apply the skills necessary to sustain abstinence and, importantly, to return to abstinence after the recurrence of use.[100] Still, the principles of cognitive–behavioral therapy are omnibus, with uptake of these concepts used in most intervention settings, including peer and social recovery and harm reduction. Their wide-scale use is the basis for cognitive–behavioral therapies as having comparatively weaker efficacy compared with contingency management, but greater effectiveness in decreasing suffering across the community of people in treatment for stimulant use disorders.

*Behavioral therapies and strategies with less consistent evidence of efficacy*
There are several behavioral therapies that have trials showing initial signals of comparative efficacy for patients trying to establish and sustain abstinence from stimulants. These include motivational interviewing[98] and 12-step facilitation approaches.[101] As with pharmacotherapies, there seems to be some additional benefit to abstinence outcomes when combining behavioral therapies, with an especially strong signal observed for the few trials that combine contingency management and cognitive–behavioral therapy.[91,98] This strategy of combining behavioral therapies underscores the notion that stimulant use disorder is difficult to treat, with best outcomes seen when interventions that address multiple targets are outlined in the treatment plan (see **Table 2**). Despite this replicated boost in efficacy for the combination, few programs incorporate contingency management. Similarly, there is increasing interest in incorporating behavioral therapies with the few medications showing signals of efficacy for stimulant use disorder to boost outcomes, particularly in those patients with severe stimulant use disorders. There are some indications that incorporating agonist medications with contingency management can boost achieving remission, with the medications reinforcing incentive salience.[102] The use of behavioral therapies for stimulant use disorders is complex for clinicians who work in primary care, emergency departments, and other settings that do not have access to behavioral health. This area is ripe for development in the field, with a notable example of the bridge to recovery movement for increasing access to medications for opioid use disorder. A parallel focus that involves increasing access to medications for stimulant use disorders is an important research direction for the near future.

## SUMMARY

For the first time there is a consistent signal of efficacy supporting use of agonists for cocaine use disorder and mirtazapine for methamphetamine use disorder as single medications in outpatient settings. A similar report on the strength and consistency of signal for combination pharmacotherapies for cocaine use disorder (mixed amphetamine salts, extended release plus topiramate) and for methamphetamine use disorder (extended release naltrexone plus high-dose bupropion) in outpatient settings can now be made. Moreover, there is now sufficient evidence to support consideration of a medication approach as a foundation for outpatient treatment for stimulant use disorders. A single approach, however, will likely be insufficient to overcome the pernicious and difficult challenges to achieving and maintaining remission from stimulants. Integrating medications with behavioral therapies (contingency management, cognitive–behavioral therapy) and social and peer support approaches (12-step groups, 12-step facilitation) represent an opportunity for helping patients to make significant decreased in stimulant use and in reaching their substance use goals.

## CLINICS CARE POINTS

- There are no FDA approved medications for stimulant use disorder; behavioral therapies are the treatment of choice for stimulant use disorder.
- Behavioral therapies differ in their focus to address patients abilities to initiate abstinence, to maintain abstinence and to re-initiate abstinence following recurrence of use.
- High quality scientific evidence documents efficacy and supports consideration of a limited set of medications for stimulant use disorder.

- No single approach of behavioral therapy, medication or social intervention is likely to produce sustained treatment outcome for persons with stimulant use disorder; integration of treatments emphasizing the whole person is optimal.

## FUNDING

The authors acknowledge funding from National Institutes of Health, National Institute of Drug Abuse, grants R01DA054190; R01DA054190; R01DA037820; U01DA036267; UG1DA020024; P30MH058107.

## DISCLOSURES

Dr Ciccarone reports consultant fees from Celero Systems and expert testimony fees from Motley Rice LLP.

## REFERENCES

1. Jalal H, Buchanich JM, Roberts MS, et al. Changing dynamics of the drug over-dose epidemic in the United States from 1979 through 2016. Science 2018; 361(6408):eaau1184.
2. Ciccarone D. The triple wave epidemic: supply and demand drivers of the US opioid overdose crisis. Int J Drug Policy 2019;71:183–8.
3. Ciccarone D. Fentanyl in the US heroin supply: a rapidly changing risk environ-ment. Int J Drug Policy 2017;46:107–11.
4. Centers for Disease Control and Prevention. 2019 Annual Surveillance Report of Drug-Related Risks and Outcomes — United States Surveillance. Special Report. Atlanta, GA: Centers for Disease Control and Prevention, U.S.; 2019. Published November 1, 2019.
5. Substance Abuse and Mental Health Services Administration. Key Substance use and Mental Health Indicators in the United States: Results from the 2019 National Survey on Drug Use and Health. Rockville, MD: Center for Behavioral Health Statistics and Quality, Substance Abuse and Mental Health Services Administration; 2020.
6. Glick SN, Burt R, Kummer K, et al. Increasing methamphetamine injection among non-MSM who inject drugs in King County, Washington. Drug Alcohol Depend 2018;182:86–92.
7. Artigiani EE, Hsu MH, Hauser W, et al. Law Enforcement Seizures of Metham-Phetamine Widespread and Increasing. College Park, MD: National Drug Early Warning System; 2020.
8. Wakeman S, Flood J, Ciccarone D. Rise in presence of methamphetamine in oral fluid toxicology tests among outpatients in a large healthcare setting in the Northeast. J Addict Med 2021;15(1):85–7.
9. US Drug Enforcement Administration. 2020 National Drug Threat Assessment. Ar-lington VA: US Drug Enforcement Administration, Department of Justice; 2021.
10. Ciccarone D. The rise of illicit fentanyls, stimulants and the fourth wave of the opioid overdose crisis. Curr Opin Psychiatry 2021;34(4):344–50.
11. Hedegaard H, Miniño AM, Warner M. Drug overdose deaths in the United States, 1999–2018. NCHS Data Brief, no 356. Hyattsville, MD: National Center for Health Statistics; 2020.
12. Han B, Cotto J, Etz K, et al. Methamphetamine overdose deaths in the US by sex and race and ethnicity. JAMA Psychiatry 2021;78(5):564–7.

13. Gladden RM, O'Donnell J, Mattson CL, et al. Changes in opioid-involved overdose deaths by opioid type and presence of benzodiazepines, cocaine, and methamphetamine - 25 states, July- December 2017 to January-June 2018. MMWR Morb Mortal Wkly Rep 2019;68(34):737–44.

14. Jones CM, Einstein EB, Compton WM. Changes in synthetic opioid involvement in drug overdose deaths in the united states, 2010-2016. J Am Med Assoc 2018; 319(17):1819–21.

15. Al-Tayyib A, Koester S, Langegger S, et al. Heroin and methamphetamine injection: an emerging drug use pattern. Substance use & misuse 2017;52(8): 1051–8.

16. Hedegaard H, Miniño AM, Warner M. Co-involvement of opioids in drug overdose deaths involving cocaine and psychostimulants. NCHS Data Brief, no 406. Hyattsville, MD: National Center for Health Statistics; 2021.

17. Strickland JC, Havens JR, Stoops WW. A nationally representative analysis of "twin epidemics": rising rates of methamphetamine use among persons who use opioids. Drug Alcohol Depend 2019;204:107592.

18. NPS stimulants & hallucinogens in the United States: trend report Q1, 2021. Available at: https://www.npsdiscovery.org/wp-content/uploads/2021/04/2021-Q1_NPS-Stimulants-and- Hallucinogens_Trend-Report.pdf. [Accessed 3 May 2021].

19. Bade R, White JM, Chen J, et al. International snapshot of new psychoactive substance use: case study of eight countries over the 2019/2020 new year period. Water Res 2021;193:116891.

20. Peacock A, Bruno R, Gisev N, et al. New psychoactive substances: challenges for drug surveillance, control, and public health responses. Lancet (London, England) 2019;394(10209):1668–84.

21. United Nations Office on Drug and Crime. World Drug Report 2020: Booklet 3, drug Supply. Vienna: United Nations; 2020. E.20.XI.6.

22. Drug Enforcement Administration. 2019 National drug threat assessment. Arlington, VA: US Drug Enforcement Administration, Department of Justice; 2020.

23. Ciccarone D. Stimulant abuse: pharmacology, cocaine, methamphetamine, treatment, attempts at pharmacotherapy. Prim Care 2011;38(1). 41-58, v-vi.

24. Erowid. Available at: https://www.erowid.org/chemicals/meth/meth_basics.shtml. [Accessed 30 April 2021].

25. Available at: Tweaker.org. [Accessed 30 April 2021] https://tweaker.org/crystal-meth/ways-guys-do-meth/.

26. Cruickshank CC, Dyer KR. A review of the clinical pharmacology of methamphetamine. *Addiction* (*Abingdon, England*) 2009;104(7):1085–99.

27. Zimmerman JL. Cocaine intoxication. Crit Care Clin 2012;28(4):517–26.

28. Volkow ND, Wang GJ, Fischman MW, et al. Effects of route of administration on cocaine induced dopamine transporter blockade in the human brain. Life Sci 2000;67(12):1507–15.

29. Ellis MS, Kasper ZA, Cicero TJ. Twin epidemics: the surging rise of methamphetamine use in chronic opioid users. Drug Alcohol Depend 2018;193:14–20.

30. Goncalves JL, Alves VL, Aguiar J, et al. Synthetic cathinones: an evolving class of new psychoactive substances. Crit Rev Toxicol 2019;49(7):549–66.

31. Fleckenstein AE, Volz TJ, Riddle EL, et al. New insights into the mechanism of action of amphetamines. Annu Rev Pharmacol Toxicol 2007;47:681–98.

32. Panenka WJ, Procyshyn RM, Lecomte T, et al. Methamphetamine use: a comprehensive review of molecular, preclinical and clinical findings. Drug Alcohol Depend 2013;129(3):167–79.

33. Paulus MP, Stewart JL. Neurobiology, clinical presentation, and treatment of methamphetamine use disorder: a review. JAMA Psychiatry 2020;77(9):959–66.

34. Courtney KE, Ray LA. Methamphetamine: an update on epidemiology, pharmacology, clinical phenomenology, and treatment literature. Drug Alcohol Depend 2014;143:11–21.

35. Schmidt HD, Pierce RC. Cocaine-induced neuroadaptations in glutamate transmission: potential therapeutic targets for craving and addiction. Ann N Y Acad Sci 2010;1187:35–75.

36. Mantsch JR, Vranjkovic O, Twining RC, et al. Neurobiological mechanisms that contribute to stress-related cocaine use. Neuropharmacology 2014;76 Pt B: 383–94.

37. Duflou J. Psychostimulant use disorder and the heart. Addiction 2020;115(1): 175–83.

38. Brody SL, Slovis CM, Wrenn KD. Cocaine-related medical problems: consecutive series of 233 patients. Am J Med 1990;88(4):325–31.

39. Weber JE, Chudnofsky CR, Boczar M, et al. Cocaine-associated chest pain: how common is myocardial infarction? Acad Emerg Med 2000;7(8):873–7.

40. Paratz ED, Cunningham NJ, MacIsaac AI. The cardiac complications of methamphetamines. Heart Lung Circ 2016;25(4):325–32.

41. Chen JP. Methamphetamine-associated acute myocardial infarction and cardiogenic shock with normal coronary arteries: refractory global coronary microvascular spasm. J Invasive Cardiol 2007;19(4):E89–92.

42. Neeki MM, Kulczycki M, Toy J, et al. Frequency of Methamphetamine Use as a Major Contributor Toward the Severity of Cardiomyopathy in Adults ≤50Years. The Am J Cardiol 2016;118(4):585–9.

43. Virmani R, Robinowitz M, Smialek JE, et al. Cardiovascular effects of cocaine: an autopsy study of 40 patients. Am Heart J 1988;115(5):1068–76.

44. Darke S, Duflou J, Kaye S, et al. Psychostimulant use and fatal stroke in young adults. J forensic Sci 2019;64(5):1421–6.

45. Lappin JM, Sara GE. Psychostimulant use and the brain. Addiction (Abingdon, England) 2019;114(11):2065–77.

46. Scott JC, Woods SP, Matt GE, et al. Neurocognitive effects of methamphetamine: a critical review and meta-analysis. Neuropsychol Rev 2007;17(3):275–97.

47. Akindipe T, Wilson D, Stein DJ. Psychiatric disorders in individuals with methamphetamine dependence: prevalence and risk factors. Metab Brain Dis 2014; 29(2):351–7.

48. Centers for Disease Control and Prevention. HIV Surveillance Report, 2018 (Preliminary). Atlanta, GA: Centers for Disease Control and Prevention, US Department of Health and Human Services; 2019.

49. AtlasPlus. Available at: https://gis.cdc.gov/grasp/nchhstpatlas/charts.html. [Accessed 29 April 2021].

50. Peters PJ, Pontones P, Hoover KW, et al. HIV Infection Linked to Injection Use of Oxymorphone in Indiana, 2014-2015. N Engl J Med 2016;375(3):229–39.

51. Evans MELS, Hogan V, Agnew-Brune C, et al. Notes from the field: HIV infection investigation in a rural area — West Virginia, 2017. Morb Mortal Wkly Rep 2018;67: 257–8.

52. Wheeling-Ohio West Virginia Health Department. HIV Cluster Identified in Ohio county 2018. Available at:http://www.ohiocountyhealth.com/news/hiv-cluster-identified-in-ohio-county/. Accessed 29 April 2021.

53. Centers for Disease Control and Prevention. Epi-2: Preliminary Epi-Aid Report: Undetermined Risk Factors and Mode of Transmission for HIV Infection Among

Persons Who Inject Drugs — Massachusetts. Atlanta, GA: Centers for Disease Control and Prevention, US Department of Health and Human Services; 2018.

54. Tyndall MW, Currie S, Spittal P, et al. Intensive injection cocaine use as the primary risk factor in the Vancouver HIV-1 epidemic. Aids 2003;17(6):887–93.

55. Patterson TL, Semple SJ, Zians JK, et al. Methamphetamine-using HIV-positive men who have sex with men: correlates of polydrug use. J Urban Health : Bull New York Acad Med 2005;82(Suppl 1):i120–6.

56. Spindler HH, Scheer S, Chen SY, et al. Viagra, methamphetamine, and HIV risk: results from a probability sample of MSM, San Francisco. Sex Transm Dis 2007; 34(8):586–91.

57. Fulcher JA, Shoptaw S, Makgoeng SB, et al. Brief report: recent methamphetamine use is associated with increased rectal mucosal inflammatory cytokines, regardless of HIV-1 serostatus. J Acquir Immune Defic Syndr 2018;78(1):119–23.

58. Fairbairn N, Kerr T, Milloy M-J, et al. Crystal methamphetamine injection predicts slower HIV RNA suppression among injection drug users. Addict Behav 2011; 36(7):762–3.

59. Lopez-Quintero C, Perez de los Cobos J, Hasin DS, et al. Probability and Predictors of Transition from First Use to Dependence on Nicotine, Alcohol, Cannabis, and Cocaine: Results of the National Epidemiologic Survey on Alcohol and Related Conditions (NESARC). Drug Alcohol Depend 2011;115(1–2):120–30.

60. American Psychiatric Association FE, DSM-5. Diagnostic and Statistical Manual of Mental Disorders. Washington DC: American Psychiatric Publishing; 2013.

61. Tang S, Jones CM, Wisdom A, et al. Adverse childhood experiences and stimulant use disorders among adults in the United States. Psychiatry Res 2021;299: 113870.

62. Richards JR, Hawkins JA, Acevedo EW, et al. The care of patients using methamphetamine in the emergency department: perception of nurses, residents, and faculty. Subst Abus 2019;40(1):95–101.

63. Zorick T, Nestor L, Miotto K, et al. Withdrawal symptoms in abstinent methamphetamine- dependent subjects. Addiction 2010;105(10):1809–18.

64. Amato L, Minozzi S, Davoli M, et al. Psychosocial and pharmacological treatments versus pharmacological treatments for opioid detoxification. Cochrane Database Syst Rev 2008;(3):CD005031.

65. Shoptaw SJ, Kao U, Heinzerling K, et al. Treatment for amphetamine withdrawal. Cochrane Database Syst Rev 2009;2009(2):CD003021.

66. Liang Y, Wang L, Yuan TF. Targeting withdrawal symptoms in men addicted to methamphetamine with transcranial magnetic stimulation: a randomized clinical trial. JAMA Psychiatry 2018;75(11):1199–201.

67. Brandt L, Chao T, Comer SD, et al. Pharmacotherapeutic strategies for treating cocaine use disorder-what do we have to offer? Addiction 2021;116:694–710.

68. Grabowski J, Rhoades H, Schmitz J, et al. Dextroamphetamine for cocaine-dependence treatment: a double-blind randomized clinical trial. J Clin Psychopharmacol 2001;21(5):522–6.

69. Schmitz JM, Rathnayaka N, Green CE, et al. Combination of modafinil and d-amphetamine for the treatment of cocaine dependence: a preliminary investigation. Front Psychiatry 2012;3:77.

70. Nuijten M, Blanken P, van de Wetering B, et al. Sustained-release dexamfetamine in the treatment of chronic cocaine-dependent patients on heroin-assisted treatment: a randomised, double-blind, placebo-controlled trial. Lancet 2016;387(10034):2226–34.

71. Levin FR, Mariani JJ, Specker S, et al. Extended-release mixed amphetamine salts vs placebo for comorbid adult attention-deficit/hyperactivity disorder and cocaine use disorder: a randomized clinical trial. JAMA Psychiatry 2015;72(6): 593–602.

72. Kampman KM, Pettinati H, Lynch KG, et al. A pilot trial of topiramate for the treatment of cocaine dependence. Drug Alcohol Depend 2004;75(3):233–40.

73. Johnson BA, Ait-Daoud N, Wang XQ, et al. Topiramate for the treatment of cocaine addiction: a randomized clinical trial. JAMA Psychiatry 2013;70(12): 1338–46.

74. Kampman KM, Pettinati HM, Lynch KG, et al. A double-blind, placebo-controlled trial of topiramate for the treatment of comorbid cocaine and alcohol dependence. Drug Alcohol Depend 2013;133(1):94–9.

75. Levin FR, Mariani JJ, Pavlicova M, et al. Extended release mixed amphetamine salts and topiramate for cocaine dependence: a randomized clinical replication trial with frequent users. Drug Alcohol Depend 2020;206:107700.

76. Mariani JJ, Pavlicova M, Bisaga A, et al. Extended-release mixed amphetamine salts and topiramate for cocaine dependence: a randomized controlled trial. Biol Psychiatry 2012;72(11):950–6.

77. Pani PP, Trogu E, Vacca R, et al. Disulfiram for the treatment of cocaine dependence. Cochrane Database Syst Rev 2010;(1):Cd007024.

78. Chan B, Freeman M, Ayers C, et al. A systematic review and meta-analysis of medications for stimulant use disorders in patients with co-occurring opioid use disorders. Drug Alcohol Depend 2020;216:108193.

79. Colfax GN, Santos G-M, Das M, et al. Mirtazapine to reduce methamphetamine use: a randomized controlled trial. Arch Gen Psychiatry 2011;68(11):1168–75.

80. Coffin PO, Santos GM, Hern J, et al. Effects of mirtazapine for methamphetamine use disorder among cisgender men and transgender women who have sex with men: a placebo-controlled randomized clinical trial. JAMA Psychiatry 2020;77(3):246–55.

81. Trivedi MH, Walker R, Ling W, et al. Bupropion and naltrexone in methamphetamine use disorder. N Engl J Med 2021;384(2):140–53.

82. Wang GJ, Smith L, Volkow ND, et al. Decreased dopamine activity predicts relapse in methamphetamine abusers. Mol Psychiatry 2011;17:918.

83. Martinez D, Carpenter KM, Liu F, et al. Imaging dopamine transmission in cocaine dependence: link between neurochemistry and response to treatment. Am J Psychiatry 2011;138:634–41.

84. Gowin JLS JL, May AC, Ball TM, et al. Altered cingulate and insular cortex activation during risk-taking in methamphetamine dependence: losses lose impact. Addiction 2013;109:237–47.

85. Lake MT, Shoptaw S, Ipser JC, et al. Decision-making by patients with methamphetamine use disorder receiving contingency management treatment: magnitude and frequency effects. Front Psychiatry 2020;11:22.

86. Skinner BF. The Behaviour of organisms: an experimental analysis. New York: Appleton-Century; 1938.

87. Stitzer M, Bigelow G, Lawrence C, et al. Medication take-home as a reinforcer in a methadone maintenance program. Addict Behav 1977;2(1):9–14.

88. Higgins ST, Budney AJ, Bickel WK, et al. Achieving cocaine abstinence with a behavioral approach. Am J Psychiatry 1993;150(5):763–9.

89. Petry NM, Bohn MJ. Fishbowls and candy bars: using low-cost incentives to increase treatment retention. Sci Pract Perspect 2003;2(1):55–61.

90. Benishek LA, Dugosh KL, Kirby KC, et al. Prize-based contingency manage-ment for the treatment of substance abusers: a meta-analysis. Addiction (Abing-don, England) 2014;109(9):1426–36.

91. Dutra L, Stathopoulou G, Basden SL, et al. A meta-analytic review of psychoso-cial interventions for substance use disorders. Am J Psychiatry 2008;165(2):179–87.

92. Griffith JD, Rowan-Szal GA, Roark RR, et al. Contingency management in outpa-tient methadone treatment: a meta-analysis. Drug Alcohol Depend 2000;58(1–2):55–66.

93. Prendergast M, Podus D, Finney J, et al. Contingency management for treat-ment of substance use disorders: a meta-analysis. Addiction 2006;101:1546–60.

94. Menza TW, Jameson DR, Hughes JP, et al. Contingency management to reduce methamphetamine use and sexual risk among men who have sex with men: a randomized controlled trial. BMC Public Health 2010;10:774.

95. DePhilippis D, Petry NM, Bonn-Miller MO, et al. The national implementation of Contingency Management (CM) in the Department of Veterans Affairs: atten-dance at CM sessions and substance use outcomes. Drug Alcohol Depend 2018;185:367–73.

96. Center for Substance Abuse Treatment. Counselor's Treatment Manual: Matrix Intensive Outpatient Treatment for People With Stimulant Use Disorders. HHS Publication No. (SMA) 13-4152. Rockville, MD: Substance Abuse and Mental Health Services Administration; 2006.

97. Carroll K. A cognitive behavioral approach: treating cocaine addiction. Rockville MD: National Institute on Drug Abuse; 1998.

98. De Crescenzo F, Ciabattini M, D'Alò GL, et al. Comparative efficacy and accept-ability of psychosocial interventions for individuals with cocaine and amphet-amine addiction: a systematic review and network meta-analysis. PLoS Med 2018;15(12):e1002715.

99. Harada T, Tsutomi H, Mori R, et al. Cognitive-behavioural treatment for amphet-amine- type stimulants (ATS)-use disorders. Cochrane Database Syst Rev 2018;12(12):Cd011315.

100. Carroll KM, Ball SA, Martino S, et al. Enduring effects of a computer-assisted training program for cognitive behavioral therapy: a 6-month follow-up of CBT4CBT. Drug Alcohol Depend 2009;100(1–2):178–81.

101. Donovan DM, Wells EA. 'Tweaking 12-Step': the potential role of 12-Step self-help group involvement in methamphetamine recovery. Addiction 2007;102(Suppl 1):121–9.

102. Schmitz JM, Lindsay JA, Stotts AL, et al. Contingency management and levodopa-carbidopa for cocaine treatment: a comparison of three behavioral targets. Exp Clin Psychopharmacol 2010;18(3):238–44.

103. Pasha AK, Chowdhury A, Sadiq S, et al. Substance use disorders: diagnosis and management for hospitalists. J Community Hosp Intern Med Perspect 2020;10(2):117–26.

# Tobacco Use Disorder

Frank T. Leone, MD, MS[a,b,*], Sarah Evers-Casey, MPH, CTTS-M[a]

## KEYWORDS

- Tobacco use • Nicotine • Smoking treatment • Pharmacotherapeutic interventions

## KEY POINTS

- Nicotine is the major reinforcing component of tobacco and exerts control over behavior by influencing the molecular mechanisms of learning and memory.
- Significant advances in product development have increased both the availability and addictive potential of tobacco products.
- Combined with counseling, pharmacologic interventions are effective and well-tolerated.
- Future treatment strategies will incorporate phenotypic information into more refined, precision decision making.

## INTRODUCTION

Plants of the genus *Nicotiana* are members of the nightshade family, originating primarily in the Central and South Americas well before the appearance of humans. Genus *Nicotiana* encompasses at least 70 naturally occurring species, but the cultivated species *N tabacum* L is of primary economic importance.[1,2] The product of chance hybridization between several other species, natural genetic drift, and agricultural selection pressures, *N tabacum* L is prized for its ability to deliver relatively high concentrations of nicotine directly to the respiratory tract.

Ancient civilizations across the Americas used tobacco in a variety of religious and cultural ceremonies. Tobacco was smoked chiefly in cigars and pipes or chewed with lime (primarily calcium oxides) to produce stimulating, then emetic, and ultimately hallucinatory effects. In the sixteenth century, European explorers disseminated and cultivated tobacco for recreational use throughout North America, systematically creating markets for trade by promoting its medicinal properties and overall salutary effects to western European society. The French ambassador to Portugal, Jean Nicot, introduced tobacco to the French royal family and methodically promoted its use throughout the world, resulting in the adoption of his name for both the plant's genus and its principle active salt, nicotine.[3] As a result, potions and salves made from the

[a] Comprehensive Smoking Treatment Program, Penn Lung Center, Suite 251 Wright-Saunders Building, 51 North 39th Street, Philadelphia, PA, USA; [b] Abramson Cancer Center, University of Pennsylvania, Perelman School of Medicine, Philadelphia, PA, USA
* Corresponding author.
*E-mail address:* frank.tleone@uphs.upenn.edu

Med Clin N Am 106 (2022) 99–112
https://doi.org/10.1016/j.mcna.2021.08.011
0025-7125/22/© 2021 Elsevier Inc. All rights reserved.

decoction of tobacco leaves have been used as diuretics, emetics, anthelmintics, and antibiotics by a variety of cultures worldwide, with an estimated use by 1.25 billion individuals scattered throughout every nation on Earth.[4–6]

Tobacco use in the United States began to transition into tobacco use disorder during the industrial revolution. During the antebellum period, agricultural tobacco production generally was part of a diversified, regionally integrated system of farming that focused on growing small allotments for local consumption alongside larger volumes of staples like wheat, corn, and oats. Following the emancipation of slaves, Southern farm owners sought ways to maintain profits within their new labor paradigm and began systematically shifting from staples to products with higher profitability per cultivated acre.[7] The arrival of an expanding network of railways through small Southern towns made distribution to a wider audience possible, transforming tobacco from local market offering to a nationally commoditized product.

In 1881, a 21-year-old James Bonsack patented the world's first automated cigarette rolling machine. The Bonsack machine was so effective, its daily output matched the output of 48 experienced, and otherwise costly, human hand-rollers. James Buchanan "Buck" Duke and his American Tobacco Company capitalized on the convergence of nascent industrial technologies and evolving social norms to market the inexpensive product to densely populated urban communities in the North. These included the bustling immigrant populations of New York City, where concern over the potential spread of tuberculous through spitting had stigmatized chewable forms of tobacco, and a blossoming suffrage movement placed a premium on tobacco forms that could be marketed as "lady-like."[8,9] By the end of the nineteenth century, Buck Duke was able to decrease the cost of production from 96 cents to just under 8 cents per 1000 cigarettes, marking the onset of the tobacco industry's golden period in the United States.[10]

## TRANSITION TO MODERN ERA TOBACCO USE DISORDER

Several nineteenth-century agricultural advances made N tabacum L increasingly popular, effective, and profitable. For example, the application of potash—high-pH potassium salts derived from the combustion of hardwoods—to the crop increased yields and improved the balance of sugars and nicotine content to make smoked tobacco delivery more palatable and ubiquitous.[11] Flue-curing—the steady application of heat to the mature green plant—resulted in a bright leaf product with increased sugar content and a reduced acridity that was more amenable to being used in cigarette form. Potash application and flue-curing arguably produced a more addictive end product by producing a more deeply inhalable smoke and a more reinforcing experience.[12]

Nineteenth-century work with mild bases like lime and potash led to twentieth-century experimentation with ammonization as a method of changing the pH of inhaled smoke. Although there are several minor alkaloids in tobacco that have known reinforcing effects, the major pharmacologically active component is nicotine.[13] Although all tobacco species contain small amounts of intrinsic ammonia-producing compounds, it was direct ammonization that allowed producers to fine-tune their product's "impact" by altering the proportion of free-base nicotine elaborated from the leaf upon heating.[14–16] Upon dissociation from the acid component of the salt, free-base nicotine is volatilizable and delivered more readily to the alveolar-capillary interface of the lungs, where a massive surface area allows for more efficient absorption.[17] Free-base nicotine quickly reacts with water in the airway to form a protonated molecule that is absorbed rapidly and carried by transport proteins across the blood-brain barrier at a rate much faster than simple diffusion.[18,19] As with other free-base stimulant substances, free-base nicotine produces rapid changes in blood concentrations and significantly amplifies the reinforcing effects of nicotine, resulting in the rather impressive pharmacodynamic effects of the modern cigarette.[20]

## EPIDEMIOLOGY OF TOBACCO USE DISORDER

Tobacco use disorder remains responsible for a majority of preventable deaths in the Western world.[21] Worldwide, approximately 1.4 billion people regularly use tobacco.[22] In 2019, the World Health Organization announced its first-ever projected reduction in the number of men who use tobacco, with a total anticipated reduction of approximately 60 million individuals who use tobacco.[22] The prevalence of tobacco use disorder varies significantly across demographic, economic, and cultural groups, but the highest burden is borne by people from lower socioeconomic groups as well as people with mental health and substance use disorders.[23–26] Several important social-environmental factors have been identified as predictors of tobacco use: higher density of tobacco retailers, peer and/or parental tobacco use modeling, and divorced marital status all have been associated with higher rates of continued tobacco use.[27–29]

Although cigarette smoking remains the most common method of tobacco use, other forms, including flavored cigars, hookah, and electronic delivery devices, increasingly have become attractive to young consumers in recent years. For example, following a long period of slowly declining prevalence, use of tobacco in any form increased considerably among US middle and high school students from 2017 to 2018, primarily due to a remarkable increase in fourth-generation electronic cigarette (e-cigarette) use.[30] Early prospective observations of US adolescent tobacco use recently were confirmed in European cohorts and seem to support concerns that early adolescent exposure to e-cigarettes confers substantially increased risk of going on to later use of combustible tobacco products.[31,32] A US Surgeon General report concluded that e-cigarette use among youths and young adults is an emerging public health concern.[33]

## NEUROBIOLOGY OF TOBACCO USE DISORDER

Like other substances, the dominant neural system affected by nicotine is the mesolimbic survival system. Nicotine's main effect is through stimulation of the nicotinic cholinergic receptors located throughout the mesolimbic system, but it also has both direct and indirect effects on noradrenergic, dopaminergic, serotonergic, vasopressin and glutamatergic systems as well as the stress response regulation of the hypothalamic-pituitary-adrenal axis.[34,35] The ventral tegmental area (VTA) of the midbrain is extensively equipped with the $\alpha 4 \beta 2$ variety of cholinergic receptor, highly sensitive to the natural acetylcholine ligand and with a high affinity for the agonist nicotine.[36–38] Stimulation of cholinergic receptors in the VTA by the exogenous ligand confers abnormal survival salience to otherwise nonsurvival sensory inputs.[39] Nicotinic stimulation of striatal pathways projecting from the VTA begins the transduction of sensory inputs into motor response.[40] Dopaminergic projections from the VTA result in an increased activation of the nucleus accumbens shell, resulting in a generalized appetitive state and an ineluctable consummatory motor drive.[41] Tobacco use behaviors that are forbidden or foregone induce a negative prediction error signal in the nucleus accumbens core, which amplifies negative affect, increases aggressiveness, and facilitates automaticity of response.[42,43] Activation of the prefrontal and orbitofrontal areas of the cortex constrain cognition so that thoughts and reactions are consistent with the instinct to act.[44]

On a molecular level, nicotine's repeated stimulation of ion-gated cholinergic channels begins the process of translocating cyclic AMP response element binding protein (CREB) to the nucleus of the cell.[45,46] Nicotine also blocks the enzymatic activity of histone deacetylase, which regulates CREB activity.[47] Through translocation and disinhibition of CREB, nicotine facilitates the expression of ΔFosB, a transcription factor known as the molecular switch of addiction, increasing expression of genes coding for endogenous opioid neurotransmitters.[48] Endogenous opioids, including endorphin, enkephalin, and dynorphin, are used to regulate the strength of connections between cells, reinforcing some striatal connections and pruning others.[49]

## PHARMACOLOGIC TREATMENT OF TOBACCO USE DISORDER

Early approaches to tobacco use disorder treatment were essentially reactive, with people encouraged to use the support after making their decision to change the behavior. This perspective inevitably led to unrealistic outcome expectations and normalized the custom of delaying cessation interventions. As a result, clinicians engage in tobacco use disorder treatment infrequently, despite the high morbidity and mortality related to tobacco use.[33,50,51] In pilot work investigating clinical decision making, primary care clinicians strongly agreed with statements suggesting a comfort with tobacco counseling and a prioritization of treatment in patients with comorbid conditions. They disagreed, however, with statements suggesting effective counseling would lead patients to quit, even if additional institutional resources were made available to address the problem. Underestimation of the probability of treatment success appears to be the result of a complex set of social motivations, including several important cognitive biases that influence clinical decision making.[52–54]

The US Surgeon General first described tobacco use as the cardinal sign of addiction to nicotine in 1988, beginning the slow clinical shift away from episodic advice to quit toward an understanding that tobacco use disorder requires long-term management due to the profound neuroadaptations that occur with long term use.[55] Ten years later, the US Public Health Service published the first comprehensive tobacco use disorder treatment guideline, providing the evidential basis for both clinical workflow change and aggressive pharmacologic treatment.[56,57] Since then, a first principle of tobacco use disorder treatment has been to both encourage behavior change and recommend pharmacotherapy for all people who use tobacco. Most recently, medication pretreatment strategies have been recommended as a means of controlling the root source of compulsive behavior even before attempting behavior change. Pharmacologic pretreatment strategies have been proposed to help patients manage impulsivity and reduce the anticipatory anxiety of predicted tobacco cessation.[58,59]

To facilitate the use of tobacco use disorder treatments in the clinical setting, tailored guideline recommendations have emerged emphasizing clinical decision making based on relative pharmacotherapeutic effectiveness.[59,60] Straightforward clinical paths help to reduce hesitancy and provide specific guidance on managing common clinical scenarios. For example, medications with different pharmacokinetic profiles are categorized into controller and reliever classes based on their dominant effect.[61] Pharmacologic agents with different mechanisms of action are no longer seen as therapeutically equivalent. Mechanistic combinations and longer duration of treatment now are preferred strategies in pursuit of improved outcomes. Perhaps most consequentially, current guidelines recommend use of medication treatments to treat the underlying tobacco use disorder, even in individuals who have not yet stopped smoking, thus facilitating long-term tobacco cessation and reducin tobacco withdrawal symptoms. This simple shift alone was estimated to result in up to 300 additional patients achieving tobacco cessation per 1000 treated.[59]

Although the exact mechanism of action remains unclear, nicotine replacement therapies (NRTs) generally are felt to work as an adjunct to behavioral management techniques by decreasing the intensity of signaling in the VTA and NA, blunting the downstream appetitive drive and anxiety response.[62–64] The transdermal nicotine patch has the slowest onset of action but provides the longest and most constant rate of delivery (**Table 1**). Blood levels of nicotine peak 2 hours to 4 hours after applying the patch, compared with 5 minutes to 10 minutes after using the nasal spray.[65] The patch is positioned best as a controller medication and used in combination with 1 or more relievers like nicotine gum, lozenge, or spray, based on patient preference.[66] For example, when used in conjunction with the nicotine patch, a piece of 4-mg gum may be used every 1 hour to 2 hours as needed to address breakthrough nicotine cravings.[67] For patients unable to use the gum properly or who cannot tolerate its taste, the nicotine lozenge also can be used to relieve withdrawal symptoms in a fashion similar to that of the gum.[68] Fear of overdose is common, and both clinicians and patients tend to underestimate how much NRT is required to produce the desired effect.[69] Concerns over acute cardiac events also undermine clinical confidence, yet NRT is considered safe even in populations at risk for coronary artery disease.[70,71] Fortunately, patients who continue to smoke while using NRT reproduce baseline blood levels of nicotine, not higher.[72]

Sustained-release bupropion is a tetracyclic antidepressant that acts in part by inhibiting uptake of dopamine from the accumbal synapse.[73] Bupropion SR is approximately equivalent in efficacy to NRT monotherapy but most effectively promotes abstinence and controls withdrawal symptoms when combined with NRT and counseling.[74,75] Patients should begin bupropion SR at least 7 days to 10 days before the anticipated quit date; however, it is not uncommon for patients to require longer pretreatment to see the full effect. Varenicline, an agonist-antagonist of the nicotinic cholinergic receptors of the mesolimbic system, is purported to work by partially stimulating the VTA while limiting the effectiveness of the nicotine ligand. Its actual mechanism of action, however, remains unclear; outcomes counterintuitively improve when varenicline is combined with NRT.[76,77] Varenicline also requires an initial pretreatment period longer than labeled, exerting maximum effect with at least 4 weeks of treatment before attempting behavior change.[30,78] Despite popular concerns, the rate of neuropsychiatric side effects with varenicline appears to be quite low. Varenicline should be considered safe and efficacious, even in patients with preexisting mental illness.[79]

### Future directions

Nicotine is metabolized primarily into its 3'hydroxycotinine (3HC) and cotinine metabolites by the liver cytochrome P450 enzyme CYP2A6.[80] Functional polymorphisms have been associated with slower nicotine clearance and are more prevalent among individuals who do not smoke and people who find it easier to quit.[81] Conversely, faster nicotine metabolism has been associated with increased cigarette consumption[82] and difficulty achieving cessation in response to nicotine pharmacotherapy.[83] The 3HC/cotinine nicotine metabolite ratio is a promising biomarker that reflects both CYP2A6 genetic variation and the gene-by-environment interactions known to influence nicotine clearance in vivo.[84,85] In a retrospective examination of clinical trial data derived from subjects randomized to receive either transdermal nicotine patches or nicotine nasal spray, individuals with slower nicotine metabolism experienced a significantly higher cessation rate when treated with nicotine patch than their counterparts who are fast-metabolizers.[86] This relationship later was confirmed in a double-blind, cohort-randomized clinical trial, where slow-metabolizers were nearly twice as likely to respond to nicotine patch, whereas no difference in clinical effectiveness was observed among subjects receiving varenicline.[87] Strategies aimed at personalizing pharmacologic

**Table 1**
Tobacco use disorder pharmacotherapy

| Medication | Dosage | Clinical Considerations | Side Effects | Cautions |
|---|---|---|---|---|
| Controller medications | | | | |
| Bupropion SR | 150 mg twice daily | • Consider starting 4–6 wk before planned quit attempt.<br>• Can cause insomnia if taken at bedtime—advise patients to take second dose with evening meal.<br>• May help prevent relapse<br>• Often useful in preventing negative affect of withdrawal in patients with history of depressed mood | • Agitation<br>• Dry mouth<br>• Vivid dreams/insomnia<br>• Can decrease seizure threshold in alcohol withdrawal | • Current use of monoamine oxidase inhibitors or other bupropion-containing medications<br>• Seizure disorder<br>• Eating disorder |
| Nicotine patch | 7–21 mg patch daily | • Most useful when used in combination with other medications<br>• Frequently underdosed—consider start with 21 mg for all patients with signs of tobacco dependence. Should be dosed for response<br>• Longer duration of treatment may be clinically beneficial. | • Local skin irritation<br>• Rarely nausea | • No absolute contraindications<br>• Consider alternative in patients with skin conditions, such as eczema. |
| Varenicline | Titrate to 1 mg twice daily | • Consider starting 4–6 wk before planned quit attempt.<br>• Can cause insomnia if taken at bedtime—advise patients to take second dose with evening meal. | • Nausea is relatively common on initiation. Encourage patients to take with food.<br>• Vivid dreams/insomnia<br>• Depressed mood—may indicate dose is too high | • Dose adjustment required for renal impairment |

| | | | | |
|---|---|---|---|---|
| | | • Can cause nausea if taken on empty stomach—advise patients to take with meals.<br>• Safe in patients with mental illness | | |
| **Reliever medications** | | | | |
| Nicotine gum or lozenge | 2 mg or 4 mg every h as needed | • Most effective when parked against oral mucosa<br>• Consider starting with 4-mg dose; reduce to 2 mg only in patients with difficulty tolerating oral irritation.<br>• Most useful as adjunct to controller medication | • Gastrointestinal symptoms usually indicate excessive saliva ingestion.<br>• Oral irritation | • No absolute contraindications<br>• Use caution in patients with dentures or significant periodontal disease. |
| Nicotine inhaler | 10-mg cartridge every 1–2 h as needed | • Flexible dosing, used in response to cravings<br>• Consider start with 5–10 puffs every h as baseline routine.<br>• Particularly useful in conjunction with patch | • Cough, if inhaled too deeply<br>• Oral irritation | • Consider alternative in patients lacking manual dexterity or hand strength necessary to load the device. |
| Nicotine nasal spray | 1 spray each nostril every h as needed | • Flexible dosing, used in response to cravings<br>• May require period of accommodation to nasal irritation/sneezing | • Nasal irritation<br>• Coughing<br>• Vivid dreams<br>• Headache | • Approximately 10% of patients develop dependence syndrome due to rapid absorption. |

treatment of tobacco use disorder have the potential to maximize pharmacotherapeutic effectiveness while minimizing adverse events.[88]

In the future, the way measuring the effect of pharmacotherapy is thought about is likely to change substantially. Given the shift to a chronic disease management paradigm, it is easy to imagine several intermediate outcomes becoming increasingly relevant to refinement of treatment strategies. For example, objective measures of the degree of control over compulsion, predictive models that quantify risk of relapse, and biomeasures of reduction in harms induced by tobacco smoke all are likely to provide clinicians with finer-grain information about the effects of their interventions.[89] Clinical phenotypes, defined by variables, such as prior response to therapy, smoking behavior topography, and biomarker status, will continue to move clinicians away from a monolithic approach to smoking and toward a more refined, precision therapeutic approach.[90]

The future also holds significant threats to achieving control over the epidemic of tobacco use. Innovations in alkaloid chemical production have resulted in tailoring of highly efficient salts that dissociate at more easily achievable pH and temperature and are increasingly palatable to the individual using tobacco.[91,92,93] The introduction of progressively more efficient electronic delivery devices also has increased the availability of nicotine to the adolescent brain, with kinetic profiles and addictive liabilities that rival, and potentially exceed, those of traditional cigarettes.[94,95] The ever-growing variety of inexpensive and available nicotine delivery devices has resulted in an unfortunate shift away from evidence-based therapies among populations of individuals who smoke seeking complete tobacco cessation.[96] Finally, innovative processes have made commercial production of synthetic nicotine more cost-effective. These synthetic products potentially fall into regulatory gaps that threaten to place them outside the purview of agencies responsible for ensuring their safety—unless new oversight frameworks can be adopted before their widespread availability.[97]

## DISCUSSION

Tobacco use disorder continues to be popularly understood from a nineteenth-century perspective. Popular assumptions regarding the euphoric requirement for drugs of abuse have at times clouded the communal perspective on the impact of tobacco use disorder, trivializing both the behavior and approach to treatment. Compared with other chronic relapsing and remitting illnesses, health care systems often lack the appropriate infrastructure and resources to treat substance use disorders in the most effective manner.[98] Unfortunately, much of the current dilemma is a derivative of public perceptions of addiction and the stigmatization of tobacco use.[99,100] There is a growing sense that stigma and inadequate public policies that limit access to treatments for tobacco use disorder are unacceptable and unethical, particularly in circumstances like lung cancer, where the afflicted suffer stigmatized tobacco-related illnesses.[101–103] Solving the seemingly intractable and tragic problem of nicotine addiction should be a core component of strategies to improve twenty-first–century public health.

## CLINICS CARE POINTS

- Though at times trivialized as a minor substance of addiction, nicotine exposure results in a compulsive motivation to continue use.
- Because nicotine impacts survival mechanisms, the potential for long-term abstinence is often experienced as "threat," manifest as anticipatory anxiety.

- Pharmacologic agents with different mechanisms of action are no longer seen as therapeutically equivalent; mechanistic combinations and prolonged duration of therapy are now seen as preferred strategies for achieving abstinence.

## FUNDING

Funded in part by the National Institute on Drug Abuse (DA045244).

## DISCLOSURE STATEMENT

The authors have nothing to disclosue.

## REFERENCES

1. Lewis RS, Nicholson JS. Aspects of the evolution of Nicotiana tabacum L. and the status of the United States Nicotiana Germplasm Collection. Genet Resour Crop Evol 2007;54(4):727–40.
2. Ćwintal M, Sawicka B, Otekunrin O, et al. Plant-derived stimulants and psychoactive substances -social and economic aspects. J Med Clin Res Rev 2020;5:313–35.
3. Kishore K. Monograph of Tobacco (Nicotiana tabacum). Indian J Drugs 2014; 2(1):5–23.
4. Nouri F, Nourollahi-Fard SR, Foroodi HR, et al. In vitro anthelmintic effect of Tobacco (Nicotiana tabacum) extract on parasitic nematode, Marshallagia marshalli. J Parasit Dis 2016;40(3):643–7.
5. Lalruatfela B. A review on tobacco and its effect on health. Sci Vis 2019;19(1):16–23.
6. World Health Organization. WHO global report on trends in prevalence of tobacco smoking 2015. Available at: http://apps.who.int/iris/bitstream/10665/156262/1/9789241564922_eng.pdf. Accessed May 23, 2021.
7. Wright G. Slavery and American Agricultural History. Agric Hist 2003;77(4):527–52.
8. Porter PG. Origins of the American Tobacco Company. Bus Hist Rev 1969;43(1):59–76.
9. Leone FT, Douglas IS. The emergence of E-cigarettes: a triumph of wishful thinking over Science. Ann Am Thorac Soc 2014;11(2):216–9.
10. Farnsworth C. Buck Duke, roller skates, and cigarettes - how one machine transformed an entire industry [Internet]. Foundation for a Smoke-Free World. 2020 [cited 2021 May 23]. Available at: https://www.smokefreeworld.org/buck-duke-roller-skates-and-cigarettes-how-one-machine-transformed-an-entire-industry/.
11. Marchand M. Effect of Potassium on the Production and Quality of tobacco Leaves. International Potash Institute; 2010. Available at: https://www.ipipotash.org/publications/eifc-145. Accessed May 23, 2021.
12. Stevenson T, Proctor RN. The secret and soul of Marlboro. Am J Public Health 2008;98(7):1184–94.
13. Caine SB, Collins GT, Thomsen M, et al. Nicotine-like behavioral effects of the minor tobacco alkaloids nornicotine, anabasine, and anatabine in male rodents. Exp Clin Psychopharmacol 2014;22(1):9–22.
14. Brunnemann KD, Hoffmann D. Chemical studies on tobacco smoke XXXIV. gas chromatographic determination of ammonia in cigarette and cigar smoke. J Chromatogr Sci 1975;13(4):159–63.
15. Henningfield JE, Pankow JF, Garrett BE. Ammonia and other chemical base tobacco additives and cigarette nicotine delivery: Issues and research needs. Nicotine Tob Res 2004;6(2):199–205.

16. Pankow JF, Mader BT, Isabelle LM, et al. Conversion of nicotine in tobacco smoke to its volatile and available free-base form through the action of gaseous ammonia. Environ Sci Technol 1997;31(8):2428–33.

17. van Amsterdam J, Sleijffers A, van Spiegel P, et al. Effect of ammonia in cigarette tobacco on nicotine absorption in human smokers. Food Chem Toxicol 2011; 49(12):3025–30.

18. Hawkins BT, Abbruscato TJ, Egleton RD, et al. Nicotine increases in vivo blood–brain barrier permeability and alters cerebral microvascular tight junction protein distribution. Brain Res 2004;1027(1):48–58.

19. Tega Y, Yamazaki Y, Akanuma S, et al. Impact of nicotine transport across the blood–brain barrier: carrier-mediated transport of nicotine and interaction with central nervous system drugs. Biol Pharm Bull 2018;41(9):1330–6.

20. Volkow ND. Stimulant medications: how to minimize their reinforcing effects? Am J Psychiatry 2006;163(3):359–61.

21. George O, Le Moal M, Koob GF. Allostasis and addiction: Role of the dopamine and corticotropin-releasing factor systems. Physiol Behav 2012;106(1):58–64.

22. Hunter RG, Bloss EB, McCarthy KJ, et al. Regulation of the nicotinic receptor alpha7 subunit by chronic stress and corticosteroids. Brain Res 2010;1325:141–6.

23. Corrigall WA, Coen KM, Adamson KL. Self-administered nicotine activates the mesolimbic dopamine system through the ventral tegmental area. Brain Res 1994;653(1–2):278–84.

24. Ikemoto S, Qin M, Liu Z-H. Primary reinforcing effects of nicotine are triggered from multiple regions both inside and outside the ventral tegmental area. J Neurosci 2006;26(3):723–30.

25. Mao D, Gallagher K, McGehee DS. Nicotine potentiation of excitatory inputs to ventral tegmental area dopamine neurons. J Neurosci 2011;31(18):6710–20.

26. Leone FT, Evers-Casey S. Developing a rational approach to tobacco use treatment in pulmonary practice. Clin Pulm Med 2012;19(2):53–61.

27. Giorguieff-Chesselet MF, Kemel ML, Wandscheer D, et al. Regulation of dopamine release by presynaptic nicotinic receptors in rat striatal slices: Effect of nicotine in a low concentration. Life Sci 1979;25(14):1257–61.

28. Cadoni C, Muto T, Di Chiara G. Nicotine differentially affects dopamine transmission in the nucleus accumbens shell and core of Lewis and Fischer 344 rats. Neuropharmacology 2009;57(5–6):496–501.

29. Fu Y, Matta SG, James TJ, et al. Nicotine-induced norepinephrine release in the rat amygdala and hippocampus is mediated through brainstem nicotinic cholinergic receptors. J Pharmacol Exp Ther 1998;284(3):1188–96.

30. Volkow ND, Koob GF, McLellan AT. Neurobiologic advances from the brain disease model of addiction. N Engl J Med 2016;374(4):363–71.

31. Volkow ND, Fowler JS. Addiction, a disease of compulsion and drive: involvement of the orbitofrontal cortex. Cereb Cortex 2000;10(3):318–25.

32. Brunzell DH, Mineur YS, Neve RL, et al. Nucleus accumbens CREB activity is necessary for nicotine conditioned place preference. Neuropsychopharmacol 2009;34(8):1993–2001.

33. Kaste K. Transcription Factors ΔFosB and CREB in Drug Addiction : Studies in Models of Alcohol Preference and Chronic Nicotine Exposure. Transkriptiotekijät ΔFosB ja CREB päihderiippuvuudessa : tutkimuksia alkoholismin ja kroonisen nikotiinialtistuksen malleissa [Internet]. 2009 May 15 [cited 2020 Jul 12]. Available at: https://helda.helsinki.fi/handle/10138/19112.

34. Kandel ER, Kandel DB. A molecular basis for nicotine as a gateway drug. N Engl J Med 2014;371(10):932–43.

35. Davenport KE, Houdi AA, Van Loon GR. Nicotine protects against μ-opioid receptor antagonism by β-funaltrexamine: Evidence for nicotine-induced release of endogenous opioids in brain. Neurosci Lett 1990;113(1):40–6.

36. Volkow ND, Baler RD. Neuroscience. To stop or not to stop? Science 2012; 335(6068):546–8.

37. Jamal A, Phillips E, Gentzke AS, et al. Current cigarette smoking among adults — United States, 2016. Morb Mortal Wkly Rep 2018;67(2):53–9.

38. WHO global report on trends in prevalence of tobacco use 2000-2025, third edition [Internet]. Available at: https://www.who.int/publications-detail-redirect/who-global-report-on-trends-in-prevalence-of-tobacco-use-2000-2025-third-edition. Accessed August 16, 2021.

39. Beyer J de, Lovelace C, Yürekli A. Poverty and tobacco. Tob Control 2001;10(3): 210–1.

40. Silva VD, Samarasinghe D, Hanwella R. Association between concurrent alcohol and tobacco use and poverty. Drug Alcohol Rev 2011;30(1):69–73.

41. Blosnich J, Lee JGL, Horn K. A systematic review of the aetiology of tobacco disparities for sexual minorities. Tob Control 2013;22(2):66–73.

42. Lee JGL, Griffin GK, Melvin CL. Tobacco use among sexual minorities in the USA, 1987 to May 2007: a systematic review. Tob Control 2009;18(4):275–82.

43. Farley SM, Maroko AR, Suglia SF, et al. The influence of tobacco retailer density and poverty on tobacco use in a densely populated urban environment. Public Health Rep 2019;134(2):164–71.

44. Burke JD, Loeber R, White HR, et al. Inattention as a key predictor of tobacco use in adolescence. J Abnorm Psychol 2007;116(2):249–59.

45. Pang S, Subramaniam M, Abdin E, et al. Prevalence and predictors of tobacco use in the elderly. Int J Geriatr Psychiatry 2016;31(7):716–22.

46. Cullen KA, Ambrose BK, Gentzke AS, et al. Notes from the field: use of electronic cigarettes and any tobacco product among middle and high school students — United States, 2011–2018. Morb Mortal Wkly Rep 2018;67(45):1276–7.

47. Khouja JN, Suddell SF, Peters SE, et al. Is e-cigarette use in non-smoking young adults associated with later smoking? A systematic review and meta-analysis. Tob Control 2020;10(30):8–15.

48. O'Brien D, Long J, Quigley J, et al. Association between electronic cigarette use and tobacco cigarette smoking initiation in adolescents: a systematic review and meta-analysis. BMC Public Health 2021;21(1):954.

49. National Center for Chronic Disease Prevention and Health Promotion (US). Office on smoking and Health. The Health Consequences of smoking—50 Years of Progress: a report of the Surgeon general. Atlanta (GA): Centers for Disease Control and Prevention (US); 2014 (Reports of the Surgeon General). Available at: http://www.ncbi.nlm.nih.gov/books/NBK179276/. Accessed April 13, 2014.

50. Bernstein SL, Yu S, Post LA, et al. Undertreatment of tobacco use relative to other chronic conditions. Am J Public Health 2013;103(8):e59–65.

51. van Eerd EAM, Risør MB, Spigt M, et al. Why do physicians lack engagement with smoking cessation treatment in their COPD patients? A multinational qualitative study. Npj Prim Care Respir Med 2017;27(1):1–6.

52. Leone FT, Evers-Casey S, Graden S, et al. Behavioral economic insights into physician tobacco treatment decision-making. Ann Am Thorac Soc 2015; 12(3):364–9.

53. Leone FT, Evers-Casey S, Graden S, et al. Academic detailing interventions improve tobacco use treatment among physicians working in underserved communities. Ann Am Thorac Soc 2015;12(6):854–8.

54. Evers-Casey S, Schnoll R, Jenssen BP, et al. Implicit attribution of culpability and impact on experience of treating tobacco dependence. Health Psychol 2019; 38(12):1069–74.

55. The Health Consequences of smoking: Nicotine Addiction: a report of the Surgeon general. Available at: http://profiles.nlm.nih.gov/NN/B/B/Z/D/. Accessed August 7, 2019.

56. Fiore M. Smoking cessation. Clinical Practice Guideline, Number 18. Rockville (MD): U.S.: Department of Health and Human Services, Public Health Service, Agency for Health Care Policy and Research; 1996.

57. Fiore M, Jaén C, Baker T, et al. Treating tobacco Use and Dependence: 2008 Update. Clinical Practice Guideline. Rockville (MD): U.S. Department of Health and Human Services. Public Health Service.; 2008.

58. Leone FT, Baldassarri SR, Galiatsatos P, et al. Nicotine dependence: future opportunities and emerging clinical challenges. Ann Am Thorac Soc 2018;15(10): 1127–30.

59. Leone FT, Zhang Y, Evers-Casey S, et al. Initiating pharmacologic treatment in tobacco-dependent adults. An Official American Thoracic Society Clinical Practice Guideline. Am J Respir Crit Care Med 2020;202(2):e5–31.

60. Barua RS, Rigotti NA, Benowitz NL, et al. 2018 ACC expert consensus decision pathway on tobacco cessation treatment: a report of the American College of Cardiology Task Force on Clinical Expert Consensus Documents. J Am Coll Cardiol 2018;72(25):3332–65.

61. Sachs D, Leone F, Farber H, et al. ACCP Tobacco Dependence Treatment Toolkit [Internet]. American College of Chest Physicians Tobacco-Dependence Treatment Tool Kit, 3rd Edition. Available at: http://tobaccodependence. chestnet.org. Accessed November 7, 2010.

62. Leone FT, Evers-Casey S. Behavioral Interventions in Tobacco Dependence. Prim Care Clin 2009;36(3):489–507.

63. Lydon-Staley DM, Schnoll RA, Hitsman B, et al. The network structure of tobacco withdrawal in a community sample of smokers treated with nicotine patch and behavioral counseling. Nicotine Tob Res 2020;22(3):408–14.

64. Lydon-Staley DM, Cornblath EJ, Blevins AS, et al. Modeling brain, symptom, and behavior in the winds of change. Neuropsychopharmacology 2021;46(1):20–32.

65. Croghan GA, Sloan JA, Croghan IT, et al. Comparison of nicotine patch alone versus nicotine nasal spray alone versus a combination for treating smokers: A minimal intervention, randomized multicenter trial in a nonspecialized setting. Nicotine Tob Res 2003;5(2):181–7.

66. Rigotti NA. Clinical practice. Treatment of tobacco use and dependence. N Engl J Med 2002;346(7):506–12.

67. Shiffman S, Sembower MA, Rohay JM, et al. Assigning Dose of Nicotine Gum by Time to First Cigarette. Nicotine Tob Res 2013;15(2):407–12.

68. Shiffman S, Dresler CM, Hajek P, et al. Efficacy of a nicotine lozenge for smoking cessation. Arch Intern Med 2002;162(11):1267–76.

69. Shiffman S, Ferguson SG, Hellebusch SJ. Physicians' counseling of patients when prescribing nicotine replacement therapy. Addict Behav 2007;32(4):728–39.

70. Rigotti NA, Pipe AL, Benowitz NL, et al. Efficacy and safety of varenicline for smoking cessation in patients with cardiovascular disease: a randomized trial. Circulation 2010;121(2):221–9.

71. Pack QR, Priya Aruna, Lagu Tara C, et al. Short-term safety of nicotine replacement in smokers hospitalized with coronary heart disease. J Am Heart Assoc 2018;7(18):e009424.

72. Foulds J, Stapleton J, Feyerabend C, et al. Effect of transdermal nicotine patches on cigarette smoking: a double blind crossover study. Psychopharmacology (Berl) 1992;106(3):421–7.
73. Stahl SM, Pradko JF, Haight BR, et al. A review of the neuropharmacology of bupropion, a dual norepinephrine and dopamine reuptake inhibitor. Prim Care Companion J Clin Psychiatry 2004;6(4):159–66.
74. Holm KJ, Spencer CM. Bupropion: a review of its use in the management of smoking cessation. Drugs 2000;59(4):1007–24.
75. Jorenby D. Clinical efficacy of bupropion in the management of smoking cessation. Drugs 2002;62(Suppl 2):25–35.
76. Ebbert JO, Burke MV, Hays JT, et al. Combination treatment with varenicline and nicotine replacement therapy. Nicotine Tob Res 2009;11(5):572–6.
77. Koegelenberg CFN, Noor F, Bateman ED, et al. Efficacy of varenicline combined with nicotine replacement therapy vs varenicline alone for smoking cessation: a randomized clinical trial. JAMA 2014;312(2):155–61.
78. Hawk LW, Ashare RL, Lohnes SF, et al. The effects of extended pre-quit varenicline treatment on smoking behavior and short-term abstinence: a randomized clinical trial. Clin Pharmacol Ther 2012;91(2):172–80.
79. Hajek P, McRobbie HJ, Myers KE, et al. Use of varenicline for 4 weeks before quitting smoking: decrease in ad lib smoking and increase in smoking cessation rates. Arch Intern Med 2011;171(8):770–7.
80. Anthenelli RM, Benowitz NL, West R, et al. Neuropsychiatric safety and efficacy of varenicline, bupropion, and nicotine patch in smokers with and without psychiatric disorders (EAGLES): a double-blind, randomised, placebo-controlled clinical trial. Lancet 2016;2507–20.
81. Hukkanen J, Jacob P, Benowitz NL. Metabolism and Disposition Kinetics of Nicotine. Pharmacol Rev 2005;57(1):79–115.
82. West O, Hajek P, McRobbie H. Systematic review of the relationship between the 3-hydroxycotinine/cotinine ratio and cigarette dependence. Psychopharmacology (Berl) 2011;218(2):313–22.
83. Strasser AA, Malaiyandi V, Hoffmann E, et al. An association of CYP2A6 genotype and smoking topography. Nicotine Tob Res 2007;9(4):511–8.
84. Schnoll RA, Patterson F, Wileyto EP, et al. Nicotine metabolic rate predicts successful smoking cessation with transdermal nicotine: a validation study. Pharmacol Biochem Behav 2009;92(1):6–11.
85. Allenby CE, Boylan KA, Lerman C, et al. Precision medicine for tobacco dependence: development and validation of the nicotine metabolite ratio. J Neuroimmune Pharmacol 2016;11(3):471–83.
86. Siegel SD, Lerman C, Flitter A, et al. The use of the nicotine metabolite ratio as a biomarker to personalize smoking cessation treatment: current evidence and future directions. Cancer Prev Res Phila Pa 2020;13(3):261–72.
87. Lerman C, Tyndale R, Patterson F, et al. Nicotine metabolite ratio predicts efficacy of transdermal nicotine for smoking cessation. Clin Pharmacol Ther 2006;79(6):600–8.
88. Lerman C, Schnoll RA, Hawk LW, et al. Use of the nicotine metabolite ratio as a genetically informed biomarker of response to nicotine patch or varenicline for smoking cessation: a randomised, double-blind placebo-controlled trial. Lancet Respir Med 2015;3(2):131–8.
89. Schnoll RA, Leone FT. Biomarkers to optimize the treatment of nicotine dependence. Biomark Med 2011;5(6):745–61.

90. Leone FT, Baldassarri SR, Galiatsatos P, et al. Nicotine dependence: future opportunities and emerging clinical challenges. Ann Am Thorac Soc 2018;15(10): 1127–30.

91. Pomerleau OF, Pomerleau CS, Mehringer AM, et al. Nicotine dependence, depression, and gender: characterizing phenotypes based on withdrawal discomfort, response to smoking, and ability to abstain. Nicotine Tob Res 2005;7(1):91–102.

92. Harvanko AM, Havel CM, Jacob P, et al. Characterization of nicotine salts in 23 electronic cigarette refill liquids. Nicotine Tob Res 2020;22(7):1239–43.

93. Gholap VV, Kosmider L, Golshahi L, et al. Nicotine forms: why and how do they matter in nicotine delivery from electronic cigarettes? Expert Opin Drug Deliv 2020;17(12):1727–36.

94. Gholap VV, Pearcy AC, Halquist MS. Potential factors affecting free base nicotine yield in electronic cigarette aerosols. Expert Opin Drug Deliv 2021; 0(0):1–11.

95. Goniewicz ML, Boykan R, Messina CR, et al. High exposure to nicotine among adolescents who use Juul and other vape pod systems ('pods'). Tob Control 2019;28(6):676–7.

96. Neto B. SCHEER (Scientific Committee on Health, Environmental and Emerging Risks), Scientific advice on "Emerging issues at the environment-social interface." 2020 Sep 23. Available at: https://ec.europa.eu/health/sites/health/files/ scientific_committees/scheer/docs/scheer_o_017.pdf. Accessed March 9, 2021.

97. Zettler PJ, Hemmerich N, Berman ML. Closing the regulatory gap for synthetic nicotine products. Boston Coll Law Rev 2018;59(6):1933–82.

98. Dackis C, O'Brien C. Neurobiology of addiction: treatment and public policy ramifications. Nat Neurosci 2005;8(11):1431–6.

99. Evans-Polce RJ, Castaldelli-Maia JM, Schomerus G, et al. The downside of tobacco control? Smoking and self-stigma: A systematic review. Soc Sci Med 2015;145:26–34.

100. Graham H. Smoking, Stigma and Social Class. J Soc Policy 2012;41(1):83–99.

101. Warren GW, Evans WK, Dresler C. Critical determinants of cancer treatment outcomes: smoking must be addressed at the highest levels in cancer care. J Thorac Oncol 2021;16(6):891–3.

102. Steuer CE, Jegede OA, Dahlberg SE, et al. Smoking behavior in patients with early-stage NSCLC: a report from ECOG-ACRIN 1505 trial. J Thorac Oncol 2021;16(6):960–7.

103. Aredo JV, Luo SJ, Gardner RM, et al. Tobacco smoking and risk of second primary lung cancer. J Thorac Oncol 2021;16(6):968–79.

# Benzodiazepines and Related Sedatives

Linda Peng, MD[a],*, Kenneth L. Morford, MD[b], Ximena A. Levander, MD, MCR[a]

## KEYWORDS

- Hypnotics and sedatives • Benzodiazepines • Substance withdrawal syndrome
- Drug tapering • Designer drugs • Substance-related disorders

## KEY POINTS

- Benzodiazepines are used most commonly as anxiolytics and hypnotics, with increasing use among women and non-Hispanic white adults and increasing misuse among young adults.
- A growing number of unregulated novel psychoactive substances, including designer benzodiazepines, are increasingly available on the recreational drug market and Internet.
- Benzodiazepines and Z-drugs both act through GABA-mediated neuronal inhibition, which affects brain reward circuitry, resulting in the addiction potential of these substances.
- Discontinuing long-term benzodiazepine use can be achieved by an outpatient benzodiazepine taper or inpatient withdrawal management at a hospital or detoxification facility.
- Benzodiazepines and Z-drugs have significant adverse effects and complications, which are compounded when used in combination with other substances.

## HISTORY AND EPIDEMIOLOGY OF SEDATIVES

The first hypnotic barbiturate, barbital, was introduced into clinical practice in 1903, followed by phenobarbital in 1912.[1] In subsequent years, multiple barbiturates were synthesized and widely used as anxiolytics and anticonvulsants.[1] Subsequently, increasing rates of barbiturate dependence and overdose resulted in laws and campaigns aimed at reducing use.[1] As a result, barbiturates were mostly replaced with benzodiazepines, a newer class of sedative medications considered to have a more favorable safety profile.[1] The first benzodiazepine was chlordiazepoxide, which was

---

[a] Department of Medicine, Division of General Internal Medicine and Geriatrics, Addiction Medicine Section, Oregon Health & Science University, 3181 SW Sam Jackson Park Road, Mail Code L475, Portland, Oregon 97239, USA; [b] Department of Internal Medicine, Section of General Internal Medicine, Program in Addiction Medicine, Yale School of Medicine, 367 Cedar Street, ES Harkness A, Room 417A, New Haven, Connecticut 06510, USA
* Corresponding author.
*E-mail address:* pengli@ohsu.edu
Twitter: @LindaPengMD (L.P.); @XimenaLevander (X.A.L.)

Med Clin N Am 106 (2022) 113–129
https://doi.org/10.1016/j.mcna.2021.08.012
0025-7125/22/© 2021 Elsevier Inc. All rights reserved.

discovered in 1955.[1] Shortly after, diazepam was introduced in 1963, followed by other benzodiazepines.[1] Benzodiazepines were marketed especially to women as a "safer" alternative to barbiturates, and their usage rapidly increased during the 1960s and 1970s.[1] In 1975, total sales in the United States of anxiolytic and hypnotic medications accounted for 10% of all prescriptions.[1]

Between 1996 and 2013, the number of US adults filling a benzodiazepine prescription increased by 67%, from 8.1 million to 13.5 million.[2] The quantity of benzodiazepines filled during this time period increased more than 3-fold, from 1.1 to 3.6 kg lorazepam equivalents per 100,000 adults.[3] Women and non-Hispanic white adults reported the highest rates of benzodiazepine use, with past year use in 15.4% of women, 9.5% of men, and 15.4% of non-Hispanic white adults.[4] Among those reporting any benzodiazepine use, a significant number did not take them as prescribed, or misused them, with misuse being highest among young adults aged 18 to 25 years old.[4] Benzodiazepine misuse among young adults is especially concerning because younger age of misuse is associated with greater risk of developing a sedative hypnotic use disorder.[5] In addition, people with substance use disorders, particularly opioid use disorder (OUD), have higher rates of benzodiazepine misuse.[6] Finally, psychiatric disorders, especially anxiety and mood disorders, are associated with both benzodiazepine misuse and sedative hypnotic use disorder.[6] In recognition of these increasing rates of benzodiazepine misuse and risk of developing sedative hypnotic use disorder, the Food and Drug Administration (FDA) required an updated boxed warning in September 2020 for the "potential for abuse, addiction, and other serious risks" of benzodiazepines.[7]

Overdose deaths involving benzodiazepines have also steadily increased by a factor of 8 from 1999 to 2015.[2] Despite the increase in benzodiazepine use and misuse, the prevalence of sedative hypnotic use disorders has remained relatively stable.[6] This is likely due to underdiagnosis and may also reflect increasing polysubstance use with benzodiazepines being combined with other substances.[6] The increase in polysubstance use is especially concerning because benzodiazepines potentiate the effects of opioids, alcohol, and other sedating substances, increasing overdose risk.[8,9] Benzodiazepine involvement in US opioid overdose deaths has nearly doubled, from 18% in 2005 to 31% in 2011.[9]

As the dangers of benzodiazepines became clearer, another class of medications, called Z-drugs (eg, zaleplon, zolpidem, and zopiclone), were developed and marketed for insomnia as a "safer" alternative to benzodiazepines starting in the early 1990s.[10] Over time, Z-drug availability has increased in parallel with a decrease in benzodiazepine prescriptions.[11] However, increasing data suggest that complications of misuse, physical dependence, and withdrawal are also associated with all Z-drugs.[11]

Over the last 10 years, there has been a growing number of unregulated novel psychoactive substances (NPS), which are increasingly available on the recreational drug market and the Internet.[12] NPS include designer benzodiazepines (DBZDs), which are also known as "new benzodiazepines" or "new research benzodiazepines." DBZDs are benzodiazepine relatives and derivatives, including benzodiazepines not FDA approved or those synthesized by a structural modification of approved benzodiazepines.[13] Data from the National Poison Data System between 2014 and 2017 found annual increases in DBZD exposures with etizolam and clonazolam being the most common DBZD compounds.[14] The Drug Enforcement Administration's Emerging Threat Report has also noted an increase in DBZDs with 62 total identifications of DBZDs in 2017, 42 in 2018, 115 in 2019, and 295 in 2020.[15] In these reports, etizolam was the most common DBZD identified from 2017 to 2019.[15] In 2020, flualprazolam became the most common, accounting for 42% of the DBZDs reported, followed by etizolam (39%) and clonazolam (12%).[15] Severe adverse effects related to DBZDs, such as respiratory depression and death, have been reported.[16]

## NEUROBIOLOGY

Benzodiazepines bind to the central $\gamma$-aminobutyric acid type A (GABA$_A$) receptor located in postsynaptic and presynaptic membranes.[17] Activation of GABA$_A$ receptors, which are ligand-gated ion channels, leads to hyperpolarization and inhibition of neurotransmission.[17] GABA$_A$ receptors are composed of 5 protein subunits, and variations in these subunits determine the subtype of GABA$_A$ receptor.[17] Benzodiazepines have different affinities for various subtypes of the GABA$_A$ receptor, and these variations result in specific clinical effects.[17] Like benzodiazepines, Z-drugs are also GABA$_A$ receptor agonists, and binding results in GABA-mediated neuronal inhibition.[11] The specific receptor binding selectivity of Z-drugs has been reported to decrease the risk of dependence and withdrawal when compared with benzodiazepines. However, Z-drugs still have a significant potential for misuse, physical dependence, and even death.[11]

GABA$_A$ receptors in the mesolimbic dopamine system play a significant role in the brain reward circuitry, contributing to the addiction potential of benzodiazepines and other substances.[18] Activation of GABA$_A$ receptors in the ventral tegmental area (VTA) causes hyperpolarization of GABAergic neurons, resulting in dopaminergic disinhibition.[18] Increased dopamine in the VTA leads to positive reinforcement and enhances the reward of substances with high addiction potential.[18]

Long-term use of GABAergic substances, including benzodiazepines, Z-drugs, and alcohol, results in compensatory changes by the brain, primarily upregulation of excitatory (glutamate) neurotransmission and downregulation of inhibitory (GABA) neurotransmission.[19] When these substances are removed, the compensatory changes are no longer opposed, and the balance shifts toward hyperexcitation resulting in withdrawal symptoms.[19]

## PHARMACOLOGY

Benzodiazepines are generally well absorbed, lipophilic, and highly protein bound, which are all properties that result in fast onset of clinical effects.[20] Benzodiazepines, such as alprazolam, that are rapidly absorbed with short half-lives and higher potencies have greater misuse potential than other benzodiazepines.[21] Although there is limited information available on DBZDs, many DBZDs likely have higher addiction potential than FDA-approved benzodiazepines because of short half-lives and high potency.[22] **Table 1** provides information on the approximate half-lives, equivalent oral dose ranges, and presence of active metabolites of benzodiazepines and Z-drugs, as well as onset, duration of action, and dose ranges of DBZDs.[23–26] Because very little information exists for DBZDs, approximations for onset, duration, and dosing are based on Internet reports.[26]

Most benzodiazepines are hepatically metabolized by microsomal oxidation or demethylation, followed by glucuronide conjugation.[20] Cytochrome P450 (CYP) 3A4 enzymes metabolize most benzodiazepines, so metabolism is slowed when combined with CYP 3A4 enzyme inhibitors.[27] Many benzodiazepines also have pharmacologically active metabolites (see **Table 1**). These active metabolites may exert additional clinical action, making estimation of half-lives challenging.[20] Some benzodiazepines already have a hydroxyl group, such as oxazepam and lorazepam. These compounds are metabolized directly by glucuronide conjugation and have a shorter elimination half-life with no active metabolites. These pharmacologic features make them safer in individuals with liver dysfunction or those taking medications that may interfere

**Table 1**
**Benzodiazepines and related sedative drugs**

| Commonly Used FDA-Approved Benzodiazepines[23,24] | | | |
|---|---|---|---|
| Generic Name (Brand Name) | Half-Life (h) | Equivalent Oral Dose (mg) | Active Metabolite |
| Alprazolam (Xanax) | 6–12 | 0.5 | Yes |
| Chlordiazepoxide (Librium) | 5–30 | 10–25 | Yes |
| Clonazepam (Klonopin) | 18–50 | 0.25–0.5 | No |
| Diazepam (Valium) | 20–100 | 5–10 | Yes |
| Lorazepam (Ativan) | 10–20 | 1 | No |
| Oxazepam (Serax) | 4–15 | 15–20 | No |
| Temazepam (Restoril) | 8–22 | 20–30 | Yes |
| Triazolam (Halcion) | 2 | 0.25–0.5 | Yes |
| Commonly Used FDA-Approved Nonbenzodiazepine Hypnotics (Z-drugs)[23,25] | | | |
| Zaleplon (Sonata) | 2 | 20 | No |
| Zolpidem (Ambien) | 2 | 20 | No |
| Zopiclone (Zimovane) | 5–6 | 15 | Yes |
| Eszopiclone (Lunesta) | 6 | 3 | Yes |
| Commonly Used Non-FDA-Approved Benzodiazepines (designer benzodiazepines)[26] | | | |
| | Onset/Duration[a] | Weak/Common/Strong Oral Doses[a] | |
| Clonazolam | 10–30 min/6–10 h | 75–200 μg/200–400 μg/500–1000 μg | |
| Flualprazolam | 10–30 min/6–14 h | 0.125–0.25 mg/0.25–0.5 mg/0.5–1 mg | |
| Etizolam | 10–40 min/5–8 h | 0.5–1 mg/1–2 mg/2–4 mg | |

Approximate half-life, equivalent oral dose ranges, and presence of active metabolite of commonly used FDA-approved benzodiazepines and Z-drugs.[22,23] Onset, duration of action, and oral doses of designer benzodiazepines.[24]

[a] Approximate onset, duration, and oral doses as reported in online forums.

with hepatic drug metabolism, with lower likelihood of oversedation compared with other benzodiazepines.[28]

Detecting benzodiazepine exposure may be challenging because of testing limitations. Most standard in-office immunoassay urine drug tests (UDT) consistently detect diazepam, oxazepam, and temazepam, but not alprazolam, lorazepam, or clonazepam.[29] In addition, most DBZDs are not detected on immunoassay UDTs.[30] Because false negatives are common with immunoassay UDTs, liquid chromatography tandem mass spectrometry (LC-MS) must be used to identify specific benzodiazepines. LC-MS can identify some DBZDs, including clonazolam and etizolam, but this method is not available in every laboratory, is more expensive, and takes longer to receive results.[31]

## PHYSIOLOGIC DEPENDENCE AND WITHDRAWAL SYMPTOMS

Physiologic dependence on benzodiazepines can occur in as little as a few weeks of regular use.[32] Rebound symptoms, such as insomnia and anxiety, can occur after stopping benzodiazepines after using them for just 2 weeks.[33] Dependence develops in about half of patients who use benzodiazepines daily for more than 1 month.[28] The onset of benzodiazepine withdrawal is mostly determined by the half-life of the medication. Withdrawal symptoms develop earlier with short-acting benzodiazepines (within 2–3 days) compared with long-acting benzodiazepines (within 5–10 days).[28] Withdrawal symptoms generally develop gradually and then reach a peak, followed by a slow decline.[34] In addition, withdrawal symptoms from short-acting benzodiazepines, including many DBZDs, are typically more severe than those from longer-acting benzodiazepines, and abrupt dose reduction or cessation is more likely to cause seizure.[21,22]

Benzodiazepine withdrawal symptoms can include symptom recurrence, rebound symptoms, and true withdrawal, which may be difficult to differentiate given their similarities.[35] Patients may also have anxiety and apprehension before dose reduction in anticipation of developing symptoms, which can exacerbate withdrawal. Symptom recurrence is a return of the original symptoms that the benzodiazepine intended to treat.[35] Rebound is an increase in the severity of the original symptoms.[35] True physiologic withdrawal is characterized by development of symptoms not experienced before initiation of benzodiazepines and can include anxiety, agitation, insomnia, sensory disturbances (eg, tinnitus, paresthesias), and motor phenomena (eg, tremor, muscle pain/cramps, spasms).[36] These true withdrawal symptoms arise in those with physiologic benzodiazepine dependence because of the increased excitatory (glutamate) neurotransmission that is no longer opposed by benzodiazepines (as referenced in the previous neurobiology section).[19] Severe withdrawal can lead to seizures, delirium, and even death.[35]

In cases whereby symptom recurrence or rebound symptoms occur following benzodiazepine dose reduction or cessation, it can be challenging to determine whether the benefits outweigh the risks of continuing benzodiazepines. Although benzodiazepines are effective at treating anxiety disorders (eg, general anxiety disorder, panic disorder, and social anxiety disorder), they are not necessarily more effective than alternative treatments and are not recommended as first-line treatment because of their potential adverse effects and inability to treat comorbid depression.[37] In addition, benzodiazepines are effective for short-term treatment of insomnia (less than 4 weeks), but long-term treatment is not recommended because of the lack of evidence and possible adverse effects.[38] A diagnosis of sedative-hypnotic disorder should be distinguished from ongoing therapeutic use of benzodiazepines whereby the risks (see section on adverse effects and other complications later) outweigh the clinical benefits. Diagnosis of a sedative-hypnotic use disorder adheres to the *Diagnostic and Statistical Manual of Mental Disorders* (Fifth Edition) (*DSM-5*) 11-point criteria and can be classified as mild, moderate, or severe. Extra caution should be used when continuing benzodiazepines in those who meet *DSM-5* criteria for sedative-hypnotic use disorder, especially in those with concomitant opioid or alcohol use, given the increased misuse potential and overdose risk.[37] However, abrupt discontinuation of benzodiazepines without tapering is not recommended given risks associated with rapid benzodiazepine withdrawal (see section on discontinuation and withdrawal management later). The authors recommend all patients receiving benzodiazepines or other sedatives who also use opioids or have potential opioid exposure be prescribed naloxone, an opioid antagonist that reverses opioid-related overdoses. In many situations, the potential adverse effects of prescribing benzodiazepines long term outweigh the benefits, although risks and benefits must be weighed carefully in order to make the best decision for each individual patient.

## DISCONTINUATION AND WITHDRAWAL MANAGEMENT

In patients seeking to discontinue long-term benzodiazepine use or in those experiencing harms related to benzodiazepines, the first consideration for withdrawal management should be determining the appropriate treatment setting (**Fig. 1**). Most importantly, it must be determined whether a patient can complete an outpatient taper or if they would benefit from inpatient withdrawal management at a hospital or detoxification facility. Inpatient withdrawal management may be limited in geographic areas where these facilities are not available or difficult to access owing to cost and lack of insurance coverage. However, inpatient withdrawal management should be considered in patients who[27]

- Were previously unable to complete an outpatient taper
- Are taking very high doses (eg, >100 mg diazepam equivalents per day)
- Have a more severe sedative hypnotic use disorder
- Are high risk of developing seizures or complicated withdrawal
- Have other substance use disorders, especially concurrent alcohol use disorder
- Have other unstable mental health diagnoses or medical conditions

If patients are candidates for an outpatient taper, most expert consensus guidelines recommend discontinuing benzodiazepines over a period of at least several weeks, with the withdrawal rate determined by tolerance of withdrawal symptoms, duration of benzodiazepine use, current dose of benzodiazepine, and the patient's specific preferences and comorbidities.[28] Recommendations vary on the rate of and method for benzodiazepine dose reduction. Although multiple tapering schedules exist (eg, the Ashton Manual), there is no clear consensus on the duration or rate of taper.[23] Most tapers reduce the total benzodiazepine dose by 10% to 25% weekly for the first 2 to 4 weeks, followed by 5% to 10% every 1 to 2 weeks, for a total of 2 to 6 months.[23,39] **Table 2** provides a sample outpatient taper. Tapering benzodiazepines can be done by reducing the patient's current benzodiazepine or by converting to a long-acting benzodiazepine and then tapering the long-acting benzodiazepine.

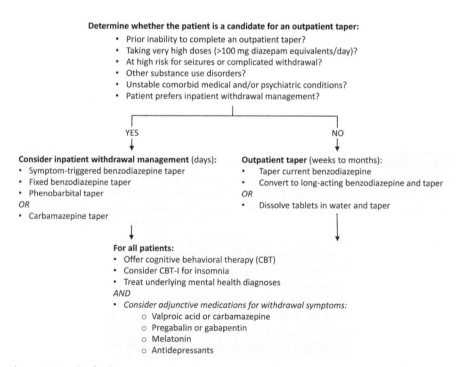

**Fig. 1.** Strategies for benzodiazepine discontinuation. Flowchart for determining the appropriate treatment setting and subsequent options and recommendations for benzodiazepine discontinuation.

Anecdotally, use of a water titration method, whereby benzodiazepine tablets are dissolved in water to taper by smaller increments, has been reported. Switching from a short half-life benzodiazepine to a longer-acting benzodiazepine is not associated with better outcomes,[28] and it is unclear which method may be the most efficacious. Ultimately, the benzodiazepine discontinuation strategy must be determined by shared decision making between the clinician and the patient.

Approximately two-thirds of patients who undergo a taper successfully discontinue benzodiazepines in the short term, and one-third maintain long-term abstinence.[40] Prior episodes of short-term abstinence, lower benzodiazepine dose at the start of the taper, and substantial dose reduction by the patient before starting the taper are most predictive of long-term abstinence.[40] Higher levels of psychiatric comorbidities, such as anxiety and depression, concurrent alcohol use, and greater severity of sedative hypnotic use disorder, are associated with lower abstinence rates.[40] Methods for rapid benzodiazepine discontinuation (3–9 days in length) without a prolonged taper have also been described.[27] More rapid tapers may be a better option in patients who are at risk for misusing prescribed benzodiazepines or may have difficulty adhering to a taper, particularly in those with more severe sedative hypnotic use disorder or other comorbid substance use disorders.[27]

Numerous medications of various classes have been studied for benzodiazepine discontinuation and withdrawal symptoms, although the quality of evidence is overall

**Table 2**
**Sample outpatient benzodiazepine taper**

| 4-mo Benzodiazepine Taper[a] | | | |
| Example: Alprazolam 2 mg bid → Convert to Diazepam 40 mg | | | |
| Timeline[b] | Morning | Evening | Total Daily Dose |
| --- | --- | --- | --- |
| Starting dose | Diazepam 20 mg | Diazepam 20 mg | Diazepam 40 mg |
| Week 1 | Diazepam 18 mg | Diazepam 18 mg | Diazepam 36 mg |
| Week 2 | Diazepam 16 mg | Diazepam 16 mg | Diazepam 32 mg |
| Week 3 | Diazepam 14 mg | Diazepam 14 mg | Diazepam 28 mg |
| Week 4 | Diazepam 12 mg | Diazepam 12 mg | Diazepam 24 mg |
| Week 5 | Diazepam 10 mg | Diazepam 10 mg | Diazepam 20 mg |
| Week 6 | Diazepam 10 mg | Diazepam 8 mg | Diazepam 18 mg |
| Week 7 | Diazepam 8 mg | Diazepam 8 mg | Diazepam 16 mg |
| Week 8 | Diazepam 6 mg | Diazepam 8 mg | Diazepam 14 mg |
| Week 9 | Diazepam 4 mg | Diazepam 8 mg | Diazepam 12 mg |
| Week 10 | Diazepam 2 mg | Diazepam 8 mg | Diazepam 10 mg |
| Week 11 | — | Diazepam 8 mg | Diazepam 8 mg |
| Week 12 | — | Diazepam 6 mg | Diazepam 6 mg |
| Week 13 | — | Diazepam 5 mg | Diazepam 5 mg |
| Week 14 | — | Diazepam 4 mg | Diazepam 4 mg |
| Week 15 | — | Diazepam 3 mg | Diazepam 3 mg |
| Week 16 | — | Diazepam 2 mg | Diazepam 2 mg |
| Week 17 | — | Diazepam 1 mg | Diazepam 1 mg |

[a] This sample outpatient taper is intended for guidance. Clinicians should observe for signs of withdrawal and adjust as needed. Can slow down taper by reducing morning dose first before reducing evening dose. Clinicians should discuss with patients the likelihood of rebound and recurrent symptoms and encourage additional support and alternative treatments.
[b] If needed, can slow down timeline of dose reduction to every 2 wk.

low.[41] There are no medications FDA approved for benzodiazepine dependence or withdrawal symptom management, and use of medications is considered off-label. Anticonvulsants may have some benefit for benzodiazepine withdrawal or as adjunctive medications for benzodiazepine tapers.[27,42] Small trials have shown that valproate (2- to 5-week taper starting at 500–1000 mg per day) may increase short-term benzodiazepine abstinence.[41] Carbamazepine (200 mg 3 times a day for 7–10 days) may reduce withdrawal symptoms, although it has not been shown to help with benzodiazepine discontinuation.[41,43] In terms of GABAergic medications, pregabalin (75–150 mg twice a day for 6–12 weeks) has been shown to reduce withdrawal symptoms and anxiety in small studies.[44,45] Although gabapentin is effective for alcohol withdrawal,[27] a small pilot study for benzodiazepine withdrawal found no significant difference between gabapentin and placebo, and further data are needed.[46] Small trials have shown that flumazenil, a competitive inhibitor at the benzodiazepine GABA receptor binding site, may improve withdrawal symptoms, although this medication carries the risk of fatal arrhythmias, seizures, and precipitating severe withdrawal.[43] Studies on tricyclic antidepressants have been mixed, with potential for benefit on benzodiazepine discontinuation.[41] Melatonin may have some benefit for insomnia related to benzodiazepine discontinuation, although not all studies demonstrated benefit.[41] Other medications with the potential to reduce withdrawal symptoms include paroxetine, an antidepressant, and captodiame, an antihistamine.[41] Clonidine and hydroxyzine are frequently used off-label for anxiety; however, both have not demonstrated clear benefit for benzodiazepine withdrawal.[43] Lithium, buspirone, and propranolol also currently have no evidence for benefit.[41] Ultimately, patients may benefit from medications targeting specific withdrawal symptoms, but more studies are needed to determine whether these medications have significant benefit on benzodiazepine withdrawal or discontinuation.

Inpatient withdrawal management protocols for benzodiazepine detoxification administered at either hospital-based or inpatient detoxification facilities vary depending on the facility. Although a prolonged benzodiazepine taper as described above has the most data, it is often challenging to find an outpatient prescriber who will continue a benzodiazepine taper once the patient discharges from the hospital or detoxification facility. As such, a short benzodiazepine withdrawal protocol is often required. In the inpatient withdrawal management setting, a comparison of symptom-triggered benzodiazepine taper method (using the Clinical Withdrawal Assessment Scale-Benzodiazepines) had no significant differences compared with a fixed-dose benzodiazepine taper method, with both being efficacious for benzodiazepine discontinuation.[47] In addition, a 3-day fixed-dose phenobarbital taper protocol (**Table 3**) has been shown to be well tolerated, safe, and effective at preventing seizures with only 1% of patients requiring readmission for withdrawal symptoms.[48] Although the phenobarbital taper protocol has the advantage of being shorter than benzodiazepine tapers, no comparison trials have been conducted to determine which method is more efficacious or better tolerated. A phenobarbital taper may be preferred in those who have a high risk for seizures or have experienced an unsuccessful prior benzodiazepine taper. Phenobarbital should be used with caution in patients prescribed opioids (especially methadone) and should be avoided in patients older than 65, those with severe liver disease, and those experiencing concomitant alcohol withdrawal. Few studies have evaluated other medications as monotherapy for benzodiazepine discontinuation. For example, carbamazepine monotherapy was successfully used in 9 hospitalized patients for benzodiazepine discontinuation,[42] but evidence is otherwise quite limited.

All patients undergoing benzodiazepine discontinuation should be evaluated and treated using evidence-based therapies for coexisting psychiatric diagnoses (eg,

| Table 3 | |
|---|---|
| Sample inpatient/hospital phenobarbital protocol for benzodiazepine withdrawal management | |
| **Phenobarbital Protocol and Dosing** | |
| Day 1 | Phenobarbital 200 mg po once, followed by 100 mg po every 4 h for 5 doses |
| Day 2 | Phenobarbital 60 mg po every 4 h for 4 doses |
| Day 3 | Phenobarbital 60 mg po every 8 h for 3 doses |

Sample phenobarbital protocol and dosing for benzodiazepine inpatient withdrawal management at a hospital or detoxification facility. This protocol should not be used for outpatient management. Phenobarbital doses should be held for sedation.

depression, anxiety, schizophrenia, or bipolar disorder) with medications as well as behavioral treatments.[28]

## BEHAVIORAL TREATMENTS FOR BENZODIAZEPINE DISCONTINUATION

Multiple behavioral interventions have been studied for benzodiazepine dependence and sedative hypnotic use disorder, with cognitive behavioral therapy (CBT) showing the most benefit.[49] CBT aims to alter behavior by changing dysfunctional cognitions and beliefs by promoting positive cognitions and motivation to change behaviors.[49] There is moderate quality evidence that CBT plus taper is more likely to result in successful discontinuation of benzodiazepines compared with taper alone, although CBT alone without a taper was not found to have benefit in 2 small trials.[49] CBT for chronic insomnia is an effective treatment for insomnia[50] and should be considered among individuals using sedative hypnotics for insomnia.

Smaller studies have shown that motivational interviewing (MI) may increase successful benzodiazepine discontinuation and reduce benzodiazepine use.[49] MI aims to help patients develop more self-motivation to make positive behavior changes and has been shown to be effective in decreasing substance use and seeking additional treatment.[51]

Other behavioral interventions for decreasing benzodiazepine use that have shown some benefit based on limited evidence include a letter sent to the patient by their general practitioner describing benefits of benzodiazepine discontinuation, risks of developing tolerance, and offering support/skills around discontinuation; standardized biweekly visits with a standardized message regarding risks of benzodiazepines plus taper; and relaxation techniques.[49] Behavioral interventions, such as contingency management, which has strong evidence for other substance use disorders,[52] have not been adequately studied for sedative hypnotic use disorder.[49]

## POSTACUTE WITHDRAWAL SYNDROME

Very little literature exists describing persistent and protracted withdrawal symptoms after discontinuing long-term benzodiazepine use, otherwise known as postacute withdrawal syndrome (PAWS). A longer duration of benzodiazepine use with high potency and short half-life benzodiazepines is more likely to result in PAWS.[53] Resolution of PAWS has been observed to take 6 to 12 months, and in rare instances even years.[53] The most persistent withdrawal symptoms attributed to PAWS include anxiety, depression, headache, paresthesias, and motor symptoms (eg, tremor, muscle twitches, weakness).[36] Patients may have difficulty maintaining long-term abstinence because of PAWS, which can be challenging to treat. Unfortunately, there are no definitive pharmacologic options for treating PAWS. Treatment with antidepressants, antihistamines, alpha-adrenergic agonists, anticonvulsants, buspirone, and melatonin has been described, but evidence is lacking for long-term benefit of these medications to relieve PAWS-related symptoms.[27]

## ADVERSE EFFECTS AND OTHER COMPLICATIONS

Benzodiazepines present several important adverse effects and other complications. In addition to the previously described risks of overdose, withdrawal symptoms from physiologic dependence, and development of sedative hypnotic use disorder, individuals may experience a range of central nervous system effects from benzodiazepine toxicity, especially at higher doses (**Table 4**).[54]

Motor vehicle accidents and falls leading to fractures, especially in older adults, are among the most serious and well-established complications of psychomotor impairment from benzodiazepine use.[55] Older adults are particularly vulnerable to adverse effects owing to age-related physiologic changes in drug metabolism and distribution resulting in increased accumulation of benzodiazepines and their active metabolites.[20] These risks appear to increase within the first few weeks of use and when using benzodiazepines with longer elimination half-lives and at higher doses.[56,57] However, increased incidence of hip fractures has been associated with any benzodiazepine exposure, suggesting cautious use of this class of medications in older adults regardless of half-life duration.[58] Given these multiple risks, the American Geriatrics Society Beers Criteria strongly recommend avoiding benzodiazepines in older adults.[59]

Although benzodiazepines have been associated with other serious medical complications, including dementia, infections, pancreatitis, respiratory disease exacerbation, and cancer, there is currently insufficient and conflicting evidence to suggest causal effects (**Table 5**).[55] Similarly, benzodiazepines may increase the risk of suicide, but further evidence is needed to clarify this association.[60,61] Of note, US veterans with posttraumatic stress disorder and benzodiazepine exposure were found to have a nearly 3-fold increase in suicide risk, suggesting this population may be particularly susceptible to psychiatric harms of benzodiazepine use.[62]

## SEDATIVES IN COMBINATION WITH OTHER SUBSTANCES

People who use benzodiazepines and other sedatives routinely combine them with or use them in close proximity to other classes of substances, including alcohol, stimulants, cannabis, and opioids.[6,63] Benzodiazepines can enhance the sensation of intoxication when consumed with alcohol.[6] Those who use stimulants, including cocaine, methamphetamine, or bath salts, may use sedatives to attenuate stimulating acute intoxication effects like stimulant-induced anxiety or psychosis, and to aid with falling asleep.[6]

| Table 4 | |
| --- | --- |
| **Central nervous system effects from benzodiazepine toxicity** | |
| **Central Nervous System Effects**[a] | |
| Sedation | Slurred speech |
| Inattentiveness | Visual disturbances |
| Impaired coordination | Mood fluctuations |
| Dizziness | Anterograde amnesia |
| Vertigo | Disinhibition |
| Ataxia | Delirium |

[a] A wide range of central nervous system effects can result from benzodiazepine toxicity, especially at higher doses.

**Table 5**

Hill causality criteria for benzodiazepine/Z-drug adverse events[55]

| | Traffic Accidents | Falls Leading to Fractures | Dementia | Infections | Pancreatitis | Respiratory Worsening | Cancer |
|---|---|---|---|---|---|---|---|
| Consistency | + | + | ± | ± | ± | – | ± |
| Strength | + | + | + | ± | + | ± | ± |
| Temporality | + | + | – | + | – | – | – |
| Specificity | – | – | – | – | – | – | – |
| Dose response | + | + | ± | – | ± | – | ± |
| Coherence | + | + | ± | ± | – | ± | – |
| Experimental evidence | + | + | – | ± | – | ± | – |
| Analogy | + | + | + | – | ± | + | – |

Summary on the evidence base for causality of benzodiazepines/Z-drugs and adverse events.

*Abbreviations:* +, criteria fulfilled; ±, criteria partially fulfilled or arguable either way; –, criteria not fulfilled.

Reprinted with permission from "Benzodiazepines and Z-Drugs: An Updated Review of Major Adverse Outcomes Reported on in Epidemiologic Research" by Brandt J & Leong C, *Drugs R D*. 2017;17(4):493-507, Copyright 2017 by Springer Nature, with permission from the author and under the terms of the Creative Commons Attribution-NonCommercial 4.0 International License (http://creativecommons.org/licenses/by-nc/4.0/).

The combination of opioids with benzodiazepines or other sedatives is of particular concern. Benzodiazepines enhance the respiratory depression of opioids, significantly increasing the risk of nonfatal and fatal overdose.[64] In the United States, involvement of benzodiazepines in opioid-related overdose deaths has been increasing.[8]

Benzodiazepines are frequently used by people who use opioids, including those taking buprenorphine or methadone, and those not engaged in OUD treatment.[65] People who use opioids may use benzodiazepines, either in combination or on their own, for various reasons (**Box 1**).[66,67]

People who use opioids can acquire benzodiazepines nonmedically (eg, from "the street" or from friends/family), or through a prescription from a clinician. From 2002 to 2014, coprescribing of opioids and benzodiazepines increased by 41%.[68] Being actively prescribed both benzodiazepines and opioids, particularly at higher doses, significantly increases risk of overdose and death,[69,70] and these patients should be prescribed naloxone and have family/friends counseled on how to use it. In 2016, the FDA announced that clinicians should not prescribe opioids along with benzodiazepines.[71] Since then, total numbers of benzodiazepine prescriptions have gone down,[72] although they remain significantly higher than in the late 1990s. With reduced benzodiazepine prescribing, there has been increased prescribing of other opioid potentiators, such as gabapentinoids.[72]

In 2017, the FDA clarified their earlier benzodiazepine warning, recommending that medications for OUD (MOUD), methadone and buprenorphine, not necessarily be withheld in patients who are taking benzodiazepines.[73] This is particularly relevant given increasing rates of addiction treatment facility admissions among patients seeking OUD treatment who are also misusing benzodiazepines.[74] The benefits of MOUD for treatment of OUD and reduced risk of opioid-related overdose may outweigh the potential risks in patients who are also using prescribed or nonprescribed benzodiazepines and other sedatives.[73] Recent evidence suggests reduced risk of nonfatal overdose in those prescribed buprenorphine for OUD who are also prescribed benzodiazepines or Z-drugs compared with those not prescribed buprenorphine with OUD.[70] However, the study found risk of nonfatal overdose was lower in those prescribed a shorter duration of benzodiazepines, prescribed a Z-drug as opposed to a benzodiazepine, or on a lower benzodiazepine dose.[70] Switching patients to a benzodiazepine with a longer half-life or to a Z-drug may be worth

---

**Box 1**
**Reasons people who use opioids use benzodiazepines**

People who use opioids frequently use benzodiazepines, either in combination with opioids or on their own, for various reasons.

Relief of untreated or uncontrolled anxiety

Enhancing or prolonging the euphoria or "high" from opioids

Assisting with insomnia/sleep difficulties

Managing opioid withdrawal symptoms, which can include medically supervised titration/withdrawal of methadone or buprenorphine

Alleviating depression or other mood symptoms

Managing other substance withdrawal

Mitigating or reducing pain

considering in those with OUD. Nonfatal and fatal overdose can occur in patients with OUD also on other sedating medications; thus, the recommendation remains to eventually taper patients off benzodiazepines and other sedatives.[2] Of note, those with OUD and concomitant benzodiazepine dependence tend to experience more severe withdrawal symptoms when tapering off both substances.[75]

Benzodiazepine use is more challenging to manage in patients using opioids or other substances, especially because of the increased overdose risk. Although all patients with OUD benefit from treatment with MOUD, those with concomitant benzodiazepine use should be educated on the risks of combined use and encouraged to dose reduce or taper off benzodiazepines using a patient-centered approach that promotes ongoing care engagement.[76]

## CLINICS CARE POINTS

- Benzodiazepines and related sedatives are frequently prescribed and misused medications with potentially serious risks including overdose, respiratory depression, over-sedation, memory disturbances, and falls/injury, particularly when combined with opioids, alcohol, and other non-related sedatives.

- Patients should be counseled in the risks of continued use of benzodiazepines regardless of duration of use given changes to hepatic metabolism with age that can affect the half-life of benzodiazepines.

- There are numerous options for benzodiazepine tapering plans with recommended use of motivational interviewing and shared decision making between clinician and patient when determining what option to use.

- Deciding between an outpatient benzodiazepine taper and inpatient withdrawal management should include consideration of prior inability to taper, medical and psychiatric co-morbidities, history of seizures, high-dose at start of taper, co-occurring substance use disorder, and patient preference.

- Cognitive behavioral therapy (CBT) has the most evidence of benefit for behavioral treatment for benzodiazepine dependence.

## DISCLOSURE

The authors have nothing to disclose.

## REFERENCES

1. Lader M. History of benzodiazepine dependence. J Subst Abuse Treat 1991; 8(1–2):53–9.

2. Lembke A, Papac J, Humphreys K. Our other prescription drug problem. N Engl J Med 2018;378(8):693–5.

3. Bachhuber MA, Hennessy S, Cunningham CO, et al. Increasing benzodiazepine prescriptions and overdose mortality in the United States, 1996-2013. Am J Public Health 2016;106(4):686–8.

4. Maust DT, Lin LA, Blow FC. Benzodiazepine use and misuse among adults in the United States. Psychiatr Serv 2019;70(2):97–106.

5. Chen C-Y, Storr CL, Anthony JC. Early-onset drug use and risk for drug dependence problems. Addict Behav 2009;34(3):319–22.

6. Votaw VR, Geyer R, Rieselbach MM, et al. The epidemiology of benzodiazepine misuse: a systematic review. Drug Alcohol Depend 2019;200:95–114.

7. FDA requiring boxed warning updated to improve safe use of benzodiazepine drug class. U.S. Food and Drug Administration; 2020. Available at: https://www.fda.gov/drugs/drug-safety-and-availability/fda-requiring-boxed-warning-updated-improve-safe-use-benzodiazepine-drug-class. Accessed February 25, 2021.

8. Tori ME, Larochelle MR, Naimi TS. Alcohol or benzodiazepine co-involvement with opioid overdose deaths in the United States, 1999-2017. JAMA Netw Open 2020; 3(4):e202361.

9. Jones CM, McAninch JK. Emergency department visits and overdose deaths from combined use of opioids and benzodiazepines. Am J Prev Med 2015; 49(4):493–501.

10. Atkin T, Comai S, Gobbi G. Drugs for insomnia beyond benzodiazepines: pharmacology, clinical applications, and discovery. Pharmacol Rev 2018;70(2): 197–245.

11. Schifano F, Chiappini S, Corkery JM, et al. An insight into Z-drug abuse and dependence: an examination of reports to the European Medicines Agency Database of suspected adverse drug reactions. Int J Neuropsychopharmacol 2019; 22(4):270–7.

12. Shapiro AP, Krew TS, Vazirian M, et al. Novel ways to acquire designer benzodiazepines: a case report and discussion of the changing role of the internet. Psychosomatics 2019;60(6):625–9.

13. The misuse of benzodiazepines among high-risk opioid users in Europe. European Monitoring Centre for Drugs and Drug Addiction; 2018. Available at: https://www.emcdda.europa.eu/system/files/publications/2733/Misuse%20of%20benzos_POD2015.pdf.

14. Carpenter JE, Murray BP, Dunkley C, et al. Designer benzodiazepines: a report of exposures recorded in the National Poison Data System, 2014-2017. Clin Toxicol 2019;57(4):282–6.

15. DEA emerging threat reports. Center for Substance Abuse Research (CESAR). Available at: https://cesar.umd.edu/publications/dea-emerging-threat-reports. Accessed February 25, 2021.

16. O'Connell CW, Sadler CA, Tolia VM, et al. Overdose of etizolam: the abuse and rise of a benzodiazepine analog. Ann Emerg Med 2015;65(4):465–6.

17. Sigel E, Ernst M. The benzodiazepine binding sites of GABAA receptors. Trends Pharmacol Sci 2018;39(7):659–71.

18. Engin E, Benham RS, Rudolph U. An emerging circuit pharmacology of GABAA receptors. Trends Pharmacol Sci 2018;39(8):710–32.

19. Valenzuela CF. Alcohol and neurotransmitter interactions. Alcohol Health Res World 1997;21(2):144–8.

20. Griffin CE 3rd, Kaye AM, Bueno FR, et al. Benzodiazepine pharmacology and central nervous system-mediated effects. Ochsner J 2013;13(2):214–23.

21. Ait-Daoud N, Hamby AS, Sharma S, et al. A review of alprazolam use, misuse, and withdrawal. J Addict Med 2018;12(1):4–10.

22. El Balkhi S, Monchaud C, Herault F, et al. Designer benzodiazepines' pharmacological effects and potencies: how to find the information. J Psychopharmacol 2020;34(9):1021–9.

23. Ashton H. The Ashton Manual (benzodiazepines: how they work and how to withdraw). Available at: https://www.benzo.org.uk/manual/index.htm. Accessed February 22, 2021.

24. Guina J, Merrill B. Benzodiazepines II: waking up on sedatives: providing optimal care when inheriting benzodiazepine prescriptions in transfer patients. J Clin Med Res 2018;7(2):20.

25. Gunja N. The clinical and forensic toxicology of Z-drugs. J Med Toxicol 2013;9(2):155–62.

26. Zawilska JB, Wojcieszak J. An expanding world of new psychoactive substances-designer benzodiazepines. Neurotoxicology 2019;73:8–16.

27. Miller SC, Fiellin DA, Rosenthal RN, et al. The ASAM principles of addiction medicine. 6th edition. Philadelphia: ASAM; 2018. p. 797–803.

28. Soyka M. Treatment of benzodiazepine dependence. N Engl J Med 2017;376(12):1147–57.

29. Kale N. Urine drug tests: ordering and interpreting results. Am Fam Physician 2019;99(1):33–9.

30. Pettersson Bergstrand M, Helander A, Hansson T, et al. Detectability of designer benzodiazepines in CEDIA, EMIT II Plus, HEIA, and KIMS II immunochemical screening assays. Drug Test Anal 2017;9(4):640–5.

31. Pettersson Bergstrand M, Helander A, Beck O. Development and application of a multi-component LC-MS/MS method for determination of designer benzodiazepines in urine. J Chromatogr B Analyt Technol Biomed Life Sci 2016;1035:104–10.

32. Gerada C, Ashworth M. ABC of mental health. Addiction and dependence–I: illicit drugs. BMJ 1997;315(7103):297–300.

33. Bixler EO, Kales JD, Kales A, et al. Rebound insomnia and elimination half-life: assessment of individual subject response. J Clin Pharmacol 1985;25(2):115–24.

34. MacKinnon GL, Parker WA. Benzodiazepine withdrawal syndrome: a literature review and evaluation. Am J Drug Alcohol Abuse 1982;9(1):19–33.

35. Pétursson H. The benzodiazepine withdrawal syndrome. Addiction 1994;89(11):1455–9.

36. Ashton H. Protracted withdrawal syndromes from benzodiazepines. J Subst Abuse Treat 1991;8(1–2):19–28.

37. Thibaut F. Anxiety disorders: a review of current literature. Dialogues Clin Neurosci 2017;19(2):87–8.

38. Riemann D, Baglioni C, Bassetti C, et al. European guideline for the diagnosis and treatment of insomnia. J Sleep Res 2017;26(6):675–700.

39. Helping patients taper from benzodiazepines. Veteran Affairs National center for PTSD; 2015. Available at: https://www.pbm.va.gov/PBM/AcademicDetailing Service/Documents/Academic_Detailing_Educational_Material_Catalog/59_PTSD_ NCPTSD_Provider_Helping_Patients_Taper_BZD.pdf. Accessed July 19, 2021.

40. Voshaar RCO, Gorgels WJ, Mol AJ, et al. Predictors of long-term benzodiazepine abstinence in participants of a randomized controlled benzodiazepine withdrawal program. Can J Psychiatry 2006;51(7):445–52.

41. Baandrup L, Ebdrup BH, Rasmussen JØ, et al. Pharmacological interventions for benzodiazepine discontinuation in chronic benzodiazepine users. Cochrane Database Syst Rev 2018;3:CD011481.

42. Ries RK, Roy-Byrne PP, Ward NG, et al. Carbamazepine treatment for benzodiazepine withdrawal. Am J Psychiatry 1989;146(4):536–7.

43. Fluyau D, Revadigar N, Manobianco BE. Challenges of the pharmacological management of benzodiazepine withdrawal, dependence, and discontinuation. Ther Adv Psychopharmacol 2018;8(5):147–68.

44. Hadley SJ, Mandel FS, Schweizer E. Switching from long-term benzodiazepine therapy to pregabalin in patients with generalized anxiety disorder: a double-blind, placebo-controlled trial. J Psychopharmacol 2012;26(4):461–70.

45. Caniff K, Telega E, Bostwick JR, et al. Pregabalin as adjunctive therapy in benzo-diazepine discontinuation. Am J Health Syst Pharm 2018;75(2):67–71.

46. Mariani JJ, Malcolm RJ, Mamczur AK, et al. Pilot trial of gabapentin for the treat-ment of benzodiazepine abuse or dependence in methadone maintenance pa-tients. Am J Drug Alcohol Abuse 2016;42(3):333–40.

47. McGregor C, Machin A, White JM. In-patient benzodiazepine withdrawal: com-parison of fixed and symptom-triggered taper methods. Drug Alcohol Rev 2003;22(2):175–80.

48. Kawasaki SS, Jacapraro JS, Rastegar DA. Safety and effectiveness of a fixed-dose phenobarbital protocol for inpatient benzodiazepine detoxification. J Subst Abuse Treat 2012;43(3):331–4.

49. Darker CD, Sweeney BP, Barry JM, et al. Psychosocial interventions for benzodi-azepine harmful use, abuse or dependence. Cochrane Database Syst Rev 2015; 5:CD009652.

50. Trauer JM, Qian MY, Doyle JS, et al. Cognitive behavioral therapy for chronic insomnia: a systematic review and meta-analysis. Ann Intern Med 2015;163(3): 191–204.

51. Smedslund G, Berg RC, Hammerstrøm KT, et al. Motivational interviewing for substance abuse. Cochrane Database Syst Rev 2011;(5):CD008063.

52. Lussier JP, Heil SH, Mongeon JA, et al. A meta-analysis of voucher-based rein-forcement therapy for substance use disorders. Addiction 2006;101(2):192–203.

53. Cosci F, Chouinard G. Acute and persistent withdrawal syndromes following discontinuation of psychotropic medications. Psychother Psychosom 2020; 89(5):283–306.

54. Buffett-Jerrott SE, Stewart SH. Cognitive and sedative effects of benzodiazepine use. Curr Pharm Des 2002;8(1):45–58.

55. Brandt J, Leong C. Benzodiazepines and Z-drugs: an updated review of major adverse outcomes reported on in epidemiologic research. Drugs R D 2017; 17(4):493–507.

56. Smink BE, Egberts ACG, Lusthof KJ, et al. The relationship between benzodiaz-epine use and traffic accidents: a systematic literature review. CNS Drugs 2010; 24(8):639–53.

57. Díaz-Gutiérrez MJ, Martínez-Cengotitabengoa M, Sáez de Adana E, et al. Rela-tionship between the use of benzodiazepines and falls in older adults: a system-atic review. Maturitas 2017;101:17–22.

58. Wagner AK, Zhang F, Soumerai SB, et al. Benzodiazepine use and hip fractures in the elderly: who is at greatest risk? Arch Intern Med 2004;164(14):1567–72.

59. By the 2019 American Geriatrics Society Beers Criteria® Update Expert Panel. American Geriatrics Society 2019 updated AGS Beers Criteria® for potentially inappropriate medication use in older adults. J Am Geriatr Soc 2019;67(4): 674–94.

60. Dodds TJ. Prescribed benzodiazepines and suicide risk: a review of the litera-ture. Prim Care Companion CNS Disord 2017;19(2):16r02037. https://doi.org/10.4088/PCC.16r02037.

61. Cato V, Holländare F, Nordenskjöld A, et al. Association between benzodiaze-pines and suicide risk: a matched case-control study. BMC Psychiatry 2019; 19(1):317.

62. Deka R, Bryan CJ, LaFleur J, et al. Benzodiazepines, health care utilization, and suicidal behavior in veterans with posttraumatic stress disorder. J Clin Psychiatry 2018;79(6):17m12038.

63. Votaw VR, McHugh RK, Vowles KE, et al. Patterns of polysubstance use among adults with tranquilizer misuse. Subst Use Misuse 2020;55(6):861–70.
64. The ASAM national practice guideline for the treatment of opioid use disorder: 2020 focused update. J Addict Med 2020;14(2S Suppl 1):1–91.
65. Lintzeris N, Nielsen S. Benzodiazepines, methadone and buprenorphine: interactions and clinical management. Am J Addict 2010;19(1):59–72.
66. Stein MD, Kanabar M, Anderson BJ, et al. Reasons for benzodiazepine use among persons seeking opioid detoxification. J Subst Abuse Treat 2016;68: 57–61.
67. Mateu-Gelabert P, Jessell L, Goodbody E, et al. High enhancer, downer, withdrawal helper: multifunctional nonmedical benzodiazepine use among young adult opioid users in New York City. Int J Drug Policy 2017;46:17–27.
68. Hwang CS, Kang EM, Kornegay CJ, et al. Trends in the concomitant prescribing of opioids and benzodiazepines, 2002-2014. Am J Prev Med 2016;51(2):151–60.
69. Park TW, Saitz R, Ganoczy D, et al. Benzodiazepine prescribing patterns and deaths from drug overdose among US veterans receiving opioid analgesics: case-cohort study. BMJ 2015;350:h2698.
70. Xu KY, Borodovsky JT, Presnall N, et al. Association between benzodiazepine or Z-drug prescriptions and drug-related poisonings among patients receiving buprenorphine maintenance: a case-crossover analysis. Am J Psychiatry 2021; 178(7):651–9.
71. FDA requires strong warnings for opioid analgesics, prescription opioid cough products, and benzodiazepine labeling related to serious risks and death from combined use. U.S. Food and Drug Administration; 2016. Available at: https://www.fda.gov/news-events/press-announcements/fda-requires-strong-warnings-opioid-analgesics-prescription-opioid-cough-products-and-benzodiazepine. Accessed February 25, 2021.
72. Rhee TG, Maust DT, Fiellin DA, et al. Trends in co-prescribing of opioids and opioid potentiators among U.S. adults, 2007-2018. Am J Prev Med 2021;60(3): 434–7.
73. FDA Drug Safety Communication: FDA urges caution about withholding opioid addiction medications from patients taking benzodiazepines or CNS depressants: careful medication management can reduce risks. U.S. Food and Drug Administration; 2017. Available at: https://www.fda.gov/drugs/drug-safety-and-availability/fda-drug-safety-communication-fda-urges-caution-about-withholding-opioid-addiction-medications. Accessed February 25, 2021.
74. The TEDS report: admissions reporting benzodiazepine and narcotic pain reliever abuse at treatment entry. Substance Abuse and Mental Health Services Administration (SAMHSA); 2012. Available at: https://www.samhsa.gov/data/sites/default/files/BenzodiazepineAndNarcoticPainRelieverAbuse/BenzodiazepineAndNarcoticPainRelieverAbuse/BenzodiazepineAndNarcoticPainRelieverAbuse.htm. Accessed February 25, 2021.
75. de Wet C, Reed L, Glasper A, et al. Benzodiazepine co-dependence exacerbates the opiate withdrawal syndrome. Drug Alcohol Depend 2004;76(1):31–5.
76. Park TW, Sikov J, dellaBitta V, et al. "It could potentially be dangerous... but nothing else has seemed to help me.": patient and clinician perspectives on benzodiazepine use in opioid agonist treatment. J Subst Abuse Treat 2021; 131:108455.

# Clinical Approaches to Cannabis: A Narrative Review

Deepika E. Slawek, MD, MPH, MS*, Susanna A. Curtis, MD, PhD,
Julia H. Arnsten, MD, MPH, Chinazo O. Cunningham, MD, MS

## KEYWORDS

- Cannabis • Marijuana • Medical cannabis • Endocannabinoid system

## KEY POINTS

- Cannabis use is rapidly growing in social acceptability and use.
- Black and Hispanic Americans have been disproportionately affected by the criminalization of cannabis.
- Cannabis and its cannabinoid constituents interact with the endocannabinoid system, located in the central and peripheral nervous system, endocrine system, gastrointestinal system, and inflammatory cells.
- Evidence for the use of medical cannabis for certain conditions is growing.
- Clinicians should be aware of potential complications of cannabis use.

## INTRODUCTION

Over the past decade, cannabis use in the United States experienced an unprecedented increase in public acceptance. As of Spring 2021, 37 states (including the District of Columbia) legalized medical cannabis use, 22 of which passed laws in the past 10 years, and 18 states (including the District of Columbia) legalized adult-use (recreational) cannabis, 16 of which passed laws in the past 5 years.[1–3] Despite this, the federal legal status of cannabis use remains heavily restricted. The US Controlled Substance Act classifies cannabis as a Schedule I substance with no currently accepted medical use and a high potential for misuse, categorizing it with other substances like heroin.[4] Regardless of its legal status, cannabis use is growing in social acceptability in the United States,[5] almost ensuring that health care professionals will increasingly encounter patients who use cannabis, whether under the guidance of a health care professional or not.

The authors have nothing to disclose.
*Funded by:* NIH National Institute on Drug Abuse (NIDA). *Grant number(s):* K23DA053997. *NIHMS-ID:* 1734362.
Department of Medicine, Albert Einstein College of Medicine/Montefiore Medical Center, 111 East 210th Street, Bronx, NY 10467, USA
* Corresponding author.
*E-mail address:* dslawek@montefiore.org
Twitter: @DeepikaSlawekMD (D.E.S.); @DrSusieC2 (S.A.C.); @DrArnsten (J.H.A.); @DrChinazo (C.O.C.)

Med Clin N Am 106 (2022) 131–152
https://doi.org/10.1016/j.mcna.2021.08.004
0025-7125/22/© 2021 Elsevier Inc. All rights reserved.

This narrative review provides a brief history of cannabis use in the United States, followed by epidemiology, pharmacology, and neurobiology of cannabis, use of cannabis for therapeutic purposes, and finally, complications of cannabis use. **Table 1** lists definitions of common terms used when discussing cannabis.

## BACKGROUND

In the late nineteenth and early twentieth centuries, cannabis in the United States was mostly restricted to medical use, including for the management of pain, migraines, and

**Table 1**
**Relevant terms**

| Term | Definition |
|---|---|
| Cannabis | A broad term describing various products and chemical compounds derived from the *Cannabis sativa* or *Cannabis indica* species[40] |
| Marijuana | Leaves, stems, seeds, and flower buds derived from the *Cannabis sativa* plant[40] |
| Hemp | *Cannabis sativa* plant with very low levels of THC (<0.3%)[114] |
| Street cannabis | Cannabis that is not obtained from a licensed cannabis dispensary and not recommended by a medical care provider |
| Dronabinol | An orally administered medication approved by the U.S. Food and Drug Administration to treat anorexia associated with weight loss in patients with HIV or nausea/vomiting associated with cancer chemotherapy who have not responded adequately to conventional antiemetic treatments. The active ingredient is synthetic THC[115] |
| Cannabinoid | One of a group of over 100 biologically active chemicals found in the *Cannabis* plant |
| delta-9-tetrahydrocannabinol (THC) | The main psychoactive constituent of cannabis[40] |
| Cannabidiol (CBD) | A constituent of cannabis traditionally considered nonpsychoactive[40] |
| THC:CBD ratio | The ratio of THC and CBD in a medical cannabis product |
| Administration method | Available administration methods vary depending on state. Some states allow patients to grow their own cannabis plants, that are then usually inhaled through a combustible method (pipe or rolled in a joint). Many dispensaries also carry vaporized oils, sublingual oils, oral capsules, edible products (candies, gummies, baked goods), and dried flower. |
| Dispensary | A retail site of an organization that dispenses medical cannabis to patients with medical cannabis certification |
| Less frequent or no cannabis use | Cannabis use on *less than 20 days* in a month[116] |
| Near-daily cannabis use | Cannabis use on *at least 20 days* of the month[116] |
| Harm reduction | In the clinical context, an approach and practical strategies are targeted to reduce the negative consequences of substance use. It is founded on respect for the rights of individuals who use drugs. |

seizures. Nonmedical use of cannabis was seen more often in Mexico, starting in the 1880s and onward. Laws regulating and restricting the use of cannabis first arose in 1914, when the border town, El Paso, Texas, banned the sale and possession of cannabis due to the prevailing ideology that cannabis use caused violent behavior and was limited to use among racial and ethnic minorities and people of low socioeconomic status (The Criminality Theory). These laws gained more prominence federally with the passage of the Narcotic Import and Export Act in 1922, which effectively outlawed the use of cannabis. In the following decades, more laws were passed that restricted use of cannabis and limited the ability to conduct medical research on cannabis, including the Marihuana Tax Act in 1937.[6,7] The drafting of these laws was deeply influenced by anti-Mexican bias.

During this period, cannabis began to be referred to as "marijuana" or "marihuana" rather than its scientific name, "cannabis." Although both terms refer to the same plant, many believe that the shift in terminology was a calculated attempt to make the drug sound foreign and associate it with the "vices" of Mexican Americans to gain support for its prohibition among xenophobic constituents.[8] This same language was used to exaggerate the harms of cannabis, describing episodes of "mania" or "violence" after using cannabis, particularly among racial and ethnic minorities.[9] Because of this history, some advocate for a shift back to using the term "cannabis," although colloquially and legally, "marijuana" is used more frequently.[8] In this narrative review, we use the term "cannabis" rather than "marijuana."

By the 1950s, The Criminality Theory had fallen out of favor, and the concept of cannabis as a "gateway drug" to other substances such as heroin or cocaine, became more popular. In the following 2 decades, adult use of cannabis became more popular, and was widely accepted, particularly among antiwar protestors and other countercultures. In this context, cannabis was categorized as a Schedule I substance by the US Controlled Substances Act in 1973. By some accounts, the drive to categorize cannabis as Schedule I, or a "drug or other substance with high potential for abuse… with no currently accepted medical use… and a lack of accepted safety for use of the drug" was a desire to criminalize communities of color rooted in racism.[6,7] Cannabis remains federally classified as a Schedule I substance; however, since 1996 many states have legalized cannabis use for medical purposes.[1–3] In December 2018, the Farm Bill was signed, which removed cannabis derivatives with low concentrations of delta-9-tetrahydrocannabinol (THC) (less than 0.3%) from the purview of the Controlled Substance Act. These low-THC products, often referred to as simply "CBD" (cannabidiol), are regulated by the Food and Drug Administration (FDA) similar to dietary supplements or cosmetics.[10] With this change, many states passed laws making it possible to sell CBD products low in THC,[11] and there has been increased demand and sale of CBD products across the United States.[12]

Criminalization of cannabis use and possession disproportionately impacts Black and Hispanic people.[13,14] Arrest rates for cannabis possession in the United States are 3.6 times higher for Black people than White people, despite similar rates of cannabis use in both groups, and laws in many states decriminalizing medical cannabis use.[13,15] Medical cannabis laws provide access to medical cannabis with lower risk of legal ramifications; however, barriers remain to providing equitable access to communities affected by the criminalization of cannabis due to high costs of medical cannabis, lack of insurance coverage for medical cannabis, and disparities in access to health care practitioners who offer medical cannabis certification.[16,17]

Medical cannabis laws vary greatly between states, including but not limited to differences in active ingredients, route of administration, types of products allowed (eg, whole plant, oil-based, capsules, edible), medical conditions for which patients are allowed to use medical cannabis, and pathways to obtaining medical cannabis.[7] Further, medical cannabis is unique from other medical therapies in that health care professionals may make recommendations on dose, frequency, or route of administration; however, in practice, medical cannabis dosing and route of administration are primarily titrated by patients based on their own symptoms, sometimes under the guidance of a pharmacist or a "budtender."

## EPIDEMIOLOGY
### Cannabis Use in the United States

Trends of cannabis use in the United States have changed with policy and public opinion. In 2019, 17.5% of the population older than 12 (or 48.2 million people) reported having used cannabis in the past year, compared with 11.0% of the population (or 25.8 million) in 2002.[18] Among adults 26 years or older, reported cannabis use rose from 7.0% to 15.2% in the same period.[18] Perception of risk of harm from smoking cannabis declined from 38.7% to 30.8% from 2015 to 2019 among adults 26 years and older and from 19.1% to 15% among adolescents aged 18 to 25.

### Variation by State

Unsurprisingly, rates of cannabis use are higher in states in which medical or adult-use cannabis is legal, whereas the rates of perceiving that it has a high risk of harm are lower. For instance, in 2013 in Washington State (where medical and adult use of cannabis have been legal since 1998),[3] 12.7% of people 12 years and older reported cannabis use in the past month, whereas in Utah (where cannabis use is illegal), 5.4% reported use in the past month.[19] States with higher rates of use also had lower perception of risk of harm from smoked cannabis. In the same report, 18.8% of those surveyed in Washington reported perceiving great risk of harm from smoking cannabis, whereas in Utah 32.8% perceived a great risk of harm.[19] Thus, it is likely that rates of use and perception of harm from cannabis use will continue to change as state and federal laws shift.

### Demographic Characteristics of People Who Use Cannabis

Rates of cannabis use vary by gender and race. Among adults 26 years and older in 2019, rate of cannabis use was similar in White people (16.4%), Black people (16.9%), and Native American people (18.0%), and less common among Asian American people (5.6%) and Pacific Island people (12.2%). Rates of cannabis use was higher among those who are not Hispanic or Latino people (15.9%) compared with Hispanic and Latino people (11.5%). Rates of cannabis use in the past year were higher in male (18.7%) than in female individuals (12.1%).[18]

### Demographic Characteristics of People Who Use Medical Cannabis

Although medical cannabis use also varies by gender and race, these variations are different from those observed among all people who use cannabis. Patients who are White, male, and earn more than $60,000 dollars per year are more likely to obtain medical cannabis.[20] For instance, in a study in Florida in 2019, although census data revealed Floridians were 53.2% White, 26.4% Hispanic, and 16.9% Black, those who used medical cannabis were 83.4% White, 7.6% Hispanic, and 1.9% Black.[21] In a study of Californians who used medical cannabis, 64.8% were employed and 73.4% had private health insurance.[17] These variations likely reflect barriers to accessing medical cannabis that exist due to issues of cost, health care professional preference, stigma among both patients and health care professionals, and racism in the health care system.

## CANNABIS PHARMACOLOGY AND NEUROBIOLOGY
### The Endocannabinoid System

Cannabis pharmacology was relatively recently discovered, with cannabinoids (see **Table 1**) being characterized first in the 1960s and further research developing in the following decades.[22] There is much to be discovered about the endocannabinoid system and it is likely that there will be more developments in upcoming years. To date, we know that cannabinoids act on an endogenous system of receptors in the human body called the endocannabinoid system.[23] The system contains 2 receptors, cannabinoid receptor type 1 (CB1) and cannabinoid receptor type 2 (CB2).[23] CB1 is located primarily in the central and peripheral nervous system, although it is also located in other tissues, including the gastrointestinal tract, endocrine glands including the pituitary and thyroid, and the reproductive system.[24] Activation of the CB1 receptor is involved in regulation of pain, fear, sleep, appetite, memory, and motor responses, as well as psychoactive effects.[24] CB2 is located primarily in the immune system, including the lymphoid tissues and on immune cells such as B and T cells, macrophages, and monocytes, as well as on immune regulatory cells in the brain (glia), the peripheral nervous system, and the gastrointestinal system.[24] Activation of the CB2 receptor is involved in up or down regulation of the inflammatory response.[24] The endocannabinoid receptors are stimulated by endogenously produced lipophilic cannabinoid receptor ligands (endocannabinoids). Two of these endocannabinoids are Anandamide, a potent CB1 agonist named after the Sanskrit word Ananda which means "bliss," and 2-Arachidonoylglycerol, which acts as a full agonist for both CB1 and CB2.

### Phytocannabinoids

Phytocannabinoids are cannabinoids produced by the cannabis plants, *Cannabis indica* and *Cannabis sativa*.[25] Phytocannabinoids act as ligands on either or both CB1 and CB2, and sometimes on other receptors as well.[25] There are more than 100 known phytocannabinoids, but the most frequently studied are THC and CBD. THC is a partial agonist for both CB1 and CB2.[25] The activity of THC on CB1 is primarily responsible for the psychoactive effects of cannabis.[26] CBD has low affinity for CB1 and CB2, and can act as an antagonist to the binding of other cannabinoids, such as THC, to these receptors.[26] CBD is nonpsychoactive and much of its activity is due to its effect as a ligand on other noncannabinoid receptors.[26] There is some evidence that the action of CBD as an antagonist can reduce the psychoactive effects of THC.[27] The remaining phytocannabinoids contribute to the therapeutic effect of cannabis,[28] and terpenes (eg, limonene, myrcene) produce the smell, taste, and appearance of the plant.

Some phytocannabinoids have been formulated as pharmaceuticals for medicinal purposes. Epidiolex is a CBD-containing liquid solution taken orally that has been approved by the FDA for the treatment of rare seizure disorders in children.[29] In the United Kingdom, Nabiximols, an oral mucosal spray containing plant-derived THC and CBD, has been approved for the treatment of spasticity and pain.[30]

### Synthetic Cannabinoids

Synthetic versions of cannabinoids have been created both for medicinal and recreational purposes. The FDA has approved the use of 2 synthetic cannabinoids. Dronabinol is a capsule taken orally that contains THC and is approved for the treatment of nausea, vomiting, and cachexia.[29] There are other synthetic versions of cannabinoids that are used at medical cannabis dispensaries and illicitly. One of the most notorious of these is a CBR1 super-agonist called K2 or Spice, which is associated with psychosis.[31]

*Pharmacokinetics/Pharmacodynamics*

The effects of cannabis vary based on the content of the cannabinoids within and the amount of each cannabinoid present.[32] Potency, duration, and time to onset of effects also vary based on the mode of delivery. Both nonmedical and medical cannabis are used in a variety of modes including inhaled (smoking or vaping), oral ingestion, absorption in the oral mucosa, and topical.[32] For example, in studies of THC use, THC levels peak at 30 minutes and subside within 1.0 to 3.5 hours when cannabis is smoked. When ingested, peak levels are not reached until 30 minutes to 2 hours and do not subside for 5 to 8 hours, due to the first-pass mechanism.[32] The effects of a cannabis product are based not only on its content but also on its mode of use. **Table 2** describes pharmacokinetics and pharmacodynamics of various administration methods of cannabis.

## MEDICAL CANNABIS

Interpreting the literature on medical cannabis can be challenging. As referenced previously, medical cannabis regulations vary by state, and there is no standardization of products from one state to the other. Several reviews summarize the evidence for the therapeutic use of cannabis.[7,33,34] Some, such as the report by the National Academies of Sciences, Engineering and Medicine[7] and Whiting and colleagues[33] evaluated evidence for the use of cannabis for many different conditions, while others, such as Nugent and colleagues,[34] evaluated the evidence for chronic pain only. In some cases, there is inconsistency in findings between different reviews. Further, the available reviews range in scientific rigor from narrative reviews to systematic reviews to meta-analyses. All of the available evidence is limited in quality by regulatory limits on cannabis research.[35] In the following, we briefly discuss the evidence for the use of cannabis for the management of qualifying conditions for medical cannabis use in most states.

### Common Conditions for Which Medical Cannabis Is Used

#### Chronic or severe pain

The most common condition for which patients are certified to take medical cannabis is chronic or severe pain.[36,37] It is also one of the most well-researched indications for the use of medical cannabis. Despite that, most studies testing the use of medical cannabis for chronic pain are considered low or moderate quality because of small study size, inconsistencies in dosing and delivery mechanisms across different studies, and short study duration.[33,34] Further, studies have focused on various types of pain, including neuropathic pain, cancer pain, fibromyalgia, and rheumatoid arthritis, among others and often did not specify the severity of pain.[7,33,34] Most studies evaluated pain with a numeric rating scale and considered a clinically significant reduction in pain to be $\geq$30% reduction in pain. In a meta-analysis of data from 8 studies, patients taking cannabinoids were more likely to report a clinically significant reduction in pain than those taking placebo (odds ratio 1.4; 95% confidence interval 0.99–2.0). This finding was reported as statistically significant; however, it borders on nonsignificant.[33] None of these studies tested medical cannabis products that are used in regular practice in the United States for the management of pain.

#### Severe or persistent muscle spasms

Cannabis use for management of spasticity has been studied primarily in people with multiple sclerosis (MS). One systematic review identified 27 studies (8 randomized controlled trials [RCTs]) examining spasticity in adults[38]; 21 of these studies included

**Table 2**
**Cannabis administration methods and their effects**

| Product, Method of Use, and Bioavailability | Onset and Duration of Effect | Advantages | Disadvantages |
|---|---|---|---|
| Combustible flower: usually smoked rolled in paper or in a pipe.<br>• Bioavailability: Varies between10%–35% due to difference in number of breaths, duration of puff, breath holding, inhalation volume.[32] | • Onset: 3–10 min[32]<br>• Duration: ≤2 h[117] | • Quick onset of action | Potential for adverse effects (short- and long-term):<br>• Intoxication[76]<br>• Chronic bronchitis[68] |
| Vaped oil: Inhaled using a battery-operated portable pen-like device<br>• Bioavailability: Varies between 2% to 56% due to difference in smoking dynamics (number of puffs, spacing of puffs, hold time, inhalation time, etc.)[117] | • Peak: 9 min[117]<br>• Duration: ≤2 h[117] | • Quick onset of action | Potential for adverse effects (short- and long-term):<br>• Intoxication[76]<br>• Chronic bronchitis[68]<br>• Vaping lung injury (vitamin E acetate additive)[99] |
| Vaped ground flower pods: Inhaled using a unique table-top device that creates vapor from plant material<br>• Bioavailability: Varies between 2% to 56% due to difference in smoking dynamics (number of puffs, spacing of puffs, hold time, inhalation time, etc.)[117] | • Peak: 9 min[117]<br>• Duration: ≤2 h[117] | • Quick onset of action | Potential for adverse effects (short- and long-term):<br>• Intoxication[76]<br>• Chronic bronchitis[68] |
| Dabbing: cannabis concentrate with high concentrations of THC (>60%) applied to a hot platform and inhaled. | • Peak: Almost immediate<br>• Duration: 2–3 h | • Quick onset of action | • Potential for lung injury[119]<br>• Exposure to solvents and pesticides (particularly if using unregulated cannabis)[120] |

(continued on next page)

**Table 2**
*(continued)*

| Product, Method of Use, and Bioavailability | Onset and Duration of Effect | Advantages | Disadvantages |
|---|---|---|---|
| • Bioavailability: Estimated to be approximately 75% in laboratory studies.[118] | | | • Intoxication – especially because doses of THC are much higher than in other administration methods<br>• Psychosis or hallucinations[121] |
| Ingested: Oral ingestion of capsules, edible candies (including gummies) or baked goods.<br>• Bioavailability: 4% to 25% depending upon the study.[71–75] Variable due to drug degradation in stomach, variable absorption in the stomach, and first-pass metabolism | • Peak: 1–5 h[71–75]<br>• Duration: ≤25 h[71–75] | • Slow onset of action, low bioavailability<br>• Avoid adverse effects of smoking | • Risk of dose stacking—repeating doses before an effect is felt by the patient. Usually attributable to a long period before onset of effect. Results in unanticipated intoxication and adverse effects[76,77] |
| Tincture and spray: Sublingual/oral<br>• Bioavailability: 87.5% to 90%[122,123] | • Onset: As early as 10 min[122–124]<br>• Duration: ≤10 h[122,123] | • Fast onset of action<br>• Avoid adverse effects of smoking | • Taste<br>• Potential for user error |
| Suppository: Rectal<br>• Bioavailability: 14% to 67%[28,125] | • Onset: 1–2 h[126]<br>• Duration: ≤8 h[126] | • Avoid first-pass effect[126]<br>• Avoid adverse effects of smoking | • Undesirable dosing method<br>• Very little supporting data for the use of suppositories |
| Lotions, gels: Transdermal<br>• Bioavailability: Dependent upon how it is formulated, only studied in animal models[28] | • Onset: 2 h[127]<br>• Duration: ≤48 h[127] | • Avoid adverse effects of smoking<br>• Helpful in patients unable to adhere to other formulations (terminal illness, etc.) | • Variability of bioavailability depending on how it is formulated[127] |

adults with MS. Spasticity improved in all 8 RCTs, although improvement was sometimes measured subjectively through self-report. Many studies used an outdated measure of spasticity that is now considered unreliable, the Modified Ashworth Scale.[38,39] In another meta-analysis, investigators conducted a pooled analysis of data from 3 studies investigating the efficacy of cannabinoids for spasticity in MS.[33] Formulations of cannabis with THC and CBD were associated with improved spasticity on a patient-reported rating scale compared with placebo, and improvements in patient-reported symptoms were greater with formulations containing both THC and CBD than those containing THC alone.

As with the research on chronic pain, these studies were all conducted with forms of medical cannabis that are not the same as those used by patients receiving medical cannabis in the United States. However, the cannabis products included in the studies contained the same main active ingredients (THC and CBD).

### Severe nausea
Few studies have examined the effect of cannabis on severe nausea.[40] Oral synthetic THC (nabilone or dronabinol) has been used for chemotherapy-induced nausea for decades. It is superior to placebo and equally efficacious to comparator antiemetics.[41] In human studies, CBD is less well studied than THC for management of nausea. In animal studies, CBD alone was an effective antiemetic.[42]

### Cachexia or wasting
The use of cannabis for cachexia or wasting has been studied primarily in either AIDS wasting syndrome or cancer-associated cachexia. In an article summarizing 4 RCTs that investigated the effect of cannabis in patients with AIDS wasting syndrome, the investigator concluded that these trials had a high risk of bias, but there is some evidence that cannabis is effective for weight gain in individuals with human immunodeficiency virus.[33] All 4 of these studies compared dronabinol (synthetic THC) with placebo or megestrol acetate. For cancer-associated cachexia, a phase III multicenter RCT compared cannabis extract (THC and CBD), THC alone, and placebo for 6 weeks. Participants were monitored for appetite, mood, and nausea. Of 243 participants enrolled, 164 completed the study, and no difference was found between groups. Recruitment was terminated early because the data review board determined that it was unlikely that differences between groups would emerge.[43] In a more recent pilot study, 17 patients with cancer-associated cachexia were enrolled and received high THC: low CBD cannabis capsules for 6 months. Only 6 participants completed the study, 3 of whom had weight gain of at least 10% from baseline; weight remained stable in the other participants.[44] There is very limited rigorous evidence that cannabis is effective in the management of cachexia or wasting.

### Seizures
In June 2018, CBD was approved by the FDA to treat 2 forms of childhood epilepsy: Dravet syndrome and Lennox-Gastaut syndrome.[45] Dravet syndrome is a complex childhood epilepsy disorder associated with treatment-resistant seizures and a high mortality rate. In a double-blind RCT, daily oral CBD reduced the frequency of convulsive seizures from 12.4 to 5.9 per month. There was a change in frequency from 14.9 to 14.1 seizures per month in the control group.[46] In another childhood syndrome with treatment-resistant seizures, Lennox-Gastaut, CBD use resulted in a 41% reduction in seizure frequency. Reduction in seizure frequency was dose-dependent.[47]

The use of cannabinoids for management of seizures in adults is not as well studied. In an open-label study of CBD in 132 adults and children with treatment-resistant epilepsy, 64% experienced at least a 50% reduction in seizure frequency. Participants also experienced reduced severity of seizures and fewer adverse events.[48] A smaller open-label study including 21 adult participants with treatment-resistant seizures receiving CBD found a 71% reduction in seizure frequency, an 80% reduction in seizure severity, and improved mood.[49] These outcomes are very encouraging but were achieved with doses of CBD alone that exceed the doses usually provided in state-run medical cannabis programs. There is little evidence for the use of other cannabinoids to manage seizures.[50]

### Posttraumatic stress disorder

The efficacy of cannabis for managing posttraumatic stress disorder (PTSD) is not well studied.[51] Several small studies have examined the effect of THC on nightmares and global functioning in patients with PTSD, most of whom were combat veterans.[52–55] In all of these studies, participants experienced improved sleep. Concern remains that cannabis use in people with PTSD may result in adverse outcomes, such as cannabis use disorder; however, this is also not well studied.[51]

### Opioid use

Medical cannabis treatment has emerged as a potential strategy for addressing the opioid epidemic; however, the evidence to support its use is mixed. In most ecological studies, legal medical cannabis laws are associated with a reduction in opioid-related deaths, opioid prescribing, and opioid use.[56–60] As the opioid epidemic has changed from opioid analgesics for pain to heroin and fentanyl indicative of opioid use disorder, more recent studies found conflicting results, with opioid overdose mortality increasing in some analyses.[61,62] As discussed earlier, cannabis has analgesic effects, which may explain why medical cannabis legalization was associated with decreased opioid overdose deaths when the opioid epidemic was fueled by opioid analgesics prescribed for pain. Because there are very limited data to support the use of cannabis for opioid use disorder, it is not surprising that when the opioid epidemic changed to one driven by heroin and fentanyl,[63] the association between legalized cannabis and opioid overdose changed. In all retrospective and observational studies, it is impossible to eliminate all possible confounders. Although these studies help us understand how the opioid epidemic and co-occurring availability of medical cannabis may contribute to population-level outcomes, they cannot determine causality. More rigorous studies at the individual patient level are needed, such as RCTs to truly understand the relationship between medical cannabis use and opioid use.

### Assessing Patients for Medical Cannabis Use

In the authors' combined experience of more than 10 years of certifying patients for medical cannabis use, we developed certain tenets for our patient assessments. In all patients being evaluated for medical cannabis certification, it is important to take a thorough history. Typically, this includes the patient's presenting symptoms, as well as a comprehensive history of comorbidities. Psychiatric and substance use histories are included in this assessment, including history of psychosis, hallucinations, or schizophrenia. A detailed history of prior and current cannabis use is also important, including the frequency, administration, and amount of cannabis use.

Assessing for absolute and relative contraindications to medical cannabis use is also important. Few states define clear contraindications to medical cannabis certification. THC exposure has been associated with tachycardia and development of worsening psychosis.[64–66] In addition, chronic THC exposure during pregnancy has been associated with preterm labor and intrauterine growth retardation.[67] Therefore, it is important to be cautious when determining whether to certify a patient for medical cannabis use who has unstable cardiac disease, risk factors for cardiac disease, a history of psychosis or hallucinations, or pregnancy. A harm reduction approach is an important guiding principle when assessing the patient for contraindications to medical cannabis use, especially in patients whose situation is complex. For example, if a patient is pregnant and is currently using nonmedical cannabis, medical cannabis could be used to reduce overall THC exposure during the course of the pregnancy as a harm reduction strategy.

### Initiating Medical Cannabis

When giving recommendations for medical cannabis dosing and administration method, there are many reasons to discourage patients from using smoked forms of cannabis, including combustible and vaped cannabis. These reasons include concerns for chronic bronchitis and airway inflammation with prolonged use,[68] risk of vape-related lung injury,[69] and risk of respiratory infection.[70] When advising patients on different administration methods, it is important to provide education on expected time of onset and duration of effect. For example, the onset of effect when cannabis is orally ingested is much longer than when it is inhaled, although the duration of effect is longer (see **Table 2**).[71–75] It is recommended that patients refrain from taking additional doses of orally ingested cannabis products while awaiting the onset of effect of their first dose (eg, dose stacking, which can lead to adverse events).[76,77]

Similar to when patients initiate new medications, when initiating medical cannabis, it is reasonable for patients to start with the lowest possible dose of THC available to them. In addition, starting the first dose before bedtime may reduce the risk of adverse events. Maintaining the initial dose for 2 to 3 days is warranted before increasing the dose in the smallest possible increment. Overall, this strategy is consistent with other published recommendations to "start low and go slow."[78]

Patients who are already using nonmedical cannabis may need to start at a higher dose to avoid potential THC withdrawal. The current dose of THC that the patient is taking can be estimated by calculating 10% of the approximate daily amount of cannabis they are using in grams. Some studies have found that most nonmedical cannabis is approximately 10% THC, although this may change over time and vary based on geographic location.[79] It is important for patients to abstain from nonmedical cannabis use 48 to 72 hours before starting medical cannabis so that they can attribute the effects of the medical cannabis (and not nonmedical cannabis) to their signs and symptoms.

In patients who start medical cannabis and are already using nonmedical cannabis, transitioning to medical cannabis offers an option that may be less harmful.[80] It is legal, more heavily regulated (depending on the state), has known THC and CBD content, and in many states is tested for potential contaminants.[3] In states where medical cannabis products are offered that have known THC and CBD doses in milligrams, patients are able to titrate the dose of cannabis more precisely than is possible with street cannabis, and under the guidance of a health care professional, like their doctors or pharmacists at dispensaries.[78]

### Cost of Medical Cannabis

Due to the Schedule I status of cannabis, medical cannabis is not covered by private insurance. Further, it must be paid for with cash or a debit card, which may pose a significant barrier to its use. Depending on the state, medical cannabis products could cost more than $150/mo. Patients and providers must weigh the risks and benefits of using medical cannabis, particularly if it poses risk of financial hardship.

### Potential Complications of Medical Cannabis

#### Medication interactions

The effects of cannabis may be additive with other agents used targeting similar areas of effect, including analgesic, sedative, and psychotropic effects. The cannabinoids THC and CBD are metabolized by the cytochrome P450 (CYP450) system and so may inhibit metabolism of other agents also metabolized by this system.[32] Further research and data on the potential medication interactions between medical cannabis and other medications are sorely needed.

#### Psychiatric symptoms

Few high-quality studies have been published examining how cannabis affects psychiatric symptoms, and few examined the specific effects of THC and CBD on psychiatric symptoms. In studies of adolescents and young adults using street cannabis, chronic cannabis use is associated with psychiatric symptoms, including anxiety,[81] depression,[81] and psychosis, and has been linked to worsening schizophrenia in those with a preexisting genetic vulnerability.[82,83] However, a direct causal relationship is difficult to establish, as a multitude of confounding factors blur the relationship between cannabis use and psychiatric illness. For example, people with symptoms such as anxiety or stress may be more likely to use cannabis.[84] In addition, preclinical and clinical studies show that CBD improves social anxiety, whereas THC worsens it.[85–87] It is reasonable to monitor for new or worsening psychiatric symptoms in patients new to medical cannabis, and to recommend termination of medical cannabis if new psychiatric symptoms are identified.

Among adolescents who use cannabis when they are still undergoing neurodevelopment, cannabis use is associated with memory deficits. This raises concerns for long-term learning deficits in this population.[88] Studies have been mostly cross-sectional in nature, and also have many confounding factors. However, some have found that in adolescents who cease cannabis use, memory impairment improves quickly.[89] In patients in this age group, limiting use of cannabis would be ideal.

#### Cannabis hyperemesis syndrome

The most common severe gastrointestinal adverse effect of cannabis use, cannabis hyperemesis syndrome (CHS),[90] presents as repeated cyclical nausea and vomiting and abdominal pain in patients with chronic, high-dose, cannabis use. It was first described in 2004, in a case series of patients with preceding chronic cannabis use presenting with cyclical vomiting illness that resolved in many after cessation of cannabis use.[90] Following, more case studies were published, but with variation in specifics of chronicity of cannabis use, cannabis use patterns, and duration of follow-up.[91] The Rome IV criteria were published in 2016 in an attempt to provide objective measures for the diagnosis of CHS (**Table 3**).[92] Even with these, there remains heterogeneity in cases described as CHS.[91] To better characterize CHS, Venkatesan and colleagues[91] proposed modifications to the Rome IV criteria. These modified criteria include the following: (1) episodic vomiting occurring at least 3 times in the past year; (2) cannabis use for at least 1 year; (3) cannabis frequency at least 4 times per week on average; and (4) resolution of symptoms following a period of abstinence from cannabis use for at least 6 months or a duration that spans 3 typical

**Table 3**
**Diagnostic criteria for cannabis hyperemesis syndrome**

| Rome IV Criteria[92] | | Venktesan et al. Criteria[91] |
|---|---|---|
| Stereotypical episodic vomiting resembling cyclical vomiting syndrome in terms of onset, duration, and frequency | Clinical features | Stereotypical episodic vomiting resembling cyclical vomiting syndrome in terms of onset, and frequency ≥3 episodes a year |
| Presentation after prolonged, excessive cannabis use | Cannabis use patterns | Duration of use >1 y preceding onset of symptoms Frequency of use >4 times a week on average |
| Relief of vomiting episodes by sustained cessation of cannabis use | Cannabis cessation | Resolution of symptoms should follow a period of cessation from cannabis for a minimum of 6 mo or at least equal to a duration that spans 3 typical cycles in an individual patient.[a] |
| Supportive remarks: May be associated with pathologic bathing behavior (prolonged hot baths or showers) | | |

[a] Patients unwilling or unable to abstain from heavy cannabis use pose a diagnostic challenge and may be considered to have presumed cannabis hyperemesis syndrome.

cyclical vomiting episodes in a patient (see **Table 3**).[91] Other supporting signs could include "pathologic bathing," or taking frequent and prolonged hot showers or baths to relieve symptoms.[93]

The heterogeneity in diagnosis of CHS makes defining the epidemiology of and describing risk factor for CHS difficult. Patients characterized in case reports are more often male gender and in their 20s and 30s.[91]

Treatment of CHS centers around complete cessation of cannabis use. This may be difficult, especially in patients who achieve relief of other symptoms with cannabis. A longitudinal approach, reducing cannabis frequency and dose over time with the ultimate goal of total cannabis cessation, is most likely to provide relief.[91,93] Antiemetics, such as ondansetron, prochlorperazine, and promethazine, are not as effective in the management of CHS symptoms.[94] Other antiemetics are being studied, including haloperidol and droperidol.[93]

### Pulmonary effects

Chronic inhaled cannabis use can lead to chronic bronchitis symptoms, including cough, sputum production, and wheezing.[95,96] Cannabis use may result in pulmonary function test changes, but, unlike tobacco, cannabis has not been associated with chronic obstructive lung disease.[95,96] The mode of consumption could be related to specific types of respiratory syndromes.

A new lung disease associated with heavy vaping, vaping-related lung injury, emerged in late 2019.[97,98] To date, it remains unclear whether the risk is limited to specific types of vaping products or oils or with specific use patterns. It is suspected that vaping lung injury is caused by a severe inflammatory response to vitamin E acetate, an oil included in some formulations of vaporized products (including nicotine and cannabinoids); however, more studies are needed to confirm that vitamin E acetate is directly responsible for vaping lung injury.[99]

For patients who choose to vape, using products from registered facilities reduces the risk that patients are exposed to toxins.[78] Cannabis smoking may predispose individuals to pneumonia through damage of central airways and local immune response changes.[100–102]

Smoked cannabis contains carcinogens, raising concerns about lung cancer. Observational studies have had inconsistent findings: one reported increased risk of lung cancer in all users,[103] another reported increased risk only among heavy users,[104] and another showed no increased risk.[104] These studies included potential confounders (e.g., tobacco use, environmental exposures) that may have affected results. Further research is needed to understand how people smoking cannabis should be monitored for cancer.

### Cannabis use disorder

Cannabis use disorder (CUD) is a potential complication of both adult-use and medical cannabis. An estimated 8% to 12% of people who use cannabis regularly will develop CUD over time.[105,106] Globally, CUD has been found to contribute to substantial disability[107] and is responsible for up 15% of all admissions into substance use treatment programs in the United States.[108]

Several psychotherapies have been studied for the management of CUD and have been shown to reduce frequency and quantity of cannabis use. These include motivational enhancement treatment, cognitive behavioral therapy, and contingency management.[109] Unfortunately, access to evidence-based psychotherapies are limited for many due to geographic and structural barriers.[110] Because of these limitations, there is an increasing interest in identifying pharmacologic treatments to supplement psychotherapies.[110] These are primarily used to address symptoms of cannabis withdrawal. For example, there is evidence that zolpidem and benzodiazepines may be useful for sleep disturbance due to cannabis withdrawal. Cannabinoids such as dronabinol and nabilone have also been studied and show promise in reducing cravings and withdrawal-related sleep disturbance.[110] N-acetylcysteine (NAC) has been studied for the management of CUD.[111] Findings show promise for the use of NAC to reduce cannabis use in adolescents aged 15 to 21 years.[112] In older samples, findings were not as promising.[111,113–127] Medical cannabis for the management of CUD has not been explored.

### SUMMARY

This review can help clinicians better understand how to approach cannabis use in the clinical setting. Cannabis policy is rapidly changing in the United States, including its legal status, availability to patients, and acceptability in medical communities and among the general public. High-quality research on medical cannabis has been difficult to complete because of federal restrictions. Nevertheless, clinicians will encounter patients using cannabis and should be familiar with the existing evidence for the management of common indications with cannabis, cannabis pharmacology, and potential complications of its use. By understanding these fundamental aspects of cannabis, clinicians can make informed recommendations to patients who use or have questions regarding use of cannabis.

## CLINICS CARE POINTS

- Cannabis use is common and is growing in acceptance and use.
- Cannabis causes its effects through the endocannabinoid system. Its full range of effects is still under investigation.
- Clinicians should be aware that cannabis is used for a range of clinical symptoms and be prepared to counsel patients on how to use it safely.

## REFERENCES

1. Hartman M. Cannabis overview 2021. Available at: https://www.ncsl.org/research/civil-and-criminal-justice/marijuana-overview.aspx. Accessed April 26, 2021.
2. Procon.org. Legal recreational states and DC 2021. Available at: https://marijuana.procon.org/legal-recreational-marijuana-states-and-dc/. Accessed April 26, 2021.
3. Procon.org. Legal medical marijuana states and DC. Available at: https://medicalmarijuana.procon.org/legal-medical-marijuana-states-and-dc/. Accessed April 26, 2021.
4. Administration DoJDE. Drug schedules. 2020. Available at: https://www.dea.gov/druginfo/ds.shtml. Accessed May 1, 2020.
5. Carliner H, Brown QL, Sarvet AL, et al. Cannabis use, attitudes, and legal status in the U.S.: a review. Prev Med 2017;104:13–23.
6. Patton DV. A history of United States cannabis law. J L Health 2020;34(1):1–29.
7. National Academies of Sciences, Engineering, and Medicine. The health effects of cannabis and cannabinoids: the current state of evidence and recommendations for research. Washington, DC: The National Academies Press; 2017.
8. Mikos RA, Kam CD. Has the "M" word been framed? Marijuana, cannabis, and public opinion. PLoS One 2019;14(10):e0224289.
9. Thompson M. The mysterious history of 'marijuana'. Code switch: word watch web site 2013. Available at: https://www.npr.org/sections/codeswitch/2013/07/14/201981025/the-mysterious-history-of-marijuana. Accessed August 2, 2021.
10. Abernethy A. Testimony: hemp production and the 2018 Farm Bill 2019. Available at: https://www.fda.gov/news-events/congressional-testimony/hemp-production-and-2018-farm-bill-07252019. Accessed August 2, 2021.
11. Schuman B, Fisher J, Radke B, et al. A survey of state CBD & hemp regulation since the 2018 farm bill. Cannabis Industry J 2020. Available at: https://cannabisindustryjournal.com/feature_article/a-survey-of-state-cbd-hemp-regulation-since-the-2018-farm-bill/. Accessed August 8, 2021.
12. LaVito A. CBD is booming. But US farmers struggle to keep up with demand for industrial hemp 2019. Available at: https://www.cnbc.com/2019/03/23/cbd-is-booming-but-us-farmers-struggle-to-keep-up-with-demand.html. Accessed August 2, 2021.
13. American Civil Liberties Union. A tale of two countries, . Racially targeted arrests in the era of marijuana reform. Available at: https://www.aclu.org/report/tale-two-countries-racially-targeted-arrests-era-marijuana-reform. Accessed April 27, 2021.
14. United States Department of Justic Office of Justin Programs BoJS. More than half of drug offenders in federal prison were serving sentences for powder or

crack cocaine. 2015. Available at: https://www.bjs.gov/content/pub/press/dofp12pr.cfm. Accessed April 27, 2021.

15. American Civil Liberties Union. The war of marijuana in black and white 2013. Available at: https://www.aclu.org/report/report-war-marijuana-black-and-white. Accessed April 27, 2021.

16. Shi Y, Meseck K, Jankowska MM. Availability of medical and recreational marijuana stores and neighborhood characteristics in Colorado. J Addict 2016;2016: 7193740.

17. Reinarman C, Nunberg H, Lanthier F, et al. Who are medical marijuana patients? Population characteristics from nine California assessment clinics. J Psychoactive Drugs 2011;43(2):128–35.

18. 2019 national survey of drug use and health (NSDUH) releases. Available at: https://www.samhsa.gov/data/release/2019-national-survey-drug-use-and-health-nsduh-releases. Accessed April 28, 2021.

19. Hughes A, Lipari RN, Williams MR. Marijuana use and perceived risk of harm from marijuana use varies within and across states. In: The CBHSQ report. Rockville (MD): 2013. p. 1–19.

20. Valencia CI, Asaolu IO, Ehiri JE, et al. Structural barriers in access to medical marijuana in the USA—a systematic review protocol. Syst Rev 2017;6(1):154.

21. Rosenthal MS, Pipitone RN. Demographics, perceptions, and use of medical marijuana among patients in Florida. Med Cannabis Cannabinoids 2020;4(1): 13–20.

22. Russo EB, Marcu J. Cannabis pharmacology: the usual suspects and a few promising leads. Adv Pharmacol 2017;80:67–134.

23. Kaur R, Ambwani SR, Singh S. Endocannabinoid system: a multi-facet therapeutic target. Curr Clin Pharmacol 2016;11(2):110–7.

24. Svizenska I, Dubovy P, Sulcova A. Cannabinoid receptors 1 and 2 (CB1 and CB2), their distribution, ligands and functional involvement in nervous system structures–a short review. Pharmacol Biochem Behav 2008;90(4):501–11.

25. Pertwee RG. The diverse CB1 and CB2 receptor pharmacology of three plant cannabinoids: delta9-tetrahydrocannabinol, cannabidiol and delta9-tetrahydrocannabivarin. Br J Pharmacol 2008;153(2):199–215.

26. Grotenhermen F. Pharmacokinetics and pharmacodynamics of cannabinoids. Clin Pharmacokinet 2003;42(4):327–60.

27. Solowij N, Broyd S, Greenwood LM, et al. A randomised controlled trial of vaporised $\Delta$(9)-tetrahydrocannabinol and cannabidiol alone and in combination in frequent and infrequent cannabis users: acute intoxication effects. Eur Arch Psychiatry Clin Neurosci 2019;269(1):17–35.

28. Huestis MA. Human cannabinoid pharmacokinetics. Chem Biodivers 2007;4(8): 1770–804.

29. Fraguas-Sanchez AI, Torres-Suarez AI. Medical use of cannabinoids. Drugs 2018;78(16):1665–703.

30. Johnson JR, Lossignol D, Burnell-Nugent M, et al. An open-label extension study to investigate the long-term safety and tolerability of THC/CBD oromucosal spray and oromucosal THC spray in patients with terminal cancer-related pain refractory to strong opioid analgesics. J Pain Symptom Manage 2013;46(2):207–18.

31. Tait RJ, Caldicott D, Mountain D, et al. A systematic review of adverse events arising from the use of synthetic cannabinoids and their associated treatment. Clin Toxicol (Phila) 2016;54(1):1–13.

32. Lucas CJ, Galettis P, Schneider J. The pharmacokinetics and the pharmacody-namics of cannabinoids. Br J Clin Pharmacol 2018;84(11):2477–82.

33. Whiting PF, Wolff RF, Deshpande S, et al. Cannabinoids for medical use: a systematic review and meta-analysis. Jama 2015;313(24):2456–73.

34. Nugent SM, Morasco BJ, O'Neil ME, et al. The effects of cannabis among adults with chronic pain and an overview of general harms: a systematic review. Ann Intern Med 2017;167(5):319–31.

35. Temple EC, Brown RF, Hine DW. The 'grass ceiling': limitations in the literature hinder our understanding of cannabis use and its consequences. Addiction 2011;106(2):238–44.

36. NYSDOH. Medical use of marijuana under the compassionate care act: two-year report. 2018. Available at: https://www.health.ny.gov/regulations/medical_marijuana/docs/two_year_report_2016-2018.pdf. Accessed December 8, 2020.

37. Boehnke KF, Gangopadhyay S, Clauw DJ, et al. Qualifying conditions of medical cannabis license holders in the United States. Health Aff (Millwood) 2019;38(2):295–302.

38. Nielsen S, Murnion B, Campbell G, et al. Cannabinoids for the treatment of spasticity. Dev Med Child Neurol 2019;61(6):631–8.

39. Ansari NN, Naghdi S, Moammeri H, et al. Ashworth scales are unreliable for the assessment of muscle spasticity. Physiother Theor Pract 2006;22(3):119–25.

40. National Academies of Sciences. The health effects of cannabis and cannabinoids: the current state of evidence and recommendations for research. Washington, DC: National Academies Press; 2017.

41. Grotenhermen F, Müller-Vahl K. The therapeutic potential of cannabis and cannabinoids. Dtsch Arztebl Int 2012;109(29–30):495–501.

42. Rock EM, Bolognini D, Limebeer CL, et al. Cannabidiol, a non-psychotropic component of cannabis, attenuates vomiting and nausea-like behaviour via indirect agonism of 5-HT(1A) somatodendritic autoreceptors in the dorsal raphe nucleus. Br J Pharmacol 2012;165(8):2620–34.

43. Strasser F, Luftner D, Possinger K, et al. Comparison of orally administered cannabis extract and delta-9-tetrahydrocannabinol in treating patients with cancer-related anorexia-cachexia syndrome: a multicenter, phase III, randomized, double-blind, placebo-controlled clinical trial from the Cannabis-In-Cachexia-Study-Group. J Clin Oncol 2006;24(21):3394–400.

44. Bar-Sela G, Zalman D, Semenysty V, et al. The effects of dosage-controlled cannabis capsules on cancer-related cachexia and anorexia syndrome in advanced cancer patients: pilot study. Integr Cancer Ther 2019;18. 1534735419881498.

45. FDA. FDA approves first drug comprised of an active ingredient derived from marijuana to treat rare, severe forms of epilepsy 2018. Available at: https://www.fda.gov/news-events/press-announcements/fda-approves-first-drug-comprised-active-ingredient-derived-marijuana-treat-rare-severe-forms. Accessed December 8, 2020.

46. Devinsky O, Cross JH, Laux L, et al. Trial of cannabidiol for drug-resistant seizures in the dravet syndrome. N Engl J Med 2017;376(21):2011–20.

47. Devinsky O, Patel AD, Cross JH, et al. Effect of cannabidiol on drop seizures in the lennox-gastaut syndrome. N Engl J Med 2018;378(20):1888–97.

48. Szaflarski JP, Bebin EM, Cutter G, et al. Cannabidiol improves frequency and severity of seizures and reduces adverse events in an open-label add-on prospective study. Epilepsy Behav 2018;87:131–6.

49. Allendorfer JB, Nenert R, Bebin EM, et al. fMRI study of cannabidiol-induced changes in attention control in treatment-resistant epilepsy. Epilepsy Behav 2019;96:114–21.

50. Perucca E. Cannabinoids in the treatment of epilepsy: hard evidence at last? J Epilepsy Res 2017;7(2):61–76.

51. Lowe DJE, Sasiadek JD, Coles AS, et al. Cannabis and mental illness: a review. Eur Arch Psychiatry Clin Neurosci 2019;269(1):107–20.

52. Jetly R, Heber A, Fraser G, et al. The efficacy of nabilone, a synthetic cannabinoid, in the treatment of PTSD-associated nightmares: a preliminary randomized, double-blind, placebo-controlled cross-over design study. Psychoneuroendocrinology 2015;51:585–8.

53. Cameron C, Watson D, Robinson J. Use of a synthetic cannabinoid in a correctional population for posttraumatic stress disorder-related insomnia and nightmares, chronic pain, harm reduction, and other indications: a retrospective evaluation. J Clin Psychopharmacol 2014;34(5):559–64.

54. Roitman P, Mechoulam R, Cooper-Kazaz R, et al. Preliminary, open-label, pilot study of add-on oral Δ9-tetrahydrocannabinol in chronic post-traumatic stress disorder. Clin Drug Investig 2014;34(8):587–91.

55. Fraser GA. The use of a synthetic cannabinoid in the management of treatment-resistant nightmares in posttraumatic stress disorder (PTSD). CNS Neurosci Ther 2009;15(1):84–8.

56. Bachhuber MA, Saloner B, Cunningham CO, et al. Medical cannabis laws and opioid analgesic overdose mortality in the United States, 1999-2010. JAMA Intern Med 2014;174(10):1668–73.

57. Bradford AC, Bradford WD, Abraham A, et al. Association between US state medical cannabis laws and opioid prescribing in the medicare part D population. JAMA Intern Med 2018;178(5):667–72.

58. Bradford AC, Bradford WD. Medical marijuana laws may be associated with a decline in the number of prescriptions for medicaid enrollees. Health Aff (Millwood) 2017;36(5):945–51.

59. Boehnke KF, Litinas E, Clauw DJ. Medical cannabis use is associated with decreased opiate medication use in a retrospective cross-sectional survey of patients with chronic pain. J Pain 2016;17(6):739–44.

60. Powell D, Pacula RL, Jacobson M. Do medical marijuana laws reduce addictions and deaths related to pain killers? J Health Econ 2018;58:29–42.

61. Shover CL, Davis CS, Gordon SC, et al. Association between medical cannabis laws and opioid overdose mortality has reversed over time. Proc Natl Acad Sci U S A 2019;116(26):12624–6.

62. Caputi TL, Humphreys K. Medical marijuana users are more likely to use prescription drugs medically and nonmedically. J Addict Med 2018;12(4):295–9.

63. Centers for Disease Control and Prevention. Understanding the epidemic. Opioid overdose. 2021. Available at: https://www.cdc.gov/drugoverdose/epidemic/index.html. Accessed May 3, 2021.

64. Sewell RA, Cohn AJ, Chawarski MC. Doubts about the role of cannabis in causing lung cancer. Eur Respir J 2008;32(3):815–6.

65. Bryson EO, Frost EA. The perioperative implications of tobacco, marijuana, and other inhaled toxins. Int Anesthesiol Clin 2011;49(1):103–18.

66. Khiabani HZ, Mørland J, Bramness JG. Frequency and irregularity of heart rate in drivers suspected of driving under the influence of cannabis. Eur J Intern Med 2008;19(8):608–12.

67. Gunn JK, Rosales CB, Center KE, et al. Prenatal exposure to cannabis and maternal and child health outcomes: a systematic review and meta-analysis. BMJ Open 2016;6(4):e009986.
68. Mancher M, Leshner AI. Medications for opioid use disorder save lives. Washington, DC: National Academies Press; 2019.
69. Centers for Disease Control and Prevention. Outbreak of lung injury associated with the use of e-cigarette, or vaping, products. 2020. Available at: https://www.cdc.gov/tobacco/basic_information/e-cigarettes/severe-lung-disease.html#cdc-recommends. Accessed May 3, 2021.
70. Gates P, Jaffe A, Copeland J. Cannabis smoking and respiratory health: consideration of the literature. Respirology 2014;19(5):655–62.
71. Perez-Reyes M, Lipton MA, Timmons MC, et al. Pharmacology of orally administered 9 -tetrahydrocannabinol. Clin Pharmacol Ther 1973;14(1):48–55.
72. Wall ME, Sadler BM, Brine D, et al. Metabolism, disposition, and kinetics of delta-9-tetrahydrocannabinol in men and women. Clin Pharmacol Ther 1983;34(3):352–63.
73. Ohlsson A, Lindgren JE, Wahlen A, et al. Plasma delta-9 tetrahydrocannabinol concentrations and clinical effects after oral and intravenous administration and smoking. Clin Pharmacol Ther 1980;28(3):409–16.
74. Goodwin RS, Gustafson RA, Barnes A, et al. Delta(9)-tetrahydrocannabinol, 11-hydroxy-delta(9)-tetrahydrocannabinol and 11-nor-9-carboxy-delta(9)-tetrahydrocannabinol in human plasma after controlled oral administration of cannabinoids. Ther Drug Monit 2006;28(4):545–51.
75. Gustafson RA, Moolchan ET, Barnes A, et al. Validated method for the simultaneous determination of Delta 9-tetrahydrocannabinol (THC), 11-hydroxy-THC and 11-nor-9-carboxy-THC in human plasma using solid phase extraction and gas chromatography-mass spectrometry with positive chemical ionization. J Chromatogr B Analyt Technol Biomed Life Sci 2003;798(1):145–54.
76. Monte AA, Shelton SK, Mills E, et al. Acute illness associated with cannabis use, by route of exposure: an observational study. Ann Intern Med 2019;170(8):531–7.
77. Monte AA, Zane RD, Heard KJ. The implications of marijuana legalization in Colorado. Jama 2015;313(3):241–2.
78. MacCallum CA, Russo EB. Practical considerations in medical cannabis administration and dosing. Eur J Intern Med 2018;49:12–9.
79. ElSohly MA, Mehmedic Z, Foster S, et al. Changes in cannabis potency over the last 2 decades (1995-2014): analysis of current data in the United States. Biol Psychiatry 2016;79(7):613–9.
80. Gittins R, Sessa B. Can prescribed medical cannabis use reduce the use of other more harmful drugs? Drug Sci Policy L 2020;6. 2050324519900067.
81. Patton GC, Coffey C, Carlin JB, et al. Cannabis use and mental health in young people: cohort study. BMJ 2002;325(7374):1195–8.
82. Caspi A, Moffitt TE, Cannon M, et al. Moderation of the effect of adolescent-onset cannabis use on adult psychosis by a functional polymorphism in the catechol-O-methyltransferase gene: longitudinal evidence of a gene X environment interaction. Biol Psychiatry 2005;57(10):1117–27.
83. Di Forti M, Sallis H, Allegri F, et al. Daily use, especially of high-potency cannabis, drives the earlier onset of psychosis in cannabis users. Schizophr Bull 2014;40(6):1509–17.
84. Volkow ND, Compton WM, Weiss SR. Adverse health effects of marijuana use. N Engl J Med 2014;371(9):879.

85. Crippa JA, Zuardi AW, Martín-Santos R, et al. Cannabis and anxiety: a critical review of the evidence. Hum Psychopharmacol 2009;24(7):515–23.

86. Zuardi AW, Cosme RA, Graeff FG, et al. Effects of ipsapirone and cannabidiol on human experimental anxiety. J Psychopharmacol 1993;7(1 Suppl):82–8.

87. Crippa JA, Derenusson GN, Ferrari TB, et al. Neural basis of anxiolytic effects of cannabidiol (CBD) in generalized social anxiety disorder: a preliminary report. J Psychopharmacol 2011;25(1):121–30.

88. Viveros MP, Llorente R, Suarez J, et al. The endocannabinoid system in critical neurodevelopmental periods: sex differences and neuropsychiatric implications. J Psychopharmacol 2012;26(1):164–76.

89. Schuster RM, Gilman J, Schoenfeld D, et al. One month of cannabis abstinence in adolescents and young adults is associated with improved memory. J Clin Psychiatry 2018;79(6):17m11977.

90. Allen JH, de Moore GM, Heddle R, et al. Cannabinoid hyperemesis: cyclical hyperemesis in association with chronic cannabis abuse. Gut 2004;53(11):1566–70.

91. Venkatesan T, Levinthal DJ, Li BUK, et al. Role of chronic cannabis use: cyclic vomiting syndrome vs cannabinoid hyperemesis syndrome. Neurogastroenterol Motil 2019;31(Suppl 2):e13606.

92. Stanghellini V, Chan FK, Hasler WL, et al. Gastroduodenal disorders. Gastroenterology 2016;150(6):1380–92.

93. Perisetti A, Gajendran M, Dasari CS, et al. Cannabis hyperemesis syndrome: an update on the pathophysiology and management. Ann Gastroenterol 2020;33(6):571–8.

94. Richards JR, Gordon BK, Danielson AR, et al. Pharmacologic treatment of cannabinoid hyperemesis syndrome: a systematic review. Pharmacotherapy 2017;37(6):725–34.

95. Ribeiro L, Ind PW. Marijuana and the lung: hysteria or cause for concern? Breathe (Sheff) 2018;14(3):196–205.

96. Tashkin DP. Marijuana and lung disease. Chest 2018;154(3):653–63.

97. Schier JG, Meiman JG, Layden J, et al. Severe pulmonary disease associated with electronic-cigarette-product use - Interim guidance. MMWR Morb Mortal Wkly Rep 2019;68(36):787–90.

98. Layden JE, Ghinai I, Pray I, et al. Pulmonary illness related to E-cigarette use in Illinois and Wisconsin - final report. N Engl J Med 2020;382(10):903–16.

99. Christiani DC. Vaping-induced acute lung injury. N Engl J Med 2020;382(10):960–2.

100. Fligiel SE, Roth MD, Kleerup EC, et al. Tracheobronchial histopathology in habitual smokers of cocaine, marijuana, and/or tobacco. Chest 1997;112(2):319–26.

101. Baldwin GC, Tashkin DP, Buckley DM, et al. Marijuana and cocaine impair alveolar macrophage function and cytokine production. Am J Respir Crit Care Med 1997;156(5):1606–13.

102. Shay AH, Choi R, Whittaker K, et al. Impairment of antimicrobial activity and nitric oxide production in alveolar macrophages from smokers of marijuana and cocaine. J Infect Dis 2003;187(4):700–4.

103. Zhang LR, Morgenstern H, Greenland S, et al. Cannabis smoking and lung cancer risk: pooled analysis in the International Lung Cancer Consortium. Int J Cancer 2015;136(4):894–903.

104. Aldington S, Harwood M, Cox B, et al. Cannabis use and risk of lung cancer: a case-control study. Eur Respir J 2008;31(2):280–6.

105. Moss HB, Chen CM, Yi HY. Measures of substance consumption among substance users, DSM-IV abusers, and those with DSM-IV dependence disorders in a nationally representative sample. J Stud Alcohol Drugs 2012;73(5):820–8.

106. Perkonigg A, Goodwin RD, Fiedler A, et al. The natural course of cannabis use, abuse and dependence during the first decades of life. Addiction 2008;103(3): 439–49 [discussion 431–50].

107. Degenhardt L, Ferrari AJ, Calabria B, et al. The global epidemiology and contribution of cannabis use and dependence to the global burden of disease: results from the GBD 2010 study. PLoS One 2013;8(10):e76635.

108. Hedden SL. Center for Behavioral Health Statistics and Quality. *Behavioral health trends in the United States: Results from the 2014 National Survey on Drug Use and Health* (HHS Publication No. SMA 15-4927, NSDUH Series H-50). 2015. Available at: http://www.samhsa.gov/data/.

109. Gates PJ, Sabioni P, Copeland J, et al. Psychosocial interventions for cannabis use disorder. Cochrane Database Syst Rev 2016;2016(5):Cd005336.

110. Brezing CA, Levin FR. The current state of pharmacological treatments for cannabis use disorder and withdrawal. Neuropsychopharmacology 2018; 43(1):173–94.

111. Tomko RL, Jones JL, Gilmore AK, et al. N-acetylcysteine: a potential treatment for substance use disorders. Curr Psychiatr 2018;17(6):30–6, 41-42, 55.

112. Gray KM, Carpenter MJ, Baker NL, et al. A double-blind randomized controlled trial of N-acetylcysteine in cannabis-dependent adolescents. Am J Psychiatry 2012;169(8):805–12.

113. Tomko RL, Baker NL, Hood CO, et al. Depressive symptoms and cannabis use in a placebo-controlled trial of N-Acetylcysteine for adult cannabis use disorder. Psychopharmacology (Berl) 2020;237(2):479–90.

114. Small E. Evolution and classification of cannabis sativa (marijuana, hemp) in relation to human utilization. Bot Rev 2015;81(3):189–294.

115. FDA. Marinol (dronabinol) capsules, for oral use 2017. Available at: https://www.accessdata.fda.gov/drugsatfda_docs/label/2017/018651s029lbl.pdf. Accessed December 8, 2020.

116. Compton WM, Han B, Jones CM, et al. Marijuana use and use disorders in adults in the USA, 2002-14: analysis of annual cross-sectional surveys. Lancet Psychiatry 2016;3(10):954–64.

117. Huestis MA, Sampson AH, Holicky BJ, et al. Characterization of the absorption phase of marijuana smoking. Clin Pharmacol Ther 1992;52(1):31–41.

118. Hädener M, Vieten S, Weinmann W, et al. A preliminary investigation of lung availability of cannabinoids by smoking marijuana or dabbing BHO and decarboxylation rate of THC- and CBD-acids. Forensic Sci Int 2019;295:207–12.

119. Stephens D, Patel JK, Angelo D, et al. Cannabis butane hash oil dabbing induced lung injury mimicking atypical pneumonia. Cureus 2020;12(2):e7033.

120. Raber JC, Elzinga S, Kaplan C. Understanding dabs: contamination concerns of cannabis concentrates and cannabinoid transfer during the act of dabbing. J Toxicol Sci 2015;40(6):797–803.

121. Rossi G, Beck M. A little dab will do: a case of cannabis-induced psychosis. Cureus 2020;12(9):e10311.

122. Hilliard A, Stott C, Wright S, et al. Evaluation of the effects of sativex (THC BDS: CBD BDS) on inhibition of spasticity in a chronic relapsing experimental allergic autoimmune encephalomyelitis: a model of multiple sclerosis. ISRN Neurol 2012;2012:802649.

123. Karschner EL, Darwin WD, Goodwin RS, et al. Plasma cannabinoid pharmaco-kinetics following controlled oral delta9-tetrahydrocannabinol and oromucosal cannabis extract administration. Clin Chem 2011;57(1):66–75.

124. Guy GW, Robson PJ. A phase I, open label, four-way crossover study to compare the pharmacokinetic profiles of a single dose of 20 mg of a cannabis based medicine extract (CBME) administered on 3 different areas of the buccal mucosa and to investigate the pharmacokinetics of CBME per oral in healthy male and female volunteers (GWPK0112). J Cannabis Ther 2004;3(4):79–120.

125. Elsohly MA, Little TL Jr, Hikal A, et al. Rectal bioavailability of delta-9-tetrahydrocannabinol from various esters. Pharmacol Biochem Behav 1991; 40(3):497–502.

126. Mattes RD, Shaw LM, Edling-Owens J, et al. Bypassing the first-pass effect for the therapeutic use of cannabinoids. Pharmacol Biochem Behav 1993;44(3): 745–7.

127. Valiveti S, Hammell DC, Earles DC, et al. In vitro/in vivo correlation studies for transdermal delta 8-THC development. J Pharm Sci 2004;93(5):1154–64.

# Prevention of Substance Use Disorders

Leah F. Nelson, MD, MS[a], Elissa R. Weitzman, ScD, MSc[b,c,d], Sharon Levy, MD, MPH[a,b],*

## KEYWORDS

- Prevention • Substance use disorder • Adolescence • Screening

## KEY POINTS

- Prevention of substance use disorders (SUDs) requires identifying those at risk, eliminating, or ameliorating risk factors, and minimizing disability caused by substances.
- Adolescents are neurologically and socially vulnerable to the effects of substances, and to developing SUDs.
- Adolescence is a critical period for the initiation of SUDs and both primary and secondary prevention efforts are needed for this age group.
- Novel preventive strategies, especially game- and technology-based interventions, are being developed for substance use prevention.

## INTRODUCTION

In this article, we begin with a brief review of 3 substance use prevention frameworks, then focus on the specific preventive needs of adolescents, as this is a critical time for the initiation of substance use. We pay special attention to interventions that intercept the development of SUD in the young person who has tried alcohol, nicotine, or illicit drugs. We conclude with a discussion of promising novel interventions for expanding prevention to new sectors of the child and adolescent populations.

Prevention of SUDs has been framed in multiple ways. The 3 most common frameworks are the public health model, the Institute of Medicine model, and the Center for Substance Abuse Prevention (CSAP) model. Each considers prevention differently based on the stages of the disease, which persons are being targeted, and the setting in which efforts decrease.

One of the most widely-used frameworks is the public health model which proposes preventive interventions for each stage of disease. The model was developed for

[a] Adolescent Substance Use and Addiction Program, Boston Children's Hospital, 300 Longwood Avenue, Boston, MA 02115, USA; [b] Harvard Medical School, Boston, MA 02115, USA; [c] Division of Adolescent/Young Adult Medicine, Boston Children's Hospital, 300 Longwood Avenue, Boston, MA 02115, USA; [d] Computational Health Informatics Program, Boston Children's Hospital, Boston, MA 02115, USA
* Corresponding author.
E-mail address: Sharon.Levy@childrens.harvard.edu

Med Clin N Am 106 (2022) 153–168
https://doi.org/10.1016/j.mcna.2021.08.005
0025-7125/22/© 2021 Elsevier Inc. All rights reserved.

slowly progressive chronic diseases such as cancers, COPD, and coronary artery disease; however, it works equally well for SUD. There are generally considered to be 3 types of prevention in the public health model: primary, secondary, and tertiary. **Fig. 1** shows examples of each level of prevention for SUDs beginning with a person who has never tried substances, through the escalation of use, to diagnosable illness with comorbidities.

- Primary prevention aims to prevent a disease from ever occurring through limiting exposure to substances and reducing exposure to the other known risk factors for addiction.
- Secondary prevention is the detection of subclinical disease and intervention before the onset of problems. For SUD, this means "uncovering potentially harmful substance use before the onset of overt symptoms or problems."[1] The methods of secondary prevention are screening and counseling.
- Tertiary prevention is the management of established clinical disease "and facilitating entry into treatment so further disability is minimized."[1]

An alternative to the public health framework is the Institute of Medicine classification system of prevention efforts as universal, selective, or indicated.[2]

- Universal - targeted at a whole population.
- Selective - designed for a specific high-risk group.
- Indicated - targeted at those already using substances or engaged in high-risk behaviors associated with substance use, but not meeting criteria for SUD.

A third method of considering SUD prevention is the CSAP model which suggests 4 social domains as possible points of intervention: society, community, relationship, and individual (**Fig. 2**).[3] Examples of substance use risk factors and preventive strategies within each domain are shown in **Table 1**. When these domains are considered, it becomes clear that 2 people with the same SUD diagnosis may have markedly different risk factors contributing to their predisposition for addiction (**Fig. 3**A). Therefore, a wide variety of prevention efforts are needed to lessen SUD risks (**Fig. 3**B). Prevention of substance use in racially minoritized populations is of special interest and the CSAP domains overlap with the levels of racism proposed

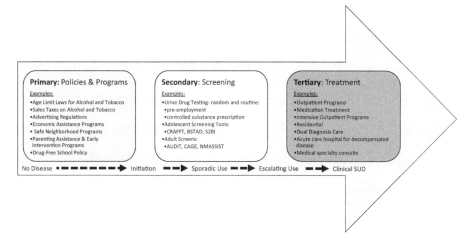

**Fig. 1.** The public health model of prevention for SUDs illustrating the progression from no disease to severe disease and examples of preventive actions available at each stage.

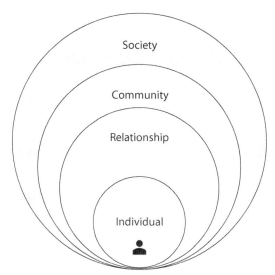

**Fig. 2.** Center for substance abuse prevention domains.

by Dr Camara Jones (institutional, personally-mediated, and internalized).[4] Recognizing experiences of racism as risk factors for SUD allow individual clinicians and organizations an opportunity to address the prevention of SUD in a structural competent manner.[5]

The 3 models—public health, Institute of Medicine (IOM), and CSAP—complement each other, allowing for prevention programs to be clearly described. For example, an increase in tobacco sales tax would be described as a universal primary prevention effort in the social domain. A screening program implemented within the juvenile court setting for youth arrested on drug charges would be an indicated secondary prevention effort in the individual domain. In the following review, we organize prevention strategies for adolescent substance use with the public health model of prevention as the disease stage model is most applicable for clinicians.

## ADOLESCENT SUBSTANCE USE

Adolescence and young adulthood, broadly defined as age 10 to 24 years, is a time of both increased risk-taking and increased vulnerability to developing SUDs. Indeed, the risk of developing SUD is inversely correlated with the age of first exposure (initiation) regardless of the choice of substance. For example, children who experience alcohol intoxication, initiate cannabis use, or have nonmedical use of opioids during early adolescence are 3 to 5 times more likely to develop SUD than individuals who initiate in early adulthood.[6–8] Therefore, preventive interventions provide an ideal opportunity to intervene and dramatically alter the entire life course—improving quality of life, promoting productive adulthood, sparing health, and decreasing financial and societal costs associated with addiction.

### Vulnerability

The developmental stage of adolescence is characterized by the progressive transition from a dependent child to an independent adult. As part of this growing independence, adolescents have increased reliance on their peers, and a desire to conform to "normal" behaviors. The desire to conform can be problematic for teens who have

**Table 1**
**Examples of risk factors and prevention efforts for each CSAP domain**

| CSAP Domain | Risk Factors | Prevention Examples |
|---|---|---|
| Society | • Availability of drugs<br>• Policies/laws<br>• Lack of enforcement of laws<br>• Social norms regarding substances<br>• Institutional racism | • Increase minimum purchase age for alcohol, nicotine, and cannabis.<br>• Increase taxes on addictive substances<br>• Social campaign to promote positive norms |
| Community | • Low neighborhood attachment<br>• Community norms<br>• Economic deprivation<br>Schools:<br>• Lack of commitment to education<br>• Negative school climate<br>• Lenient or harsh school policies regarding substances | • Improve neighborhood safety<br>• Address poverty<br>• School development<br>• Student support services |
| Relationship | • Peer use<br>• Peer norms favorable toward use<br>• Participation in social activities whereby use takes place<br>• Family history of SUD<br>• Poor parenting skills/family management<br>• Family conflict/violence<br>• Lax parental attitudes toward substances<br>• Lack of parental involvement<br>• Low family bonding<br>• Personally-mediated racism | • Provide education in schools:<br>  ○ Normative education - correction of misperceived substance use norms, students often believe substance use as being more common than it actually is.<br>  ○ Perceived harm understand the risks and short- and long-term consequences of alcohol, tobacco, and other drug use.<br>  ○ Recognize and resist external pressure from advertising, role models, and peers<br>• Increase the availability of healthy social opportunities<br>• Parental education and support starting in early childhood and extending through adolescence |
| Individual | • Genetics/epigenetics<br>• Earlier age at first exposure to substances<br>• Attitude toward substances<br>• Poor grades<br>• Chronic physical health problems requiring ongoing care, especially painful, and life-limiting diagnoses<br>• Experiences of trauma (eg, ACEs, PTSD, internalized racism)<br>• Behavioral traits:<br>  ○ Aggressive behavior in childhood<br>  ○ Sensation seeking<br>  ○ Low harm avoidance<br>  ○ Lack of impulse control | • General social and emotional skills training:<br>  ○ Self-control<br>  ○ Emotional awareness<br>  ○ Social problem solving<br>  ○ Academic support<br>  ○ Peer relationships<br>• Improve medical care to alleviate suffering<br>• Educational support<br>• SUD-specific skills training:<br>  ○ Refusal skills with role play<br>  ○ Self-efficacy and assertiveness<br>  ○ Re-enforcement of antidrug attitudes, personal commitments against substance use |

(continued on next page)

| Table 1 (*continued*) | | |
|---|---|---|
| **CSAP Domain** | **Risk Factors** | **Prevention Examples** |
| | ○ Low resiliency<br>• Psychiatric disorders:<br>　○ ADHD<br>　○ Anxiety<br>　○ Depression<br>　○ Schizophrenia<br>　○ Conduct/antisocial personality<br>　○ Borderline personality<br>　○ Autism spectrum disorders | ○ Stigma reduction teaches students skills to seek help and help their peers who may be struggling with substance use and/or mental health issues<br>• Access to counseling and psychiatric care. |

*Abbreviations*: ACEs, Adverse Childhood Experiences; ADHD, Attention Deficit Hyperactivity Disorder; PTSD, Post Traumatic Stress Disorder.

friends who use substances, which increases the initiation of substance use up to 1.5- to 2-fold.[9–11] Adolescents also are extremely sensitive to the influences of substance use behaviors and perceived norms portrayed by social media, celebrities, and advertisements.[12–16]

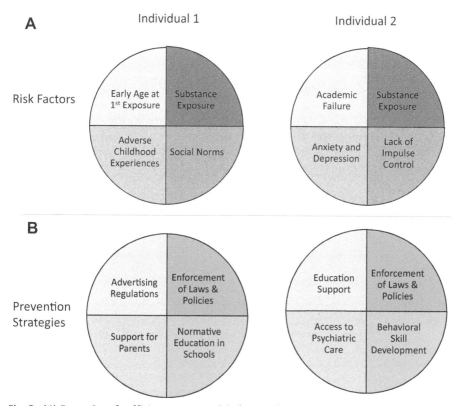

**Fig. 3.** (*A*) Examples of sufficient cause models for 2 individuals with substance use disorder illustrating how multiple risk factors combine to lead to the development of clinical disease. (*B*). Illustrates primary prevention strategies targeted at each risk factor in the sufficient cause model. Through multifaceted prevention efforts, the number of risk factors can be reduced, thus decreasing the probability of SUD.

In addition to social vulnerability, the adolescent brain is undergoing a period of rapid neurologic maturation, especially in the regions for executive functioning/impulse control (prefrontal cortex).[17] A useful metaphor is to consider the brain to be like a car, the reward pathway is the gas pedal encouraging the repetition of a feel-good behavior, and the prefrontal cortex is the brake pedal allowing the individual to stop and think about the consequences. In the adolescent brain, the reward pathway (gas pedal) is fully developed, appearing adult on fMRI, and is tuned to seek highly stimulating experiences; but the prefrontal cortex (brakes), is still developing, seems more like a child than an adult on imaging.[18] The use of psychoactive substances results in unnatural supraphysiologic levels of reward neurotransmitters, especially dopamine, and the prefrontal cortex has not developed the needed strength to overcome the signal to repeat the unhealthy behavior.

## PRIMARY PREVENTION FOR ADOLESCENTS

The goal of primary prevention is to help individuals avoid or delay the initiation of substance use. Every person who develops a SUD has exposure to an addictive substance. Thus, a fundamental part of all SUD prevention is reducing substance exposure. Most primary prevention interventions are universal and selective public health efforts including: community and family programs, policies and laws, and education for families and in schools (see **Fig. 1**).

- Community and family programs help build up people, places, and prosperity and reduce substance initiation.[19] Interventions in racially and ethnically minoritized communities are especially important as these youth often experience added harms of systemic racism and incarceration.[20,21]
- Policies and laws can make it more difficult to acquire substances and/or increase the cost. Examples include: age-limit laws, sales taxes, retail density regulations, retailer training requirements, and penalties for adults supplying minors with substances.[22,23]
- Family education programs coach communication skills between parents and children, provide structure for conversations about substance use and family values, and give strategies for monitoring the youth's activities.[24,25]
- In schools, high-quality antisubstance programs are longitudinal, usually starting in late elementary or middle school, and emphasize general social and academic skill building, normative education regarding the true prevalence of substance use, refusal skills, and stigma reduction for substance and mental health. Older programs that relied primarily on fear such as Drug and Alcohol Resistance Education (DARE) failed to achieve their goals.[26]

In addition to public health interventions, all caring adults in the lives of adolescents can be critical players in primary prevention. Hearing consistent messages from parents, teachers, coaches, mentors, counselors, and clinicians, all reiterating that "choosing not to use is best for your health and development" provides counteraction against strong prosubstance advertising and culture. Clinicians in primary care and school-based settings can provide this individual preventive counseling as part of routine care. Primary care providers (PCPs) are especially valuable as they may have a long-term ongoing relationship with the child that allows for the discussion of these topics in a way that feels safe and are in an important position to know about the child's unique risk factors such as family history, home environment, and behavioral problems at school.

## SECONDARY PREVENTION FOR ADOLESCENTS

For the adolescent who has already tried substances, more intensive and individualized efforts are needed to prevent the escalation of use and progression to SUD. This is the realm of secondary prevention (the detection of preclinical disease and early intervention) and indicated prevention (targeted at individuals not meeting SUD criteria, but using substances or engaging in high-risk activities). For addiction, preclinical disease is the period spanning the initial use of a substance and sporadic use/escalation, but before the physical, social, and behavioral manifestations of severe SUD (see **Fig. 1**).

In a medical setting, the screening, brief intervention, and referral to treatment (SBIRT) model has been well-validated as a strategy to quickly identify and respond to substance use problems and disorders. As shown in **Fig. 4**, the SBIRT model allows trained providers to screen for substance use, provide education, and, if needed, connect adolescents to treatment. Adolescent SBIRT seems to be gaining traction in primary care settings and more recently has been expanded in school-based health centers and emergency departments.[27–29]

Despite the utility of universal screening during routine medical visits, fewer than 50% of adolescents receive annual well-child care visits.[30] Therefore, secondary prevention must attempt to reach at-risk youth in other locations. A review of screening and brief intervention programs outside of medical offices are listed later in the discussion. These programs use caring adults outside the medical profession such as coaches, teachers, foster parents, mentors, caseworkers, judges, probation officers, and correctional officers.

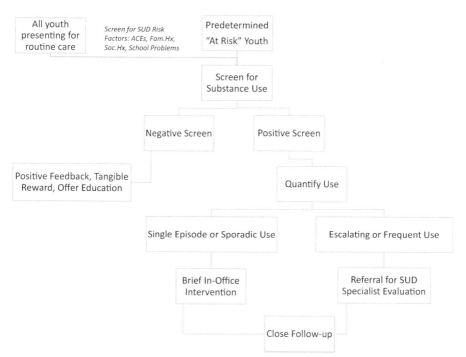

**Fig. 4.** Flow diagram for secondary prevention in a primary care, school-based, emergency department, or pediatric medical specialty setting.

### Clubs and Sports

About 57.4% of adolescents participate in team sports through schools and clubs in the United States (US).[31] The benefits of sports involvement for social, physical, and academic success are well-known. However, the data regarding sports and substance use are mixed and sometimes contradictory. Student athletes often have higher reported use of alcohol than nonathletic peers, but are less likely to use tobacco, cannabis, and illicit drugs.[32,33] Team sports can be an excellent venue for substance use prevention. Coaches who provide consistent messages about the importance of a drug-free lifestyle and have a no-play policy for substance use have lower substance use among their athletes.[34] In the US, some school districts are beginning to require athletic coaches take professional development training in the identification of substance use and referral for their student athletes.[35]

### Child Protective Services/Foster Care

As of 2018, an estimated 437,000 children and adolescents were in foster care in the US.[36] Adolescents in foster care are up to 5 times more likely to have a diagnosis of SUD than children who live with their parents.[37] The American Academy of Child and Adolescent Psychiatry and the Child Welfare League of America recommend all children be screened for substance use and mental health needs within 24 hours of being placed in out-of-home care.[38] A secondary prevention program that shows promise in foster care settings is KEEP SAFE. This 16-week support group and educational program improve the caregiving environment and the youth–caregiver relationship, teaches parenting techniques (eg, positive reinforcement, increased supervision), and coaches communication skills. A randomized controlled trial showed that adolescents participating in KEEP SAFE had significantly less substance use than those in the group receiving standard services.[39] Clearly, the thousands of children involved in foster care represent a critical population to address for all levels of substance use prevention.

### Mentoring Programs

One way to increase the number of caring adults in a youth's life is through engagement with a quality mentoring program. These programs are commonplace in today's society, with more than 5000 such programs in the US serving an estimated 4.5 million young people.[40] Programs frequently focus on children and adolescents who are perceived to be at risk. The focus of mentoring is the development of a healthy adult–child relationship, with minimal structured interaction. As such, they generally do not provide routine screening for substance use or guide adult mentors in asking and addressing this issue. Several analyses of the effectiveness of mentoring with respect to substance use have been published and concluded that mentoring programs do not show a consistent benefit.[41,42] Despite the paucity of evidence, mentoring programs have the potential to reach millions of at-risk youth and could be a key location for both primary and secondary prevention of SUDs. Mentors would need to receive training and support in how to discuss substances with children and adolescents, when to suspect substance use, and how to appropriately address it with the youth, including a protocol to follow when substance use is revealed.

### Disciplinary Settings

Teens who are already in trouble at school, home, or the community are connected to multiple adults who could provide secondary prevention services, such as school counselors, parents/foster parents, or juvenile justice officials.

a. School discipline. Schools historically have been punitive toward students suspected or confirmed to use substances, with "zero tolerance" policies causing youth to be suspended or expelled, thereby missing educational days.[43] Youth from minoritized communities (race, ethnicity, gender, sexuality, special needs, and so forth) often receive harsher punishments for the same offense.[44] Recently, many schools have initiated discipline programs that are less punitive toward substance use and focus on education and behavior change.[45]

b. Juvenile court/family court programs. As of 2018, there were more than 31 million adolescents involved in the criminal justice system,[46] of which up to 67% have initiated substance use.[47] The most common substances among court-involved, nonincarcerated (CINI) youth are cannabis (48%), alcohol (32%), and tobacco (21%).[48,49] Despite the prevalence of substance use among CINI youth, fewer than 60% of youth courts used standardized or validated instruments to provide universal substance use screening,[47] and only 33% provide substance use prevention programming (Funk 2020). The SBIRT model and other brief intervention strategies are currently being tested in juvenile justice settings with preliminary reports promising for decreased substance use among this high-risk group.[50,51]

c. Youth detention centers. Once a youth has been sentenced to a detention center, preventive efforts at all levels (primary, secondary, and tertiary) can be initiated based on the adolescent's prior experience with substances. If a youth has a positive screen for substance use, the detention setting provides a unique opportunity to provide intensive services including full assessment, counseling, medical and psychiatric physician services, and evidence-informed educational sessions.[52]

## TERTIARY PREVENTION

Once an adolescent has escalated substance use and developed the physical, social, and behavioral symptoms of addiction, they are likely to be diagnosed with SUD. According to National Institute on Drug Abuse (NIDA), tertiary prevention is "treating the medical consequences of [substance use] and facilitating entry into treatment so further disability is minimized."[1] Here we will review challenges of tertiary prevention for adolescents, key features of successful treatment, and aftercare.

### Challenges and Strategies

After an adolescent has been diagnosed with SUD, the primary challenge for the clinician is finding appropriate treatment. Depending on the substance, it can be impossible to access an addiction specialist comfortable with working with adolescents or willing to prescribe medications. Similarly, it can be difficult to find age-specific group therapy, counselors experienced with adolescents, or residential programs that accept people less than 18 years old. Because of poor access, the most effective long-term strategy is to encourage PCPs to treat most adolescents with SUD. This scope-of-practice expansion can be conducted via specialist outreach programs such as Project Echo and the Prescriber's Clinical Support System (PCSS) Mentoring Platform. These platforms allow PCPs to directly contact pediatric addiction specialists with questions and case consultations. Provider-to-provider support has the potential to empower PCPs to care for most adolescents with mild-to-moderate SUD, thereby lowering the burden on addiction specialists who are then able to focus their attention on youth with severe SUD or who have complicated coexisting conditions, while also serving as consultants to primary care colleagues.

## CLINICS CARE POINTS

Keys for treating an adolescent with substance use in primary care

1. Cultivating trust: Working with adolescents requires the youth to trust the provider. Teens are experts at finding information online and may come to the clinic with a detailed set of "facts" based on their own extensive research. Debunking myths with real information can be a challenge. Adolescent-specific sources of information are preferred. Good sources include: NIDA for Teens (https://teens.drugabuse.gov), TeensHealth (https://kidshealth.org/en/teens/know-about-drugs.html), and JustThinkTwice (https://www.justthinktwice.gov).

2. Confidentiality. Most adolescents worry that their parents will find out everything discussed in a medical visit. Explaining state laws and clinic policies regarding confidentiality and disclosure is critical. In general, if a teen is more than 13 years of age, a private interview for substance use and other risky behavior is recommended. Although confidentiality is the goal, adolescents can be encouraged to use the clinician as a mediator for a discussion with their parents about their substance use and treatment planning. Family support for adolescent SUD treatment improves outcomes.[53] For adolescents who request total confidentiality allowable within state law, it is important to inform youth who use a parent's health insurance, that insurers may send an explanation of benefits or a bill containing details of the diagnosis.

3. Promoting the dependence–independence transition. Adolescence is defined by the gradual transition from an identity based on family and parents to an independent identity largely shaped by peers. It is important to identify whereby the youth is in this transition and adjust treatment planning as the youth matures. We recommend partnering with youth in treatment planning and allowing them to express their opinions and make choices to the extent possible regarding medications, types of therapy, measurable goals, and rewards. Success in treatment can be used to help promote their developing independence. For example, when a teen has a sustained period of negative drug screening they can earn back privileges such as driving, a later curfew, or permission to attend an event.

### Aftercare

Like other chronic diseases, SUD's are remitting/relapsing and warrant ongoing monitoring and treatment even after remission has been achieved. Diabetes is a useful analogy: after the A1c goal is reached, the patient is not considered cured and discharged from care. Rather, they remain in care long-term to monitor control of their blood sugar and diabetes-related pathology. In addiction, *aftercare* is the period of time after a person achieves sustained remission of their SUD, but continues to receive services to prevent a return to use and monitor for negative health impacts of the SUD. It is a type of tertiary prevention. Usually, 2 of the 3 pillars of SUD treatment (medical/psychiatric, counseling, peer support) continue indefinitely, with a gradually decreasing frequency of visits. For adolescents, maintaining a connection to the SUD treatment team allows the patient to be supported during the inevitable high-stress experiences of transitioning to adulthood (eg, relationships, break-ups, housing transitions, starting college, new jobs) and prevent them from reinitiating substance use. Medications, especially anticraving medications (naltrexone, buprenorphine-naloxone, bupropion), are continued long-term, usually for several years.

### NOVEL PREVENTIVE INTERVENTIONS

New strategies are being developed to increase the reach and acceptability of substance use prevention to wider audiences. Examples of novel prevention strategies with evidence supporting their efficacy are shown in **Table 2**. Starting in early

**Table 2**
Novel preventive interventions for substance use

| Prevention Level | Name of the Program | Age (years) | Comments | Ref. |
|---|---|---|---|---|
| Primary | Good Behavior Game | 6–10 | Teaches self-control, delayed gratification, teamwork, and problem-solving. | 54 |
| | AlcholFX from SAMHSA | 10–12 | Games explore brain science and allow practice responding to difficult social situations involving alcohol. | 55 |
| | *PlayForward: smokeSCREEN* | 10–16 | Encourages decision-making and risk analysis of e-cigarette and vaping. | 56 |
| | Line Up Live Up | 13–18 | A "sports-based life skills training curriculum" aiming to reduce violence, crime, and drug use among at-risk and marginalized youth. | 57 |
| Secondary | SBIRTOregon.org Screening App | 10+ | Guides the patient through self-administered substance and depression screening using validated tools based on their age, summarizes the results for the provider, and provides handouts and guidance for a brief intervention | 58 |
| | iHELP | 16–20 | A smartphone-based motivational interviewing intervention to reduce substance use among foster youth transitioning to independent living | 59 |
| Tertiary | ThisIsQuitting | 13–24 | Text-to-quit vaping service with real-time messaging for managing cravings and triggers. | 60 |
| | reSET and reSET-O | 18+ | CBT-based app to be used in combination with treatment for nonopioid or opioid-SUD. FDA approved prescription only. | 61 |

elementary school, children can be introduced to the skills taught as part of evidence-based primary prevention curricula in schools in the form of games. The Good Behavior Game in early elementary school, for example, have been shown to reduce substance use and mental illness decades later.[54] As children reach middle school, primary prevention games can continue to be used for general life skills and also to help them learn to evaluate advertisements for alcohol and nicotine products, choose strategies to refuse substances, and demonstrate knowledge about the harms of specific substances.[55–57] For secondary prevention, app-based SBIRT[58] can be taken into multiple setting such as mentoring programs, foster care, and so forth to widen the availability of screening and brief intervention. For people with SUD, there are dozens of novel smartphone apps claiming to support people who have SUD. Most apps do not have data to support their efficacy. However, some newer apps are based on validated psychological models often used in addiction treatment and have promising preliminary data.[59–61]

## SUMMARY

Prevention of SUD is of critical importance and the adolescent age group needs to receive consistent messaging about the importance of avoiding substance use. Prevention activities can take place in multiple settings with the aim of addressing individual risk factors that lead to addiction. The uniform provision of high-quality primary and secondary prevention for youth has the potential to lower rates of adult substance use disorders, and address the epidemic of drug overdoses at its roots. Expanding treatment availability for youth who with SUD will allow them to achieve earlier remission and greater success long-term. The development of scalable, evidence-based technologic support for primary, secondary, and tertiary prevention warrants further exploration.

## ACKNOWLEDGMENTS

The authors have a couple of grants that supported this work. HRSA: 1T25HP37594-01-00 SAMHSA/ASAP-PC: 1H79TI081137-01 Conrad N. Hilton Foundation: 18455.

## DISCLOSURE

The authors have nothing to disclose.

## REFERENCES

1. National Institute on Drug Abuse. diagnosis and treatment of drug abuse in family practice - American family physician monograph. Available at: https://archives.drugabuse.gov/publications/diagnosis-treatment-drug-abuse-in-family-practice-american-family-physician-monograph/prevention. Accessed February 23, 2021.
2. Mrazek P, Haggerty R. Reducing risks for mental disorders: frontiers for preventive intervention research. Washington (DC): National Academies Press; 1994.
3. Substance Abuse and Mental Health Services Administration. A guide to SAMHSA's strategic prevention framework. Center for Substance Abuse Prevention. Rockville, MD: Substance Abuse and Mental Health Services Administration; 2019. Available at: https://www.samhsa.gov/sites/default/files/20190620-samhsa-strategic-prevention-framework-guide.pdf.
4. Jones C. Levels of racism: a theoretic framework and a gardener's tale. Am J Public Health 2000;90(8):1212–5.

5. Metzl JM, Hansen H. Structural competency: theorizing a new medical engagement with stigma and inequality. Soc Sci Med 2014;103:126–33.

6. Hingson RW, Zha W. Age of drinking onset, alcohol use disorders, frequent heavy drinking, and unintentionally injuring oneself and others after drinking. Pediatrics 2009;123(6):1477–84.

7. Le Strat Y, Dubertret C, Le Foll B. Impact of age at onset of cannabis use on cannabis dependence and driving under the influence in the United States. Accid Anal Prev 2015;76:1–5.

8. McCabe SE, West BT, Morales M, et al. Does early onset of non-medical use of prescription drugs predict subsequent prescription drug abuse and dependence? Results from a national study. Addict Abingdon Engl 2007;102(12):1920–30.

9. Cruz JE, Emery RE, Turkheimer E. Peer network drinking predicts increased alcohol use from adolescence to early adulthood after controlling for genetic and shared environmental selection. Dev Psychol 2012;48(5):1390–402.

10. Liu J, Zhao S, Chen X, et al. The influence of peer behavior as a function of social and cultural closeness: a meta-analysis of normative influence on adolescent smoking initiation and continuation. Psychol Bull 2017;143(10):1082–115.

11. Johnson EC, Tillman R, Aliev F, et al. Exploring the relationship between polygenic risk for cannabis use, peer cannabis use, and the longitudinal course of cannabis involvement. Addict Abingdon Engl 2019;114(4):687–97.

12. Davis JP, Pedersen ER, Tucker JS, et al. Long-term associations between substance use-related media exposure, descriptive norms, and alcohol Use from adolescence to young adulthood. J Youth Adolesc 2019;48(7):1311–26.

13. Loukas A, Paddock EM, Li X, et al. Electronic nicotine delivery systems marketing and initiation among youth and young adults. Pediatrics 2019;144(3). https://doi.org/10.1542/peds.2018-3601.

14. Tanski SE, McClure AC, Li Z, et al. Cued recall of alcohol advertising on television and underage drinking behavior. JAMA Pediatr 2015;169(3):264–71.

15. Weitzman M, Lee L. Similarities between alcohol and tobacco advertising exposure and adolescent use of each of these substances. J Stud Alcohol Drugs Suppl 2020;(s19):97–105. https://doi.org/10.15288/jsads.2020.s19.97.

16. Primack BA, Nuzzo E, Rice KR, et al. Alcohol brand appearances in US popular music. Addiction 2012;107(3):557–66.

17. Arain M, Haque M, Johal L, et al. Maturation of the adolescent brain. Neuropsychiatr Dis Treat 2013;9:449–61.

18. Galvan A, Hare TA, Parra CE, et al. Earlier development of the accumbens relative to orbitofrontal cortex might underlie risk-taking behavior in adolescents. J Neurosci 2006;26(25):6885–92.

19. Van Ryzin MJ, Fishbein D, Biglan A. The promise of prevention science for addressing intergenerational poverty. Psychol Public Policy Law 2018;24(1):128–43.

20. Unger JB. Preventing substance use and misuse among racial and ethnic minority adolescents: why are we not addressing discrimination in prevention programs? Subst Use Misuse 2015;50(8–9):952–5.

21. Xie TH, Ahuja M, McCutcheon VV, et al. Associations between racial and socioeconomic discrimination and risk behaviors among African-American adolescents and young adults: a latent class analysis. Soc Psychiatry Psychiatr Epidemiol 2020;55(11):1479–89.

22. Elder R, Lawrence B, Janes G, et al. Enhanced enforcement of laws prohibiting sale of alcohol to minors: systematic review of effectiveness for reducing sales

and underage drinking. Transp Res E-circ 2007;E-C123:181–8. https://doi.org/10.17226/22012.

23. Zaza S, Briss P, Harris K. Task force on community preventive services. tobacco. In: Zaza S, Briss PA, Harris KW, editors. The guide to community preventive services: what works to promote health?. 2005. p. 3–79. Available at: https://www.thecommunityguide.org/sites/default/files/assets/Tobacco-Community-Mobilization.pdf.

24. Foxcroft DR, Tsertsvadze A. Universal family-based prevention programs for alcohol misuse in young people. Cochrane Database Syst Rev 2011;(9):CD009308. https://doi.org/10.1002/14651858.CD009308.

25. Petrie J, Bunn F, Byrne G. Parenting programmes for preventing tobacco, alcohol or drugs misuse in children <18: a systematic review. Health Educ Res 2006; 22(2):177–91.

26. West SL, O'Neal KK, Project DARE. outcome effectiveness revisited. Am J Public Health 2004;94(6):1027–9.

27. Levy S, Ziemnik RE, Harris SK, et al. Screening adolescents for alcohol use: tracking practice trends of massachusetts pediatricians. J Addict Med 2017; 11(6):427–34.

28. Ramos MM, Sebastian RA, Murphy M, et al. Adolescent substance use: assessing the knowledge, attitudes, and practices of a school-based health center workforce. Subst Abuse 2017;38(2):230–6.

29. Barata IA, Shandro JR, Montgomery M, et al. Effectiveness of SBIRT for alcohol use disorders in the emergency department: a systematic review. West J Emerg Med 2017;18(6):1143–52.

30. Adams SH, Park MJ, Twietmeyer L, et al. Association between adolescent preventive care and the role of the affordable care act. JAMA Pediatr 2018; 172(1):43.

31. U.S. Centers for Disease Control and Prevention. High School YRBS - 2019 Results. Available at: https://nccd.cdc.gov/youthonline/App/Results.aspx?TT=B&OUT=0&SID=HS&QID=H82&LID=LL&YID=2019&LID2=&YID2=&COL=S&ROW1=N&ROW2=N&HT=QQ&LCT=LL&FS=S1&FR=R1&FG=G1&FA=A1&FI=I1&FP=P1&FSL=S1&FRL=R1&FGL=G1&FAL=A1&FIL=I1&FPL=P1&PV=&TST=False&C1=&C2=&QP=G&DP=1&VA=CI&CS=Y&SYID=&EYID=&SC=DEFAULT&SO=ASC. Accessed February 10, 2021.

32. Lisha NE, Sussman S. Relationship of high school and college sports participation with alcohol, tobacco, and illicit drug use: a review. Addict Behav 2010; 35(5):399–407.

33. Mays D, DePadilla L, Thompson NJ, et al. Sports participation and problem alcohol use. Am J Prev Med 2010;38(5):491–8.

34. Pitts M, Chow GM, Yang Y. Athletes' perceptions of their head coach's alcohol management strategies and athlete alcohol use. Addict Res Theor 2018;26(3): 174–82.

35. County Executive Bellone. Majority leader Hahn Announce program providing substance Abuse Awareness training for high school athletic coaches: Innovative program teaches coaches and training Staff to identify Signs and symptoms to prevent addiction. Suffolk County Government. Available at: https://suffolkcountyny.gov/News/county-executive-bellone-majority-leader-hahn-announce-program-providing-substance-abuse-awareness-training-for-high-school-athletic-coaches. Accessed March 2, 2021.

36. Child Welfare Information Gateway. Foster care Statistics 2018. Department of Health and Human Services, Administration for Children and Families, Children's Bureau; 2020. Available at: https://www.childwelfare.gov/pubPDFs/foster.pdf.

37. Pilowsky DJ, Wu L-T. Psychiatric symptoms and substance use disorders in a nationally representative sample of American adolescents involved with foster care. J Adolesc Health 2006;38(4):351–8.

38. American Academy of Child and Adolescent Psychiatry, Child Welfare League of America. AACAP/CWLA Statement on use of alcohol/drugs, screening/assessment of children in foster care *. 2003. Available at: https://www.aacap.org/aacap/policy_statements/2003/Mental_Health_and_Use_of_Alcohol_and_Other_Drugs_Screening_and_Assesment_of_Children_in_Foster_Care.aspx. Accessed March 4, 2021.

39. Kim HK, Buchanan R, Price JM. Pathways to preventing substance use among youth in foster care. Prev Sci 2017;18(5):567–76.

40. MENTOR, Office of Juvenile Justice and Delinquency Prevention. MENTOR: The national mentoring partnership. Available at: https://nationalmentoringresource center.org/index.php/component/k2/item/63-mentor-the-national-mentoring-partnership.html. Accessed March 4, 2021.

41. DuBois DL, Portillo N, Rhodes JE, et al. How effective are mentoring programs for youth? a systematic assessment of the evidence. Psychol Sci Public Interest 2011;12(2):57–91.

42. Thomas RE, Lorenzetti D, Spragins W. Mentoring adolescents to prevent drug and alcohol use. Cochrane Database Syst Rev 2011;11. https://doi.org/10.1002/14651858.CD007381.pub2.

43. Heitzeg NA. Education or incarceration: zero tolerance policies and the school to prison pipeline. Forum Publ Pol Online 2009;2009(2):1–102. Available at: https://eric.ed.gov/?id=EJ870076. Accessed March 2, 2021.

44. Gregory A, Skiba RJ, Mediratta K. Eliminating disparities in school discipline: a framework for intervention. Rev Res Educ 2017;41(1):253–78.

45. Neese AW. Discipline or education? Schools rethinking how they deal with vaping problem. The Columbus Dispatch. Available at: https://www.dispatch.com/news/20191115/discipline-or-education-schools-rethinking-how-they-deal-with-vaping-problem. Accessed March 11, 2021.

46. Hockenberry S, Puzzanchera C. Juvenile court statistics 2018. Milton Park, Oxfordshire: National Center for Juvenile Justice; 2020.

47. Chassin L. Juvenile justice and substance use. Future Child 2008;18(2):165–83.

48. Harrison A, Ramo D, Hall S, et al. Cigarette smoking, mental health, and other substance use among court-involved youth. Subst Use Misuse 2020;55(4):572–81.

49. Tolou-Shams M, Brown LK, Marshall BDL, et al. The behavioral health needs of first-time offending justice-involved youth: substance use, sexual risk, and mental health. J Child Adolesc Subst Abuse 2019;28(5):291–303.

50. Dauria EF, McWilliams MA, Tolou-Shams M. Substance use prevention and treatment interventions for court-involved, non-incarcerated youth. In: Brief interventions for adolescent alcohol and substance Abuse. The Guilford Press; 2018. p. 213–41.

51. Soto D, Lipkin M. SBIRT evaluation final report: successes, challenges, and lessons. Impact Justice: Research and Action Center; 2018. Available at: https://impactjustice.org/wp-content/uploads/SBIRT-Evaluation-Final-Report.pdf. Accessed March 2, 2021.

52. Belenko S, Knight D, Wasserman GA, et al. The juvenile justice behavioral health services cascade: a new framework for measuring unmet substance use treatment services needs among adolescent offenders. J Subst Abuse Treat 2017; 74:80–91.

53. Hogue A, Henderson CE, Becker SJ, et al. Evidence base on outpatient behavioral treatments for adolescent substance use, 2014–2017: outcomes, treatment delivery, and promising horizons. J Clin Child Adolesc Psychol 2018;47(4): 499–526.

54. Kellam SG, Mackenzie ACL, Brown CH, et al. The good behavior game and the future of prevention and treatment. Addict Sci Clin Pract 2011;6(1):73–84.

55. SAMHSA. AlcoholFX Mobile App. Available at: https://store.samhsa.gov/product/alcoholfx. Accessed March 2, 2021.

56. Pentz MA, Hieftje KD, Pendergrass TM, et al. A videogame intervention for tobacco product use prevention in adolescents. Addict Behav 2019;91:188–92.

57. U.N. Office. On drugs and crime. youth crime prevention through sport: Insights from the UNODC line up live up pilot programme. 2020. Available at: https://www.unodc.org/dohadeclaration/en/news/2021/01/unodcs-new-line-up-live-up-publication-unveils-four-years-of-data-and-research–showcasing-sport-as-a-critical-tool-for-youth-crime-prevention.html. Accessed March 5, 2021.

58. Department of Family Medicine at Oregon Health and Science University. Screening app. SBIRT Oregon. Available at: https://www.sbirtoregon.org/screening-app/. Accessed March 2, 2021.

59. Braciszewski JM, Tzilos Wernette GK, Moore RS, et al. A pilot randomized controlled trial of a technology-based substance use intervention for youth exiting foster care. Child Youth Serv Rev 2018;94:466–76.

60. Graham AL, Jacobs MA, Amato MS. Engagement and 3-month outcomes from a digital E-cigarette cessation program in a cohort of 27 000 teens and young adults. Nicotine Tob Res 2020;22(5):859–60.

61. U.S. Food and Drug Administration. FDA clears mobile medical app to help those with opioid use disorder stay in recovery programs. FDA. Available at: https://www.fda.gov/news-events/press-announcements/fda-clears-mobile-medical-app-help-those-opioid-use-disorder-stay-recovery-programs. Accessed March 10, 2021.

# Perioperative Buprenorphine Management

## A Multidisciplinary Approach

Thomas Hickey, MS, MD[a,b,]*, Audrey Abelleira, PharmD[a],
Gregory Acampora, MD[c], William C. Becker, MD[d,e],
Caroline G. Falker, MD[a], Mitchell Nazario, PharmD[f],
Melissa B. Weimer, DO, MCR[e,g]

## KEYWORDS

- Buprenorphine • Partial opioid agonists • Pain • Postoperative
- Opioid-related disorders • Analgesia

## KEY POINTS

- Pain from surgical procedures necessitates careful management of formulations of buprenorphine, an increasingly prescribed treatment of opioid use disorder.
- A simultaneous administration strategy using continuation of buprenorphine with full agonist opioids can provide effective postoperative analgesia, although data are limited.
- Perioperative pain should be treated appropriately in patients with addiction, and adoption of a perioperative buprenorphine strategy leveraging a multidisciplinary hospital-based team ideally involving addiction medicine and/or addiction psychiatry, anesthesia acute pain, nursing, pharmacy, and surgery is recommended, with particular attention given to care transitions at hospital discharge.

## CASE PRESENTATION

A 66-year-old man with severe left hip osteoarthritis and severe opioid use disorder (OUD) in remission on buprenorphine 24 mg/d presented to an anesthesiology preoperative clinic for evaluation 10 days before elective total hip arthroplasty. The

[a] VA Connecticut Healthcare System, 950 Campbell Avenue, West Haven, CT 06516, USA;
[b] Department of Anesthesiology, Yale School of Medicine, 950 Campbell Avenue, West Haven, CT 06516, USA; [c] MGH/Harvard Center for Addiction Medicine, Pain Management Center at MGH, Harvard Medical School, Massachusetts General Hospital, 55 Fruit Street, Boston, MA 02114, USA; [d] Pain Research, Informatics, Multimorbidities and Education Center, VA Connecticut Healthcare System; [e] Program in Addiction Medicine, Yale School of Medicine; [f] National PBM Clinical Program Manager, VHA Pharmacy Benefits Management (12PBM), 1st Avenue – 1 Block North of Cermak (Building 37), Hines, IL 60141, USA; [g] Yale School of Public Health
* Corresponding author. VA Connecticut Healthcare System, 950 Campbell Avenue, West Haven, CT 06516.
E-mail address: thomas_hickey@post.harvard.edu

Med Clin N Am 106 (2022) 169–185
https://doi.org/10.1016/j.mcna.2021.09.001
0025-7125/22/© 2021 Elsevier Inc. All rights reserved.

anesthesiologist made note of a recent addiction psychiatry recommendation that the patient take his last buprenorphine dose 24 hours before surgery and then receive a single dose of a long-acting full agonist opioid (FAO) on the day of the procedure. The addiction psychiatrist noted that both his recommendations and the reference supporting them had been e-mailed to the surgical team. The anesthesiologist's stated plan included "off buprenorphine as recommended." This statement was not further clarified, and there was no communication between the addiction psychiatrist and the anesthesiologist.

On the day of the surgery the patient presented having taken buprenorphine the prior evening. Another anesthesiologist assigned the case postponed the surgery due to concern for difficult-to-control acute postoperative pain. The case was rescheduled, and a plan for a 72-h period off buprenorphine was implemented at the anesthesiologist's recommendation. Multiple visits and calls with the patient and his wife were documented in the medical record, the majority by addiction psychiatry, to clarify the plan and provide reassurance. During the preoperative period off buprenorphine, tramadol was prescribed for pain and opioid withdrawal syndrome management.

On the day of surgery, a multimodal strategy was used, including methadone, intravenous (IV) fentanyl, a ketamine infusion, and IV acetaminophen. A hydromorphone patient-controlled analgesia (PCA) was used until the morning of postoperative day 2 along with scheduled IV ketorolac. On discontinuation of the PCA, oral hydromorphone and scheduled ibuprofen and acetaminophen were ordered. The total length of hospital stay was 6 days. Notably, the analgesics administered, both in number and amount, and length of stay were greater than for the average hip arthroplasty at the institution. The patient was discharged on a 7-day prescription of oral hydromorphone as needed with instructions to taper, but he ran out of this prescription in 4 days, with overuse due to pain. Buprenorphine reinitiation took place in the outpatient setting 9 days after hospital discharge. The patient then ran out of his buprenorphine prescription 4 days before its scheduled renewal, with overuse again due to pain. He was stabilized on his preoperative buprenorphine dose 30 days after discharge.

## INTRODUCTION

The vignette illustrates a timely clinical scenario, because buprenorphine is increasingly prescribed for the treatment of OUD and surgery is increasingly performed on patients with OUD.[1,2] The case demonstrates the critical needs for practice standardization and streamlined communication among health care providers, particularly when patients with OUD are made vulnerable by changes to their medication treatment of OUD (MOUD). The case also demonstrates the rapidly changing practices in perioperative buprenorphine management. In the following discussion, we provide a framework for perioperative buprenorphine management for multidisciplinary clinician teams who care for patients who are prescribed buprenorphine.

### Buprenorphine Treatment of Opioid Use Disorder and Chronic Pain

Opioid overdoses are at epidemic proportions in the United States, and treatment access to MOUD is of utmost importance to address this crisis.[3] Despite recent increased use of MOUD, opioid overdose events are high and increased in 2020 during the coronavirus disease 2019 pandemic, with overdose-related cardiac arrest elevated by 50% in the last year.[4]

Chronic pain is highly prevalent in patients with OUD. Uncontrolled pain is associated with OUD treatment disengagement and return to nonprescribed opioid use.[5–8] Management of perioperative pain is often complicated by the concern that postoperative opioids can increase the risk of OUD recurrence; however, patients treated with methadone for OUD who were prescribed postoperative opioids did not have significant differences in return to nonprescribed opioid use.[5–7] Indeed, undertreatment of pain in a patient with OUD has the potential to encourage recurrence of opioid use as the patient may seek nonprescribed opioids for pain relief and may disengage from MOUD treatment, thus increasing mortality risk.[9] Particularly in controlled environments, all patients, including those with OUD, should have their pain assessed and treated.

In addition to increased use as MOUD, certain buprenorphine formulations are indicated for the treatment of chronic pain (**Table 1**). These buprenorphine formulations offer an alternative to long-term opioid therapy (LTOT) involving full mu-opioid receptor ($\mu$OR) agonists, as well as an ideal analgesic for individuals requiring both MOUD and chronic pain management.[10] For these reasons, it is important that clinicians feel well-equipped to manage patients' buprenorphine treatment when they present on buprenorphine in the perioperative period.

### Acute Postoperative Pain for Patients with Opioid Tolerance

Surveys of patients undergoing surgery have found that most experience significant acute postoperative pain and many describe pain as a top perioperative concern.[11,12] Poorly controlled acute postoperative pain is a risk factor for persistent postsurgical pain. Each 10% increase in severe postoperative pain is associated with a 30% increase in persistent postoperative pain a year from surgery.[13] Persistent postoperative pain is prevalent, ranging from 10% following inguinal hernia repair to 30% to 40% after thoracotomy.[13]

Although acute postoperative pain control is important, management in the setting of chronic pain for patients receiving LTOT or for patients with OUD poses a challenge for both clinicians and patients. Pain in this patient population is often underestimated and undertreated, and opioid-tolerant patients report increased pain compared with patients without prior opioid exposure.[14,15] In addition, increased opioid requirements for opioid-tolerant individuals may be negatively interpreted as opioid misuse, further contributing to undertreatment of acute postoperative pain.[14,15]

### Buprenorphine

Buprenorphine, a US Drug Enforcement Administration schedule III opioid, was initially approved by the US Food and Drug Administration (FDA) as an injectable formulation in 1981, indicated for the treatment of moderate to severe pain.[10,16] In 2002, buprenorphine was subsequently developed in sublingual (SL) formulations (eg, buprenorphine and buprenorphine/naloxone) approved for the treatment of OUD, for a time falling out of favor as an analgesic due to misconceptions concerning the perceived futility of FAO in the setting of buprenorphine and equating *partial* $\mu$OR agonism to *partial* analgesic efficacy.[10,16–18] Since 2002, other formulations of buprenorphine—transdermal patch, buccal film, injectable, implantable—have been specifically approved by the FDA for either OUD or pain treatment (see **Table 1**).

Buprenorphine is a lipophilic opioid with a high volume of distribution, facilitating its penetration of the central nervous system.[17,18] Buprenorphine is metabolized by the liver, undergoing extensive first pass metabolism when administered orally. However, buccal and SL administration results in sufficient levels as venous drainage from the mouth bypasses first pass metabolism.[16–18] CYP3A4-mediated N-dealkylation

**Table 1**
**United States Food and Drug Administration-approved buprenorphine formulations and indications (as of 2021)**

| Name, Approval year | Route | t½ (h) | Bioavailability | Considerations for Clinicians |
|---|---|---|---|---|
| **FDA indication for pain** | | | | |
| Buprenorphine HCl injection (Buprenex), 1981 | IV/IM | IV: 2.2–3 | IM: 70%<br>IV: 100% | Available in 0.3 mg/mL ampules<br>Dosing: 0.3 mg every 6–8 h as needed |
| Buprenorphine transdermal system (Butrans), 2010 | Topical patch | 26 | ~ 15% | Available in 5, 7.5, 10, 15, and 20 μg/h patches<br>Max dose: 20 μg/h every week |
| Buprenorphine buccal film (Belbuca), 2015 | Buccal | 27.6 + 11.2 | 46% to 65% | Available in 75, 150, 300, 450, 600, 750, 900 μg films<br>Max dose: 900 μg every 12 h |
| **FDA indication for opioid dependence/opioid use disorder[a]** | | | | |
| Buprenorphine SL tab (Subutex), 2002 | SL | 31–35 | ~ 30% | Available in 2 mg and 8 mg SL tablets<br>Target maintenance dose for OUD is 16–24 mg/d |
| Buprenorphine/naloxone SL tab, SL film (Suboxone, generics), 2002 (tab), 2010 (film) | SL | 24–42 | ~ 30% | Available in 2-0.5 and 8-2 mg SL tabs and 2-0.5, 4-1, 8-2, and 12-3 mg SL films<br>Target maintenance dose for OUD is 16–24 mg/d |
| Buprenorphine/naloxone SL tab (Zubsolv), 2013 | SL | 24–42 | One Zubsolv 5.7 mg/1.4 mg tablet provides equivalent buprenorphine exposure and 12% lower naloxone exposure to 1 Suboxone 8 mg/2 mg tablet | Available in 0.7 mg/0.18 mg, 1.4 mg/0.36 mg, 2.9 mg/0.71 mg/ 5.7 mg/1.4 mg, 8.6 mg/2.1 mg, and 11.4 mg/2.9 mg buprenorphine/naloxone combination |
| Buprenorphine implant (Probuphine), 2016 | SD | 6-month SD implant; 24–48 h for buprenorphine | 31.3% (compared with 16 mg sublingual buprenorphine at steady state, day 28 of therapy) | No longer available in the United States. Consists of 4 individual implants containing 80 mg buprenorphine. The 4 implants are inserted subdermally in the upper arm and removed after 6 mo |

| | | | | |
|---|---|---|---|---|
| Buprenorphine extended-release injection (Sublocade), 2017 | SC depot | 43–60 d | 100 mg/mo steady state is comparable to 24 mg/d SL buprenorphine | SC administration, available in prefilled syringes containing 100 mg/0.5 mL and 300 mg/1.5 mL for every 28-d administration |
| Buprenorphine sustained-release injection (Brixadi), 2018 | SC depot | 3 (8 mg every 1 wk dose) to 21 d (128 mg every 28 d dose) | 32 mg every 1 wk or 160 mg every 4 wk comparable to 24 mg SL buprenorphine | FDA approved, market launch pending. For weekly or monthly administration. Dosage strengths: weekly 8, 16, 24, and 32 mg/injection; and monthly 64, 96, 128, and 160 mg/injection |

All parameters obtained from individual product prescribing information.

*Abbreviations:* IM, intramuscular; SC, subcutaneous; SD, subdermal.

[a] ICD-10 F11.2x Opioid dependence or DSM-5 Opioid Use Disorder (OUD).

converts buprenorphine to norbuprenorphine. Both buprenorphine and norbuprenorphine subsequently undergo glucuronidation to buprenorphine-3-glucuronide and norbuprenorphine-3-glucuronide. Buprenorphine half-life is variable based on the route of administration, ranging from 24 to 42 hours with transmucosal administration compared with 3 hours with IV administration.[16] The clearance of buprenorphine does not significantly differ between routes of administration; however, it is thought that transmucosal dosing results in a depot effect leading to the longer terminal half-life.

The pharmacology of buprenorphine is distinct from that of other opioids. Buprenorphine has been classified as a partial agonist at $\mu$OR primarily due to its lower intrinsic activity compared with full $\mu$OR agonists.[10,17–19] Buprenorphine has high affinity for the $\mu$OR compared with other opioids, though, allowing buprenorphine to preferentially occupy available $\mu$ORs, thereby competitively displacing other FAOs and antagonizing their activity.[10,16–18] The high affinity, efficacy, and slow dissociation of buprenorphine contribute to its clinical effectiveness in treating both pain and OUD.

Buprenorphine has demonstrated similar analgesic efficacy to FAO when evaluated for use in both acute and chronic pain.[10,16–18] Compared with other FAOs, buprenorphine demonstrates a ceiling on respiratory depression, receptor phosphorylation and $\beta$-arrestin recruitment, endocytosis-mediated receptor internalization, downregulation of $\mu$OR receptor signaling, and $\beta$-arrestin-mediated adverse effects including opioid overdose.[18] Buprenorphine acts as an agonist at the opioid receptor-like 1 (ORL1), which may contribute to secondary analgesia. Antagonism at the kappa-opioid receptor ($\kappa$OR) and delta-opioid receptor ($\delta$OR) may further reduce the risk of opioid-related adverse effects, such as dysphoria, depression, and constipation.[10,16–18] Some studies have found that buprenorphine is an inverse agonist at the $\kappa$OR, inducing a pharmacologic response opposite to that of an agonist.[20] In addition, buprenorphine's metabolites provide unique multimechanistic analgesia. Norbuprenorphine represents a bioactive metabolite of buprenorphine with full agonist activity at the $\mu$OR, but with approximately one-quarter the analgesia. The glucuronide metabolites, buprenorphine-3-glucuronide and norbuprenorphine-3-glucuronide, act at the $\mu$OR and the $\kappa$OR, respectively, and provide limited, if any, clinical analgesia.[17,21]

It is important that clinicians are familiar with the buprenorphine products available. To date buprenorphine can be delivered as the mono product or as a combined product with naloxone, typically in a 4:1 ratio; the combination product is meant to deter parenteral administration, taking advantage of naloxone's poor SL and buccal bioavailability. **Table 1** describes various currently FDA-approved and available formulations found in clinical use for either the treatment of pain or OUD.[16,22,23] Given the many buprenorphine formulations available, clinicians must understand their different clinical indications and be comfortable converting between formulations. Although we do not purport to offer exact conversions between buprenorphine formulations, approximate SL equivalencies are provided in **Table 2** taking into account the different bioavailability between formulations.[24,25]

### Rationale for Perioperative Buprenorphine Continuation

The use of buprenorphine is intended to reduce opioid cravings and recurrence of opioid use, thereby helping patients participate in their addiction recovery, resume regular daily activities, and reduce risk of morbidity and mortality. The perioperative period is a particularly vulnerable time for patients with OUD because inadequate pain control and discontinuation of MOUD elevate the potential for OUD treatment disengagement and mortality.

Buprenorphine's high $\mu$OR affinity has generated concern from clinicians who provide perioperative care who cite concern about inadequate or complicated analgesia

**Table 2**
**Sublingual dosing approximations for alternative buprenorphine formulations[a]**

| Buprenorphine Formulation | Dose | Approximate Buprenorphine SL Tablet Equivalency | Conversion Determinants |
|---|---|---|---|
| Transdermal patch | 5 μg/h | 0.25 mg | PK modeling predicts equivalency of 20 μg/h patch and 600 μg buccal film and has been used to extrapolate SL equivalencies |
| | 10 μg/h | 0.5 mg | |
| | 15 μg/h | 0.75 mg | |
| | 20 μg/h | 1 mg | |
| Buccal film | 75 μg | 0.25 mg | Buccal absorption 2 times greater than SL absorption, thus doubling buccal dose may approximate the SL dose equivalent |
| | 150 μg | 0.5 mg | |
| | 300 μg | 0.75 mg | |
| | 450 μg | 1 mg | |
| | 600 μg | 1.25 mg | |
| | 750 μg | 1.5 mg | |
| | 900 μg | 2 mg | |
| Long-acting injection | 100 mg | 24 mg | PK data suggest 100 mg monthly steady-state dose similar to 24 mg SL |
| | 300 mg | >24 mg | |

*Abbreviation:* PK, pharmacokinetic.
[a] Conversions provided are approximations and should always take clinical information into account.

management from competitive interference at the μOR. However, evidence supporting simultaneous administration of FAO with buprenorphine has been accumulating[26]; notable studies are listed in **Tables 3** and **4**.

Two significant clinical observations emerged from this evidence: (1) buprenorphine alone provided adequate analgesia after many procedures and (2) buprenorphine could be use simultaneously with FAO for adequate postoperative analgesia. Multiple investigators, while acknowledging a lack of robust prospective data, have advocated for a simultaneous strategy of buprenorphine use with FAO for treatment of pain in the perioperative period, particularly for procedures anticipated to produce mild pain such as dental procedures, cystoscopy, and surficial skin procedures.[7,26,34–39] Furthermore, there is increasing support for continuing buprenorphine perioperatively for larger-scale surgery like cardiac surgery or joint arthroplasty.[26] Inherent in this strategy is that as buprenorphine administration is not ceased but adjusted through the perioperative period, it provides an opportunity to continue buprenorphine postoperatively, therefore minimizing the risk of OUD recurrence and discontinuation of OUD treatment.

### Moving Toward a Full Agonist Opioid Simultaneous Administration Strategy

To date there is limited research on managing intraoperative and postoperative pain in patients prescribed buprenorphine. Proposed strategies being implemented often take 4 main factors into account: the historic pain burden of the procedure, baseline buprenorphine dose, applicability of a multimodal analgesia strategy including regional blocks and PCA, and the stability of the patient in OUD treatment. A critical question remains how to manage buprenorphine for patients in a way that minimizes opioid withdrawal risk and OUD recurrence risk while facilitating buprenorphine and FAO-mediated analgesia. There are data that may inform an evidence-based approach to buprenorphine dosing and timing.

**Table 3**
Evidence for the concomitant use of buprenorphine with full opioid agonist treatment

| Study | Study Design | Population | Intervention | Outcome |
|---|---|---|---|---|
| Mercandante et al,[27] 2006 | Prospective cohort | 29 patients with cancer treated with TD buprenorphine for cancer-related pain | IV morphine for breakthrough pain | IV morphine was safe and effective (92.4% of episodes treated successfully with IV morphine, with 88% of these achieving more than 50% pain decrease in pain intensity within 15 min) |
| Jones et al,[28] 2009 | Case series | 8 women treated with buprenorphine for OUD undergoing vaginal delivery | Routine pain management | Routine analgesics effective, pain scores consistent with those reported separately for non-opioid-dependent patients |
| Oifa et al,[29] 2009 | RCT | 120 patients who were non-opioid-dependent undergoing major abdominal surgery | Divided into 4 infusion + bolus arms involving buprenorphine (BUP) and morphine (MO), alone or in combination as infusion and PCA bolus: BUP/BUP, MO/MO, MO/BUP, BUP/MO | Acute postoperative pain was lowest in the BUP/BUP group, demand:delivery ratio was lowest in the BUP/BUP group, patient satisfaction was highest in the BUP/BUP group, and BUP did not inhibit morphine analgesia when used in combination |
| Kornfeld & Manfredi,[30] 2010 | Case series | 7 patients treated with buprenorphine for chronic pain, several with remote history of OUD, undergoing major surgery | Continuation of daily standard buprenorphine dose perioperatively | Postoperative pain control was effective; full agonist opioids were deemed "central" to postoperative analgesia |
| Jalili et al,[31] 2012 | RCT | Adults presenting to emergency department with acute bone fractures | 44 patients treated with buprenorphine (0.4 mg SL) and 45 patients with morphine (5 mg IV) | "Buprenorphine is as effective and safe as morphine" for acute pain from bone fractures |

| Macintyre et al,[32] 2013 | Retrospective cohort | 29 patients treated with buprenorphine for OUD who underwent surgery | Routine pain management over the first 24 h postoperatively | Patients required more postoperative opioid than would be expected of opioid-naive patients. Patients NOT given buprenorphine on the day of surgery had significantly higher opioid requirements, more time on PCA, and more time on the acute pain service |
| Quaye et al,[33] 2020 | Retrospective cohort | 55 patients treated with buprenorphine for OUD who underwent surgery | 38 patients continued buprenorphine vs 17 held | Patients continued on buprenorphine experienced reduced PACU pain scores, opioid prescriptions dispensed, and MME dispensed |

*Abbreviations:* MME, morphine milligram equivalents; PACU, RCT, randomized controlled trial; TD, transdermal.

Table 4
Best practices for multidisciplinary clinicians caring for patients undergoing surgery who are prescribed buprenorphine

| Clinician | Recommendation |
| --- | --- |
| Outpatient clinicians | • Provide patient education, including hospital algorithm as available<br>• Document patient buprenorphine dose and indication for use<br>• Document patient goals, expectations, and concerns about surgery<br>• Document patient instructions<br>• Communicate directly with the surgeon and/or anesthesiologist |
| Inpatient clinicians | • Review outpatient records<br>• Provide patient education<br>• Review patient goals, expectations, and concerns about surgery<br>• Consider specialty consultation from addiction medicine, addiction psychiatry, or anesthesia<br>• Offer multimodal analgesic approaches |
| Clinical pharmacists | • Provide patient education<br>• Address regulatory issues<br>• Assist with buprenorphine dose conversions and equivalencies<br>• Assist with admission and discharge medication reconciliation<br>• Daily postoperative rounding for analgesic optimization<br>• Care coordination between multiple providers |
| Discharging clinicians | • Provide patient education<br>• Identify patient support for monitoring of buprenorphine and opioids<br>• Communicate hospital outcomes to the outpatient clinician<br>• Provide a bridge prescription for buprenorphine or opioids as needed<br>• Document nonopioid analgesic, buprenorphine, and opioid management plan |

$\mu$OR occupancy is buprenorphine dose dependent, with 59% of $\mu$ORs available at a 2 mg dose of buprenorphine; meanwhile 16% of $\mu$ORs are available at 32 mg dose of buprenorphine.[10] Occupancy is also time dependent. Multiple studies guided by PET imaging demonstrate the gradual increase in central nervous system $\mu$OR binding potential after buprenorphine cessation.[40,41] For example, 40% of $\mu$OR receptors are clinically available for analgesia at 24 hours after omission of a 16 mg buprenorphine dose. Meanwhile symptoms of opioid withdrawal syndrome are generally suppressed with $\mu$OR availability of 50% to 60%.[42] These data help explain how concomitant use of buprenorphine and FAO can achieve analgesia in the perioperative period.

The approach of concomitant buprenorphine and FAO use in the perioperative period has been adopted by several institutions and has been recommended by many clinical experts.[26] More data are needed, but one institution found that using this approach reduced total FAO use and shortened hospital length of stay.[35] Fig. 1 shows a comprehensive and flexible algorithm instituted by one health system, which was developed with input from multiple different stakeholders.

Perioperative management of subcutaneous buprenorphine injection depot (Sublocade™) is complicated by its long half-life. We expect that management strategies for these long-acting formulations will attempt to recapitulate a simultaneous administration strategy by scheduling surgery at the expected steady state trough serum concentration, with or without SL buprenorphine supplementation. For example, by scheduling surgery 4-6 weeks after a 100mg SC dose and prescribing 8mg SL buprenorphine BID from 28 days after last SC dose, reduced to 4mg on the day of surgery.

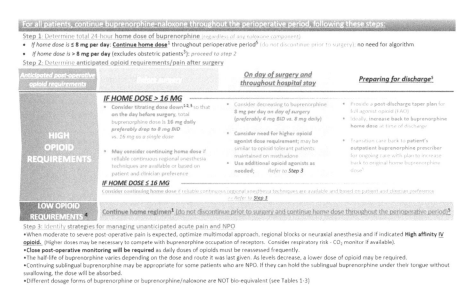

**Fig. 1.** Perioperative buprenorphine management algorithm. (*Modified from* Mass General Brigham Substance Use Steering Committee. Full document is available to MGB® internally *http://handbook.partners.org/content/pdf/PeriopOpioidTolerantPatients.pdf.* Used with permission of Mass General Physicians Organization.)

## Care Coordination and Treatment Planning

Communication among clinicians caring for patients with OUD in the perioperative period is imperative to create a unified patient-centered perioperative pain management plan. The perspective of varied specialists is largely based on their training: outpatient clinicians caring for patients with OUD tend to emphasize OUD recurrence prevention and are inclined to higher dosing of buprenorphine, whereas proceduralists, anesthesiologists, and hospitalists tend to be more focused on uncomplicated anesthesia, adequate analgesia, and length of stay. A mutually agreed upon management plan will benefit the patient by avoiding contradictory instructions on buprenorphine and pain management. A preoperative evaluation may be the ideal time to provide education to the patient and the multidisciplinary hospital team to ensure a mutually agreed upon approach for buprenorphine and pain management. Institutional algorithms or guidelines that support the continuation of buprenorphine and FAO will limit confusion and ensure engagement from surgeons and anesthesiologists. In addition, institutions are encouraged to ensure that all buprenorphine formulations are available for patient use and continuation.

## Multimodal Analgesia

Published guidelines on the management of postoperative pain made 32 recommendations, 4 of which were assessed to be supported by high-quality evidence: use of a multimodal regimen, use of acetaminophen and/or nonsteroidal anti-inflammatory drugs (NSAIDs) (**Table 5**), use of regional anesthetic techniques, and consideration of neuraxial analgesia for major thoracic and abdominal procedures.[43] These recommendations are particularly important for patients who may have more challenging perioperative pain management needs and for whom opioid-sparing techniques may be especially important.

Table 5
Suggested perioperative dosing of acetaminophen and common nonsteroidal anti-inflammatory drugs

| Adjunct | Dose Range | Comments |
|---|---|---|
| Acetaminophen | 3–4 g/d | Most sources allow for low-dose therapy (ie, ≤2 g/d) in even advanced liver disease, provided there is not active alcohol use |
| NSAID | Ibuprofen PO≤3200 mg/d<br>Naproxen PO≤1500 mg/d<br>Ketorolac IV≤120 mg/d<br>Celecoxib PO≤400 mg/d | Reduced dose may mitigate risk of GI complication; use with caution in patients with CKD and avoid if CKD is severe; doses can be reduced for patients <50 kg or ≥65 y |

*Abbreviations:* CKD, chronic kidney disease; GI, gastrointestinal; PO, oral.

Any patient undergoing surgery with anticipated moderate or severe postoperative pain should receive multimodal analgesia unless contraindicated, particularly in the patient with history of chronic pain and/or OUD. However, there is no "one size fits all" strategy, and the risk versus benefit profiles of the various agents, patient comorbidities, and surgical factors such as bleeding risk must be considered in each case. In all cases, a thorough medication reconciliation should be performed and regular home analgesics continued. The care team should recognize that muscle relaxants, alpha agonists, benzodiazepines, anticonvulsants, and antidepressants have often been prescribed as adjuncts for treatment of chronic pain and should be continued perioperatively. Premedication can be considered with acetaminophen and NSAID; indeed, these medications are additive in their benefit when given together.[44] Clonidine premedication (ie, 3 μg/kg orally) is also likely to improve postoperative pain control.[45] Evidence on premedication with gabapentinoids is mixed, with a recent meta-analysis showing no clear benefit in both acute and persistent postoperative pain.[46] Regional and neuraxial blocks should be used where appropriate for procedures such as total joint arthroscopy, major intra-abdominal surgeries, and thoracotomy; surgeons should infiltrate local anesthetic before surgical incision if neither is used.

Intraoperatively, IV dexamethasone given at 0.1 mg/kg between induction of anesthesia and incision is likely to reduce postoperative pain and opioid consumption.[47] High-affinity FAO such as sufentanil, fentanyl, or hydromorphone may be preferable for intraoperative use due to increased competitive binding at the μOR[48]; IV methadone may also be considered for patients with high opioid tolerance. Intraoperative subanesthetic ketamine, for example, as a 0.5 mg/kg IV bolus preincision and/or intraoperative infusion at 0.2 mg/kg/h, may also reduce postoperative pain. This benefit may be most apparent when severe postoperative pain is anticipated, although there is possible harm including hallucinations and nightmares, particularly in the older patient.[49–51] IV lidocaine infusion, for example, 1.5 mg/kg bolus at induction followed by 2 mg/kg/h intraoperatively and up to 24 hours postoperatively may be useful, particularly for early acute postoperative pain after intraperitoneal surgery when an epidural is not used.[52] However, this therapy should only be implemented after review and approval by the relevant hospital committee given the need for appropriate patient monitoring and the ability to obtain a serum lidocaine level in the event local anesthetic systemic toxicity were suspected. Intraoperative IV magnesium has also shown modest benefit in a variety of surgeries for healthy patients, for example, as 30 mg/kg slow bolus and/or 15 mg/kg/h infusion.[53] However, providers should be aware of the possibility of hypotension, bradycardia, and potentiation of neuromuscular blocking drugs.

Postoperatively, admitted patients should receive standing acetaminophen and NSAID unless contraindicated and home analgesics should be continued. Opioids such as hydromorphone and fentanyl may be most effective for concomitant use with buprenorphine because of their competing affinity at the μOR.[48] Patients with severe pain may benefit from scheduled over as-needed opioids due to high opioid tolerance. A clonidine patch can be considered, for example, 0.2 mg/d. Muscle relaxants may be administered if spasm is suspected. Anxiolytics may be useful if anxiety contributes to the patient's pain.

Nonpharmacologic interventions can also enhance acute postoperative pain management and may be particularly helpful for patients with OUD. Cognitive behavioral therapy (CBT), a well-established treatment of chronic pain, has emerging evidence for use in postsurgical populations.[54–57] A meta-analysis of randomized trials found moderate-quality evidence for the efficacy of psychological interventions with active components such as relaxation training and CBT in reducing persistent postsurgical pain.[56] Furthermore, a recent study of a single 15-min session of mindfulness or hypnotic suggestion has been shown to reduce pain by 23% to 29% in adult inpatients experiencing significant pain.[58] In addition to psychological interventions, transcutaneous electrical nerve stimulation has been shown in meta-analysis to reduce acute postoperative pain and promoted functional recovery.[59]

Enhanced Recovery After Surgery (ERAS) strategies seek to bundle evidence-based practices to improve surgical outcomes and standardize an opioid-sparing, multimodal analgesia technique. Pursuing a standardized approach to buprenorphine management fits within the goals and objectives of ERAS as well.

## SUMMARY

Emerging data and clinical practice support a coordinated and competent approach to the perioperative management of patients prescribed buprenorphine. In the absence of this approach, patients are at risk for poor outcomes, including OUD recurrence and poor pain treatment. A patient-centered, multidisciplinary strategy that considers the risks and benefits of the various perioperative management strategies is most likely to succeed. Although evidence is not conclusive, clinical experience supports a simultaneous administration strategy of buprenorphine and FAOs. This approach will require a shared understanding by patients, outpatient and inpatient clinicians, and surgical teams, and has the potential to better support patients with OUD, improve perioperative analgesia, reduce risks of OUD recurrence, reduce FAO use in the hospital setting, reduce health care utilization, and lead to improved perioperative pain outcomes.

## CLINICS CARE POINTS

- Buprenorphine is a partial opioid agonist with several different formulations used for the treatment of pain or OUD and has important analgesic properties.

- Continuation of buprenorphine with concomitant use of high-affinity FAOs is a promising strategy for the perioperative pain management for patients who are prescribed buprenorphine for pain or OUD.

- Coordination and a shared understanding for buprenorphine management among a diverse clinician team (eg, Anesthesia, Surgery, Internal Medicine and/or Primary Care, Addiction Medicine or Addiction Psychiatry) is critical for patients prescribed buprenorphine who are undergoing surgery.

> • Multimodal analgesia should be maximized for patients who are prescribed buprenorphine as a standard of care and to help spare overall FAO needs and adequately treat perioperative pain.

## ATTRIBUTION

T. Hickey wrote the initial draft including Clinical Vignette, Introduction, Acute Postoperative Pain, Multimodal Analgesia, and Summary sections and incorporated other authors' contributions into various revised manuscripts. G. Acampora drafted the section on Simultaneous Administration Strategy and contributed to the Buprenorphine section. A. Abelleira and M. Nazario drafted the section on Buprenorphine. C.G. Falker drafted the section on Clinical Care Points. A. Abelleira drafted the section on the possible role of clinical pharmacology. W.C. Becker developed concept and provided revisions. M.B. Weimer helped develop concept, writing for all sections, and extensive revisions. All authors were involved with the revision of the manuscript.

## ACKNOWLEDGMENTS

Katherine Hadlandsmyth, PhD, and Adam Gordon, MD, provided valued contributions to manuscript revisions. Dr Hadlandsmyth contributed to the sections on clinical pharmacology and nonpharmacologic postoperative pain management. Dr Gordon provided useful feedback on the manuscript throughout its development.

## DISCLOSURE

Dr M.B. Weimer discloses an advisory role with Path CCM, Inc. The other authors have nothing to disclose. The views and opinions of authors expressed herein do not necessarily state or reflect those of the US government or any agency thereof.

## REFERENCES

1. Weiser TG, Haynes AB, Molina G, et al. Estimate of the global volume of surgery in 2012: an assessment supporting improved health outcomes. Lancet 2015; 385(Suppl 2):S11.
2. Roehler DR, Guy GP Jr, Jones CM. Buprenorphine prescription dispensing rates and characteristics following federal changes in prescribing policy, 2017-2018: a cross-sectional study. Drug Alcohol Depend 2020;213:108083.
3. Jones CM, Campopiano M, Baldwin G, et al. National and state treatment need and capacity for opioid agonist medication-assisted treatment. Am J Public Health 2015;105(8):e55–63.
4. Friedman J, Beletsky L, Schriger DL. Overdose-related cardiac arrests observed by emergency medical services during the US COVID-19 epidemic. JAMA Psychiatry 2020;78(5):562–4.
5. Alford DP, Compton P, Samet JH. Acute pain management for patients receiving maintenance methadone or buprenorphine therapy. Ann Intern Med 2006;144(2): 127–34.
6. Kantor TG, Cantor R, Tom E. A study of hospitalized surgical patients on methadone maintenance. Drug Alcohol Depend 1980;6(3):163–73.
7. Karasz A, Zallman L, Berg K, et al. The experience of chronic severe pain in patients undergoing methadone maintenance treatment. J Pain Symptom Manag 2004;28(5):517–25.

8. Ellis MS, Kasper Z, Cicero T. Assessment of chronic pain management in the treatment of opioid use disorder: gaps in care and implications for treatment outcomes. J Pain 2021;22(4):432–9.
9. Pearce LA, Min JE, Piske M, et al. Opioid agonist treatment and risk of mortality during opioid overdose public health emergency: population based retrospective cohort study. BMJ 2020;368:m772.
10. Webster L, Gudin J, Raffa RB, et al. Understanding buprenorphine for use in chronic pain: expert opinion. Pain Med 2020;21(4):714–23.
11. Apfelbaum JL, Chen C, Mehta SS, et al. Postoperative pain experience: results from a national survey suggest postoperative pain continues to be undermanaged. Anesth Analg 2003;97(2):534–40, table of contents.
12. Gan TJ, Habib AS, Miller TE, et al. Incidence, patient satisfaction, and perceptions of post-surgical pain: results from a US national survey. Curr Med Res Opin 2014;30(1):149–60.
13. Kehlet H, Jensen TS, Woolf CJ. Persistent postsurgical pain: risk factors and prevention. Lancet 2006;367(9522):1618–25.
14. Mehta V, Langford RM. Acute pain management for opioid dependent patients. Anaesthesia 2006;61(3):269–76.
15. Rapp SE, Ready BL, Nessly ML. Acute pain management in patients with prior opioid consumption: a case-controlled retrospective review. Pain 1995;61(2):195–201.
16. Coe MA, Lofwall MR, Walsh SL. Buprenorphine pharmacology review: update on transmucosal and long-acting formulations. J Addict Med 2019;13(2):93–103.
17. Khanna IK, Pillarisetti S. Buprenorphine - an attractive opioid with underutilized potential in treatment of chronic pain. J pain Res 2015;8:859–70.
18. Gudin J, Fudin J. A narrative pharmacological review of buprenorphine: a unique opioid for the treatment of chronic pain. Pain Ther 2020;9(1):41–54.
19. Dahan A, Yassen A, Romberg R, et al. Buprenorphine induces ceiling in respiratory depression but not in analgesia. Br J Anaesth 2006;96(5):627–32.
20. Grinnell SG, Ansonoff M, Marrone GF, et al. Mediation of buprenorphine analgesia by a combination of traditional and truncated mu opioid receptor splice variants. Synapse 2016;70(10):395–407.
21. Brown SM, Holtzman M, Kim T, et al. Buprenorphine metabolites, buprenorphine-3-glucuronide and norbuprenorphine-3-glucuronide, are biologically active. Anesthesiology 2011;115(6):1251–60.
22. Sullivan JG, Webster L. Novel buccal film formulation of buprenorphine-naloxone for the maintenance treatment of opioid dependence: a 12-week conversion study. Clin Ther 2015;37(5):1064–75.
23. Saal D, Lee F. Rapid induction therapy for opioid-use disorder using buprenorphine transdermal patch: a case series. Perm J 2020;24:19–124.
24. Priestley T, Chappa AK, Mould DR, et al. Converting from transdermal to buccal formulations of buprenorphine: a pharmacokinetic meta-model simulation in healthy volunteers. Pain Med 2018;19(10):1988–96.
25. Davis MP, Pasternak G, Behm B. Treating chronic pain: an overview of clinical studies centered on the buprenorphine option. Drugs 2018;78(12):1211–28.
26. Buresh M, Ratner J, Zgierska A, et al. Treating perioperative and acute pain in patients on buprenorphine: narrative literature review and practice recommendations. J Gen Intern Med 2020;35(12):3635–43.
27. Mercadante S, Villari P, Ferrera P, et al. Safety and effectiveness of intravenous morphine for episodic breakthrough pain in patients receiving transdermal buprenorphine. J Pain Symptom Manag 2006;32(2):175–9.

28. Jones HE, O'Grady K, Dahne J, et al. Management of acute postpartum pain in patients maintained on methadone or buprenorphine during pregnancy. Am J Drug Alcohol Abuse 2009;35(3):151–6.

29. Oifa S, Sydoruk T, White I, et al. Effects of intravenous patient-controlled analgesia with buprenorphine and morphine alone and in combination during the first 12 postoperative hours: a randomized, double-blind, four-arm trial in adults undergoing abdominal surgery. Clin Ther 2009;31(3):527–41.

30. Kornfeld H, Manfredi L. Effectiveness of full agonist opioids in patients stabilized on buprenorphine undergoing major surgery: a case series. Am J Ther 2010; 17(5):523–8.

31. Jalili M, Fathi M, Moradi-Lakeh M, et al. Sublingual buprenorphine in acute pain management: a double-blind randomized clinical trial. Ann Emerg Med 2012; 59(4):276–80.

32. Macintyre PE, Russell RA, Usher KA, et al. Pain relief and opioid requirements in the first 24 hours after surgery in patients taking buprenorphine and methadone opioid substitution therapy. Anaesth Intensive Care 2013;41(2):222–30.

33. Quaye A, Potter K, Roth S, et al. Perioperative continuation of buprenorphine at low-moderate doses was associated with lower postoperative pain scores and decreased outpatient opioid dispensing compared with buprenorphine discontinuation. Pain Med 2020;21(9):1955–60.

34. Mehta D, Thomas V, Johnson J, et al. Continuation of buprenorphine to facilitate postoperative pain management for patients on buprenorphine opioid agonist therapy. Pain Physician 2020;23(2):E163–74.

35. Quaye AN, Zhang Y. Perioperative management of buprenorphine: solving the conundrum. Pain Med 2019;20(7):1395–408.

36. Lembke A, Ottestad E, Schmiesing C. Patients maintained on buprenorphine for opioid use disorder should continue buprenorphine through the perioperative period. Pain Med 2019;20(3):425–8.

37. Acampora GA, Nisavic M, Zhang Y. Perioperative buprenorphine continuous maintenance and administration simultaneous with full opioid agonist: patient priority at the interface between medical disciplines. J Clin Psychiatry 2020;81(1): 19com12810.

38. Martin YN, Deljou A, Weingarten TN, et al. Perioperative opioid requirements of patients receiving sublingual buprenorphine-naloxone: a case series. BMC Anesthesiol 2019;19(1):68.

39. Jonan AB, Kaye AD, Urman RD. Buprenorphine formulations: clinical best practice strategies recommendations for perioperative management of patients undergoing surgical or interventional pain procedures. Pain Physician 2018;21(1): e1–12.

40. Greenwald MK, Comer SD, Fiellin DA. Buprenorphine maintenance and mu-opioid receptor availability in the treatment of opioid use disorder: implications for clinical use and policy. Drug Alcohol Depend 2014;144:1–11.

41. Greenwald MK, Johanson CE, Moody DE, et al. Effects of buprenorphine maintenance dose on mu-opioid receptor availability, plasma concentrations, and antagonist blockade in heroin-dependent volunteers. Neuropsychopharmacology 2003;28(11):2000–9.

42. Greenwald M, Johanson C-E, Bueller J, et al. Buprenorphine duration of action: mu-opioid receptor availability and pharmacokinetic and behavioral indices. Biol Psychiatry 2007;61(1):101–10.

43. Chou R, Gordon DB, de Leon-Casasola OA, et al. Management of postoperative pain: a clinical practice guideline from the American Pain Society, the American

Society of Regional Anesthesia and Pain Medicine, and the American Society of Anesthesiologists' Committee on Regional Anesthesia, Executive Committee, and Administrative Council. J pain 2016;17(2):131–57.

44. Derry CJ, Derry S, Moore RA. Single dose oral ibuprofen plus paracetamol (acetaminophen) for acute postoperative pain. Cochrane Database Syst Rev 2013; 2013(6):Cd010210.

45. Sanchez Munoz MC, De Kock M, Forget P. What is the place of clonidine in anesthesia? Systematic review and meta-analyses of randomized controlled trials. J Clin Anesth 2017;38:140–53.

46. Kharasch ED, Clark JD, Kheterpal S. Perioperative gabapentinoids: deflating the bubble. Anesthesiology 2020;133(2):251–4.

47. De Oliveira GS Jr, Almeida MD, Benzon HT, et al. Perioperative single dose systemic dexamethasone for postoperative pain: a meta-analysis of randomized controlled trials. Anesthesiology 2011;115(3):575–88.

48. Volpe DA, McMahon Tobin GA, Mellon RD, et al. Uniform assessment and ranking of opioid μ receptor binding constants for selected opioid drugs. Regul Toxicol Pharmacol 2011;59(3):385–90.

49. Laskowski K, Stirling A, McKay WP, et al. A systematic review of intravenous ketamine for postoperative analgesia. Can J Anaesth 2011;58(10):911–23.

50. Jouguelet-Lacoste J, La Colla L, Schilling D, et al. The use of intravenous infusion or single dose of low-dose ketamine for postoperative analgesia: a review of the current literature. Pain Med 2015;16(2):383–403.

51. Avidan MS, Maybrier HR, Abdallah AB, et al. Intraoperative ketamine for prevention of postoperative delirium or pain after major surgery in older adults: an international, multicentre, double-blind, randomised clinical trial. Lancet 2017; 390(10091):267–75.

52. Kranke P, Jokinen J, Pace NL, et al. Continuous intravenous perioperative lidocaine infusion for postoperative pain and recovery. Cochrane Database Syst Rev 2015;(7):Cd009642.

53. De Oliveira GS Jr, Castro-Alves LJ, Khan JH, et al. Perioperative systemic magnesium to minimize postoperative pain: a meta-analysis of randomized controlled trials. Anesthesiology 2013;119(1):178–90.

54. Ehde DM, Dillworth TM, Turner JA. Cognitive-behavioral therapy for individuals with chronic pain: efficacy, innovations, and directions for research. Am Psychol 2014;69(2):153–66.

55. Nicholls JL, Azam MA, Burns LC, et al. Psychological treatments for the management of postsurgical pain: a systematic review of randomized controlled trials. Patient Relat Outcome Meas 2018;9:49–64.

56. Wang L, Chang Y, Kennedy SA, et al. Perioperative psychotherapy for persistent post-surgical pain and physical impairment: a meta-analysis of randomised trials. Br J Anaesth 2018;120(6):1304–14.

57. Dindo L, Zimmerman MB, Hadlandsmyth K, et al. Acceptance and commitment therapy for prevention of chronic postsurgical pain and opioid use in at-risk veterans: a pilot randomized controlled study. J Pain 2018;19(10):1211–21.

58. Garland EL, Baker AK, Larsen P, et al. Randomized controlled trial of brief mindfulness training and hypnotic suggestion for acute pain relief in the hospital setting. J Gen Intern Med 2017;32(10):1106–13.

59. Zhu Y, Feng Y, Peng L. Effect of transcutaneous electrical nerve stimulation for pain control after total knee arthroplasty: a systematic review and meta-analysis. J Rehabil Med 2017;49(9):700–4.

# Infectious Complications of Injection Drug Use

Laura R. Marks, MD, PhD[a],*, Nathanial S. Nolan, MD, MPH[a],
Stephen Y. Liang, MD, MPHS[a,b], Michael J. Durkin, MD, MPH[a],
Melissa B. Weimer, DO, MCR[c]

## KEYWORDS

- Endocarditis • Osteomyelitis • Harm reduction • Lipoglycopeptides
- Substance use disorder

## KEY POINTS

- Persons who inject drugs (PWIDs) are at increased risk of invasive bacterial and fungal infections.
- Hospitalizations for infectious complications of injection drug use (IDU) should prompt harm reduction education targeted toward the exposures and risk factors likely to have facilitated the entry of specific pathogens.
- With an increasing array of antimicrobial treatment options available, clinicians should make every attempt to ensure that PWIDs are provided with flexible antimicrobial options to complete infectious diseases treatment and achieve clinical cure.
- A presentation for one infectious complication of IDU should prompt comprehensive screening for other transmissible infections and immunization for vaccine-preventable diseases.

## INTRODUCTION

The opioid overdose epidemic is one of the leading causes of death in adults.[1] Its devastating effects have included not only a burgeoning overdose crisis but also multiple converging infectious diseases epidemics. The use of both opioids and other substances through intravenous (IV) administration places individuals at increased risks of infectious diseases ranging from invasive bacterial and fungal infections[2] to human immunodeficiency virus (HIV) and viral hepatitis.[2–5] In 2012, there were 530,000 opioid use disorder (OUD)-related hospitalizations in the United States (US), with $700 million in costs associated with OUD-related infections.[2] The scale of the crisis has continued to increase since that time, with hospitalizations for

[a] Division of Infectious Diseases, Washington University in St. Louis School of Medicine, Campus Box 8051, 4523 Clayton Avenue, St. Louis, MO 63110-1093, USA; [b] Division of Emergency Medicine, Washington University in St. Louis School of Medicine; [c] Program in Addiction Medicine, Department of Medicine, Yale School of Medicine, E.S. Harkness Memorial Building A, 367 Cedar Street, Suite 417A, New Haven, CT 06510, USA
* Corresponding author:
*E-mail address:* marks@wustl.edu

Med Clin N Am 106 (2022) 187–200
https://doi.org/10.1016/j.mcna.2021.08.006
0025-7125/22/© 2021 Elsevier Inc. All rights reserved.

medical.theclinics.com

injection drug use-related infective endocarditis (IDU-IE) increasing by as much as 12-fold from 2010 to 2015.[6] Deaths from IDU-IE alone are estimated to result in over 7,260,000 years of potential life lost over the next 10 years.[7] There have been high-profile injection-related HIV outbreaks,[5,8] and injection drug use (IDU) is now the most common risk factor for hepatitis C virus (HCV).[9] As this epidemic continues to grow, clinicians in all aspects of medical care are increasingly confronted with infectious complications of IDU. This review will describe the pathogenesis, clinical syndromes, epidemiology, and models of treatment for common infectious complications among persons who inject drugs (PWIDs).

## PATHOGENESIS OF INFECTIONS

Care of the hospitalized patient with an IDU-related infection should include a thorough history of substances used and preparation steps.[10] Many different drugs may be injected including heroin, fentanyl, cocaine, methamphetamine, ecstasy, ketamine, and phencyclidine. Preparation steps between drugs may differ, and influence the risk of development of different infectious syndromes. A careful substance use history may form the basis for (1) immediate medical care of the patient, (2) differential diagnosis of potential pathogens to target empiric antimicrobial therapy, and (3) discussion of harm reduction techniques.

Infectious complications of IDU can occur through several mechanisms (**Fig. 1**). Direct inoculation of pathogens into the bloodstream can occur if either the substances, preparation materials (cotton filter, water, acidification agents), or injection equipment (needles, syringes, cookers) are contaminated with infectious pathogens. Contaminated drugs are a well-described cause of infection with spore-forming bacteria.[11–13] Bacterial spores are resistant to heat and desiccation, and studies have cultured *Bacillus* spp and *Clostridium* spp from confiscated heroin supplies.[14,15] Outbreaks of toxin-mediated diseases resulting from spore-producing organisms can occur in clusters or sporadically.[13] Outbreaks resulting from direct contamination of

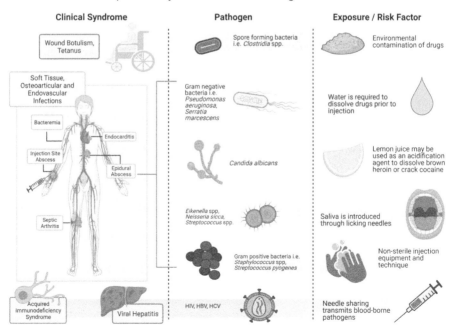

**Fig. 1.** Pathogenesis of injection drug use associated infections. Image created using BioRender©.

drugs have included large clusters of anthrax, tetanus, and *Clostridium* infections.[13] Lemon juice is often used as a solvent for brown heroin found commonly on the west coast of the US or crack cocaine and can support the growth of *Candida* species at room temperature.[16] The use of lemon juice in heroin preparation has been identified as a cause of disseminated candidiasis, infective endocarditis, osteomyelitis, and endophthalmitis in multiple case series.[17] Direct injury from injected substances can also predispose to endovascular infections. Injected particulate matter causes endothelial damage from repeated use which, when combined with infection from the direct inoculation of bacterial or fungal pathogens, leads to an increased risk of IDU-IE.[18]

Nonsterile injection technique increases the risk of injection site infection with skin flora including *Staphylococcus aureus,* coagulase-negative staphylococci, and *Streptococcus pyogenes.*[19,20] With limited access to clean injection spaces, some people may inject drugs in less sterile locations such as restrooms and other areas with a preponderance of gastrointestinal pathogens.[21] Nonsterile injection techniques in these areas may lead to the contamination and injection of pathogens such as *Escherichia coli, Enterobacter* species, and *Pseudomonas aeruginosa.* In some cases, saliva used to lubricate dull needles may lead to the direct inoculation of oral pathogens into the bloodstream.[22] Saliva may also come into contact with injection equipment when participants lick needles or other equipment to gauge the strength of the drug preparation.[23] Saliva contains several aerobic and anaerobic pathogens such as *Eikenella, Haemophilus, Prevotella,* and viridans group streptococci which cause bloodstream infections and associated endovascular and osteoarticular complications. For patients hospitalized with injection-related infections caused by these pathogens, it is crucial that clinicians adopt a harm-reduction approach which includes education on skin cleaning and the use of sterile equipment. PWIDs should discard any injection equipment that was used at sites with localized skin or soft tissue infections as *S. aureus* can remain viable on environmental surfaces for a prolonged period of time.[24]

The presence of residual blood in shared needles or works can allow for the transmission of blood-borne viral infections such as HIV, hepatitis B virus (HBV), or HCV.[2–4] Shared needles, syringes, or other paraphernalia propagate outbreaks of blood-borne pathogens within the IDU community.

Clinicians should be aware of these associations between specific pathogens and the most common risk factors for introduction during IDU to provide patients with harm reduction techniques appropriate to their current presentation (**Table 1**). Harm reduction counseling for PWIDs presenting with an acute infectious complication should focus on education about the mechanism of infection and discussion of methods to reduce the risk of recurrent infections in the future including the initiation of medication for opioid use disorder (MOUD) for patients with OUD. For many PWIDs, this may include the discussion of standard hygiene practices such as handwashing, disinfecting injection sites with alcohol, avoiding the introduction of saliva into the injection process, and referral to nearby needle exchange facilities whereby available. Providing harm reduction education interventions to reduce the development of IDU-related bacterial and fungal infections, and MOUD for patients with OUD may reduce the risk of drug-use-related mortality by greater than 90%, even among patients who cannot or are not interested in reducing their frequency of use.[7]

## CLINICAL SYNDROMES
### Skin and Soft Tissue Infections

The most frequently described infectious complication of IDU is skin and soft tissue infection, including abscess.[25,26] IDU-related infections are commonly caused by

**Table 1**
**Common pathogens and targeted harm reduction practices**

| Pathogen | Recommended Harm Reduction Practice |
|---|---|
| *Eikenella corrodens, Haemophilus parainfluenzae, Neisseria spp. Prevotella spp, Streptococcus spp.* | • Avoid introducing saliva into the injection process<br>• Avoid reuse of needles |
| *Staphylococcus spp, Streptococcus pyogenes,* | • Clean injection sites with alcohol swabs before injection<br>• Discard any used injection paraphernalia, particularly if materials were injected into a site with active infection |
| *Pseudomonas aeruginosa, Serratia marcescens,* | • Inquire about the use of tripelennamine and pentazocine.<br>• Encourage the use of sterile water |
| *Clostridia spp.* | • Provide tetanus vaccine/booster<br>• Avoid injecting into the muscle |
| *Candida spp.* | • Encourage the use of sterile acidification agents such as ascorbic acid (available at many needle exchange facilities) |
| Human Immunodeficiency Virus (HIV)<br>Hepatitis B virus (HBV)<br>Hepatitis C virus (HCV) | • Avoid sharing needles<br>• Link patients to nearest needle exchange facility<br>• Immunize against HBV if nonimmune<br>• Offer pre-exposure prophylaxis for HIV |

gram-positive organisms related to nonsterile injection techniques such as *S. aureus* and *Streptococcus* spp.[27] Empiric first-line antimicrobial therapy for skin and soft tissue infections among PWIDs should be primarily directed toward the coverage for methicillin-resistant *S. aureus* and *S. pyogenes* with the coverage of additional organisms as indicated by substance use history. However, clinicians should have a low threshold to broaden antimicrobial therapy in settings whereby patients are not responding to first-line antimicrobial regimens given higher risk of polymicrobial and gram-negative organisms among PWIDs.[27] Necrotizing fasciitis and toxic-shock syndromes may also occur and present with pain out of proportion to examination. Early recognition and surgical debridement with appropriate antimicrobial coverage are critical.

Clinicians should be aware of the increased risk of uncommon pathogens, particularly toxin-mediated infections caused by bacillus and clostridium species. The anaerobic environment provided by subcutaneous IDU or skin popping is a risk factor for toxin-mediated infections, particularly wound botulism and tetanus.[11,28] Patients infected with these pathogens will often present with systemic symptoms, dependent on the specific infecting pathogen. Wound botulism will appear several days after injecting drugs contaminated with *Clostridium botulinum* spores and causes diplopia and/or blurred vision, speech and/or swallowing difficulties, muscle weakness, and possible respiratory collapse.[29] Surgical debridement of the wound with adequate irrigation is critical to treatment accompanied by the prompt administration of antibiotics. In severe cases, early administration of antitoxin has been associated with improved outcomes.[30] Although uncommon in the general population, PWIDs are at increased risk for tetanus from the direct inoculation of contaminated drugs.[12,31] Tetanus presents with muscle spasms, often affecting the jaw muscles (ie, trismus) and autonomic instability. Tetanus is a vaccine-preventable illness and all PWIDs should be immunized.

## Osteoarticular Infections

Osteomyelitis and septic arthritis are important infectious complications among PWIDs. These infections generally start as a bloodstream infection with hematogenous seeding of distal sites in the axial skeleton. However, the absence of bacteremia at presentation does not exclude the possibility of an osteoarticular infection. The most common sites of osteoarticular infections among PWIDs include the spine, knees, and hips, although less common locations such as sternoclavicular, sacroiliac, and spinal facet joints are also observed.[32]

PWIDs are also at increased risk for spinal epidural abscess.[33] Epidural abscesses among PWIDs occur via hematogenous spread. *S. aureus* is the most common isolated organism, followed by other gram-positive cocci. However, gram-negative organisms such as *P. aeruginosa*, *Serratia marcescens*, and *E. coli* have also been described in PWIDs.[34] Treatment of osteoarticular infections including septic arthritis, osteomyelitis, and epidural abscesses require prolonged courses of antibiotics and may additionally require surgical debridement to achieve clinical cure.

## Endocarditis

One of the most serious infectious complications of IDU is the development of IE. In the US, IDU-IE now comprises almost 30% of overall IE cases.[35] IDU-IE should be considered a unique clinical entity given its distinct pathogenesis, microbiology, and patient demographics. Compared with non–IDU-IE, those who inject drugs and develop endocarditis are younger and have fewer comorbidities, such as congestive heart failure, hypertension, diabetes, and renal disease, though they are more likely to have viral-mediated liver disease.[35] Right-sided endocarditis is more common among PWIDs as peripheral venous blood encounters the tricuspid and pulmonic valves first on return to the heart and is more susceptible to damage from injected particulate matter and bacteria.[18] Clinicians caring for febrile PWIDs must maintain a high suspicion for IE, as classic signs and symptoms (eg, heart murmur, peripheral embolic phenomena) may be delayed or absent making the diagnosis of IDU-IE challenging.[36] Recent studies have highlighted the critical importance of incorporating substance use disorder treatment into IDU-IE care, including addiction medicine consultation and MOUD.[37,38]

## Viral Infections

Transmission of HIV and viral hepatitis outbreaks within IDU networks is well-described.[3–5,8] All PWIDs should receive routine screening for HIV, and be offered pre-exposure prophylaxis for HIV.[5] Screening for viral hepatitis should also be performed routinely and PWIDs should be immunized against HBV. Linkage to care for PWIDs diagnosed with HIV, HBV, or HCV should be initiated at the time of a positive test result. Importantly, neither a history of substance use nor current substance use should be considered a contraindication to treatment for HIV, HBV, or HCV. Although there has previously been reluctance among health care providers to initiate HCV treatment for PWIDs, guidelines from the American Association for the Study of Liver Diseases and the Infectious Diseases Society of America (IDSA) now recommend the consideration of HCV treatment within this population.[39] Studies show that PWIDs are motivated to complete treatment and successfully adhere to medication plans[40] and posttreatment re-infection rates among PWIDs low.[41]

## MODELS OF ANTIMICROBIAL TREATMENT

Models of treatment vary based on infection severity, surgical debridement, and patient factors. Skin and soft tissue infections can frequently be managed with short hospitalizations or outpatient treatment with oral antibiotics. Prolonged antimicrobial courses are generally required to treat osteoarticular and endovascular infections, which can present unique challenges. Clinicians should be aware of standard of care approaches to PWIDs with injection-related infections, but also be able to offer alternative antimicrobial options should patients decline the current standard of care treatment.[42–44]

For patients who elect not to continue standard antibiotic treatment regimens, clinicians are encouraged to offer an alternative option for infection treatment to prevent morbidity and mortality.[45] A patient-centered approach to this complex decision making has been described and has shown positive outcomes.[45,46] Additionally, for patients with OUD and injection-related infections, it is of the utmost importance that they are offered MOUD in addition to antimicrobial treatment. A summary of antimicrobial options is presented in **Table 2**.

### Intravenous Antibiotics

Current IDSA guidelines for both bacterial and fungal infections causing endocarditis, septic arthritis, epidural abscess, or osteomyelitis recommend IV antibiotics for a period of between 4 and 6 weeks.[47] Full details of antimicrobial regimens for specific conditions are delineated in professional guidelines and are generally not unique for PWIDs.[47] For patients without a history of substance use disorder, these antibiotic courses are typically completed at home or in skilled nursing facilities through outpatient parenteral antibiotic treatment (OPAT). However, most US health care facilities and home health agencies are reluctant to accept PWIDs into OPAT programs leading to treatment dilemmas for the practicing clinician.[48] As a result, the standard 4 to 6-week course of IV antibiotics for most PWIDs will necessarily be completed in a monitored setting such as a skilled nursing facility or an inpatient hospitalization. Although this treatment modality is well studied and considered the gold standard for infection management, this option presents particular challenges for many patients and represents a significant economic strain on the health care system. These hospitalizations result in longer lengths of stay and higher costs than non–PWIDs with similar infections.[49] Patients may be clinically stable and suitable for discharge (other than the need for continuing parenteral antibiotics) weeks before planned antimicrobial end dates. Prolonged hospitalization for patients with injection-related infection can be challenging. Clinicians are encouraged to offer supportive care, counseling, and other services to help patients tolerate prolonged hospitalization. Whenever possible, less restrictive environments such as skilled nursing facilities or OPAT via home infusion should be sought as safe alternatives. Clinicians are discouraged from applying punitive approaches such as visitor restrictions and mobility restrictions while patients are hospitalized. For all patients, evidence-based approaches to support patients' substance use disorder and mental health should be provided. As above, if patients decline prolonged hospitalization for parental antibiotics, they should be offered a safe alternative.

### Outpatient Parenteral Antibiotic Therapy

With high rates of noncompletion of IV antibiotic courses among PWIDs, there has been a renewed interest in treatment models for OPAT among PWIDs. A recent review by Suzuki and colleagues covered much of the available literature on the safety and efficacy of OPAT among PWIDs.[50] An important common theme among successful programs offering OPAT for PWIDs is the ability to reduce barriers, initiate, and link patients to ongoing outpatient substance use disorder care and medication treatments, and offer patient-centered discharge options to assist patients in completing antimicrobial therapy.[51] Jafari and colleagues evaluated a community model of OPAT care that

**Table 2**
**Antimicrobial strategies for endovascular and osteoarticular infections in PWIDs**

| Antimicrobial Strategy | Benefit | Challenges |
|---|---|---|
| Supervised parenteral antibiotics | • Allows for the completion of gold standard (prolonged course of intravenous antibiotics) as recommended by clinical guidelines.<br>• Supervised setting may limit the return to substance use. | • Requires patients to remain hospitalized or in a skilled nursing facility (SNF).<br>• Costly to the health care system and challenging for patients and health care teams.<br>• There is well-documented limited access to SNFs for PWIDs or who are treated with medication for OUD<br>• Some patients may leave before completing these antibiotic courses resulting in incomplete antimicrobial courses and high risks of hospital readmission. |
| Outpatient parenteral antibiotic therapy (OPAT) | • Allows for the completion of gold standard (prolonged course of intravenous antibiotics) as recommended by clinical guidelines.<br>• Allows patients to return home to resume social and work obligations. | • Risk of misuse and/or tampering with a peripherally inserted central catheter.<br>• Many home health agencies may have policies restricting the eligibility of PWIDs for OPAT programs.<br>• Patients with at-risk housing or homelessness may not have access to these programs. |
| Long-acting lipoglycopeptides | • Decreases the length of inpatient hospitalization.<br>• Medications administered in the hospital or clinic setting once per week.<br>• Patients do not need to take any medications at home (useful for patients with unstable housing) | • Limited outcomes data for both endovascular and osteoarticular infections in PWIDs.<br>• Medications are expensive and may not be covered by health insurance. |
| Partial oral antibiotic therapy | • Decreases the length of inpatient hospitalization.<br>• Medications can be taken by patients in any setting (useful for patients with unstable housing) | • Limited outcomes data with both endovascular and osteoarticular infections.<br>• Requires patient adherence to daily (or often twice daily) medication regimen |

*Abbreviation:* PWIDs, person who injects drugs.

provided a residence whereby patients could receive OPAT in a medically and socially supportive environment as an alternative to hospitalization.[52] This program allowed for mental health support staff to provide substance use counseling, along with wound care, medication management, and IV antimicrobial therapy.[52] Further supporting the importance of multidisciplinary care, the Improving Addiction Care Team (IMPACT) at Oregon Health Sciences University developed and implemented a novel tool for use at the multidisciplinary conference between infectious diseases and addiction medicine providers which systematically addressed the components of postdischarge care that may predict treatment success while emphasizing patient preference and harm reduction. Core areas emphasized include substance use history, home environment (access to electricity, phone, water, and refrigeration), access to postdischarge care, as well as different infectious diseases treatment options.[45] In a recent randomized clinical trial, patients with OUD who were treated with MOUD and outpatient parenteral antibiotic therapy (OPAT) showed high rates of treatment success. No participants in the OPAT arm (compared with the inpatient IV antibiotic arm) expressed any desire to inject into their PICC line and no participants in either group reported catheter misuse.[53] To address potential safety concerns surrounding the placement of peripherally inserted central catheter (PICC) lines in PWIDs discharged from health care facilities, Eaton and colleagues published a risk assessment which identifies PWIDs at low risk of ongoing substance use while receiving antibiotics by focusing on 9 factors such as cravings, home environment, dual psychiatric diagnoses, history of overdose, relapse, trauma, use of multiple drugs, family history of addiction, and willingness to change.[46] Evidence suggests that high rates of treatment success can also be achieved in patients with adequate housing, a reliable support person, and willingness to adhere to appropriate IV catheter use.[44]

### Long-Acting Lipoglycopeptides

Lipoglycopeptides are promising alternatives to traditional OPAT. These agents allow patients to receive a therapeutic level of antibiotics for weeks after a single IV infusion.[54] The 2 commercially available drugs, dalbavancin and oritavancin, are based on the chemical structure of vancomycin.[55] These drugs should only be used for gram-positive infections, particularly *S. aureus*. At the time of publication, both of these agents only have US Food and Drug Administration approval for the treatment of complex acute bacterial skin and skin structure infections. However, there is an emerging area of research demonstrating successful off-label use for IDU associated infections, including IDU-IE.[56–58] More research is needed in this area as this remains the largest barrier to their routine use in clinical practice.

### Transitions to Oral Antibiotics

The use of oral antibiotics as an alternative to IV antibiotics and long-acting lipoglycopeptides is an active area of research. Three randomized clinical trials in infective endocarditis have demonstrated that oral step-down therapy is at least as effective as IV antimicrobial therapy in right-sided, left-sided, or prosthetic valve IE.[59–61] A recent large multicenter prospective study found that among patients who have had source control, step down to oral therapy was noninferior to IV antibiotics for osteomyelitis.[62] While neither trials were focused on the PWIDs population, a recent retrospective study demonstrated similar outcomes for PWIDs.[63] Combined with multiple observational studies evaluating the effectiveness of oral antibiotics for treating IE (typically after an initial course of IV therapy), this body of evidence demonstrates the therapeutic effectiveness of oral step-down therapy for patients who have achieved clinical stability with IV regimens.[64]

**Table 3**
**Recommendations for comprehensive care of PWIDs admitted with IDU-related infections**

| | Recommendations |
|---|---|
| **Screening Tests** | |
| Human Immunodeficiency Virus (HIV) | HIV ½ Ab + P24 Ag at initial visit, screen every 3 mo if ongoing substance use. |
| Hepatitis B Virus (HBV) | HBV surface Ag at initial visit. Evaluate immunity with HBV surface antibody and core antibody. Immunize if nonimmune. Link patients with active HBV to infectious diseases care. |
| Hepatitis C Virus (HCV) | HCV Ab at initial visit. If positive, obtain HCV RNA and link to HCV treatment for viremic patients. |
| Syphilis | RPR or T pallidum (as determined by hospital syphilis algorithm testing protocols) should be assessed at initial visit. Additional testing as indicated by sexual health history. |
| Gonorrhea and Chlamydia | Gonorrhea and chlamydia nucleic acid amplification testing (urine) at initial visit. Additional testing (throat and rectum) can be considered based on sexual health history. Consider testing for other infections such as Trichomonas, bacterial vaginosis |
| Tuberculosis | Assess for latent infection at initial visit with periodic rescreening based on individual risk. |
| **Immunizations and Preventative Health Care** | |
| Pre-exposure Prophylaxis (PrEP) for HIV | All PWIDs are eligible for PrEP. Uninsured PWIDs can access PrEP through the US Department of Health and Human Services' "Ready, Set, PrEP" program |
| Hepatitis A and B | Immunize all PWIDs against hepatitis A and B |
| Influenza | Offer yearly |
| SARS-CoV-2 (COVID-19) | Assist patients with signing up for COVID-19 immunizations if eligible under local regulations |
| Tetanus | Immunize at initial visit and then every 10 y, or every 5 y for patients with necrotizing skin and soft tissue infections |
| **Substance Use Disorder Interventions** | |
| Overdose Education | Provide take-home naloxone and education on opioid overdose prevention |
| Harm Reduction Counseling | Educate on safer injection techniques including cleaning injection sites, use of sterile works, and location of needle exchange facilities |
| Offer medications for opioid use disorder (MOUD) | All PWIDs with opioid use disorder should offer initiation of MOUD (methadone, intramuscular naltrexone, or buprenorphine) and linkage to ongoing outpatient care |

*Abbreviations:* IDU, injection drug use; PWIDs, persons who inject drugs; RPR, rapid plasma reagin.

Oral antibiotic therapy avoids the need for long hospital admissions and the requirement for prolonged IV access, with both its concurrent risks of infection and potential for misuse. Administration of oral therapy, however, comes with the requirement for excellent patient adherence. Ideally, oral treatment could be administered with close monitoring and follow-up programs similar to OPAT programs that have been established for non–PWIDs with endocarditis or osteomyelitis. Although optimal oral regimens for PWIDs with invasive bacterial and fungal infections are not fully established, and there are limited data on the treatment of invasive MRSA IDU-IE, it is clear that providing antibiotics to PWIDs who leave the hospital prematurely improve patient outcomes than no antibiotics.[63]

## RECOMMENDED TESTING AND INTERVENTIONS FOR PATIENTS WHO PRESENT WITH INFECTIOUS COMPLICATIONS OF INJECTION DRUG USE

A hospital presentation for the evaluation of an IDU-related bacterial or fungal infection represents a critical opportunity to screen for potential cotransmitted infections, as well as to engage PWIDs with substance use disorder care. Hospitalization has been described as a "reachable moment" and can be transformative for some patients when their acute medical care is paired with highly effective treatments for their substance use disorders.[65] All patients who are hospitalized for an injection-related infection should be offered these evidence-based SUD treatments while hospitalized and transitioned to ongoing treatment. For many PWIDs who have limited access to routine preventative medical care, this interaction with the health care system may also represent the only opportunity for preventative health care measures such as immunizations. A comprehensive list of testing and care measures recommended for PWIDs presenting with IDU-related infections is outlined in **Table 3**.

## SUMMARY

Infectious complications of IDU represent some of the most common reasons for presentation to medical attention for PWIDs. Identification of an underlying substance use disorder is a critical first step in addressing both the acute infection, preventing future complications, and reducing mortality. Harm reduction efforts should be tailored to a patient's substance use practices to prevent future infectious complications. With an increasing array of antimicrobial treatment options available, clinicians should make every attempt to ensure that PWIDs are provided with flexible antimicrobial options to complete infectious diseases treatment and achieve clinical cure. Clinicians should be attuned to the unique risks for comorbid infections among PWIDs and prepared to offer comprehensive screening, as well as the initiation of substance use disorder treatment and linkage to outpatient treatment resources.

## CLINICS CARE POINTS

- Patients with injection drug use related infections may have difficulty accessing or completing prolonged courses of IV antibiotics. Alternative strategies including partial oral antibiotics or long acting lipoglycopeptides should always be offered if patients are not able to complete a standardized course of guideline directed IV antibiotics.

- A hospitalization for an infectious complication of substance use is an important opportunity to screen for other communicable diseases and link patients to treatment.

## DISCLOSURE

Dr M. Weimer has an advisory role with Path CCM, Inc. that does not pertain to the current work.

## REFERENCES

1. Prevention CfDCa. National Vital statistics system - drug overdose deaths.. 2017. Available at: https://www.cdc.gov/nchs/nvss/drug-overdose-deaths.htm. Accessed January 25, 2021.
2. Ronan MV, Herzig SJ. Hospitalizations related to opioid abuse/dependence and associated serious infections increased sharply, 2002-12. Health Aff (Millwood) 2016;35(5):832–7.
3. Massachusetts Department of Public Health. CDC joins Department of Public Health in investigating HIV cluster among people who inject drugs. 2018. Available at: https://www.mass.gov/news/cdc-joins-department-of-public-health-in-investigating-hiv-cluster-among-people-who-inject. Accessed January 20, 2021.
4. Northern Kentucky Health Department. As HIV cluster investigation moves into second month, health officials increase opportunities for HIV testing. 2018. Available at: https://nkyhealth.org/2018/02/22/as-hiv-cluster-investigation-moves-into-second-month-health-officials-increase-opportunities-for-hiv-testing/. Accessed January 18, 2021.
5. Centers for Disease Control and Prevention HAN. Recent HIV clusters and outbreaks across the United States among people who inject drugs and considerations during the COVID-19 pandemic-CDCHAN-00436. 2020. Available at: https://emergency.cdc.gov/han/2020/han00436.asp. Accessed Accessed 1/18/2021.
6. Fleischauer AT, Ruhl L, Rhea S, et al. Hospitalizations for endocarditis and associated health care costs among persons with diagnosed drug dependence - North Carolina, 2010-2015. MMWR Morb Mortal Wkly Rep 2017;66(22):569–73.
7. Barocas JA, Eftekhari Yazdi G, Savinkina A, et al. Long-term infective endocarditis mortality associated with injection opioid use in the United States: a modeling study. Clin Infect Dis 2020.
8. Alpren C, Dawson EL, John B, et al. Opioid use fueling HIV transmission in an urban setting: an outbreak of hiv infection among people who inject drugs-Massachusetts, 2015-2018. Am J Public Health 2020;110(1):37–44.
9. Hagan H, Pouget ER, Des Jarlais DC. A systematic review and meta-analysis of interventions to prevent hepatitis C virus infection in people who inject drugs. J Infect Dis 2011;204(1):74–83.
10. Seval N, Eaton E, Springer SA. Beyond antibiotics: a practical guide for the infectious disease physician to treat opioid use disorder in the setting of associated infectious diseases. Open Forum Infect Dis 2020;7(1):ofz539.
11. Peak CM, Rosen H, Kamali A, et al. Wound botulism outbreak among persons who use black Tar Heroin — San Diego County, California, 2017–2018. MMWR Morb Mortal Wkly Rep 2019;67:1415–8.
12. Centers for Disease C, Prevention. Tetanus among injecting-drug users–California, 1997. MMWR Morb Mortal Wkly Rep 1998;47(8):149–51.
13. Palmateer NE, Hope VD, Roy K, et al. Infections with spore-forming bacteria in persons who inject drugs, 2000-2009. Emerg Infect Dis 2013;19(1):29–34.
14. Benusic MA, Press NM, Hoang LM, et al. A cluster of Bacillus cereus bacteremia cases among injection drug users. Can J Infect Dis Med Microbiol 2015;26(2):103–4.

15. Mc LJ, Mithani V, Bolton FJ, et al. An investigation into the microflora of heroin. J Med Microbiol 2002;51(11):1001–8.
16. Collignon PJ, Sorrell TC. Disseminated candidiasis: evidence of a distinctive syndrome in heroin abusers. Br Med J (Clin Res Ed) 1983;287(6396):861–2.
17. Bisbe J, Miro JM, Latorre X, et al. Disseminated candidiasis in addicts who use brown heroin: report of 83 cases and review. Clin Infect Dis 1992;15(6):910–23.
18. Wurcel AG, Anderson JE, Chui KK, et al. Increasing infectious endocarditis admissions among young people who inject drugs. Open Forum Infect Dis 2016; 3(3):ofw157.
19. Phillips KT, Anderson BJ, Herman DS, et al. Risk factors associated with skin and soft tissue infections among hospitalized people who inject drugs. J Addict Med 2017;11(6):461–7.
20. Murphy EL, DeVita D, Liu H, et al. Risk factors for skin and soft-tissue abscesses among injection drug users: a case-control study. Clin Infect Dis 2001;33(1): 35–40.
21. Adamson K, Jackson L, Gahagan J. Young people and injection drug use: is there a need to expand harm reduction services and support? Int J Drug Policy 2017;39:14–20.
22. Kannangara DP, Dhyanesh. Infections in injection drug users: the significance of oral bacteria and a comparison with bacteria originating from skin and environmental sources. Drug Drug Abuse 2020;1–5.
23. Oh S, Havlen PR, Hussain N. A case of polymicrobial endocarditis caused by anaerobic organisms in an injection drug user. J Gen Intern Med 2005; 20(10):C1–2.
24. Desai R, Pannaraj PS, Agopian J, et al. Survival and transmission of community-associated methicillin-resistant Staphylococcus aureus from fomites. Am J Infect Control 2011;39(3):219–25.
25. Larney S, Peacock A, Mathers BM, et al. A systematic review of injecting-related injury and disease among people who inject drugs. Drug Alcohol Depend 2017; 171:39–49.
26. See I, Gokhale RH, Geller A, et al. National public health burden estimates of endocarditis and skin and soft-tissue infections related to injection drug use: a review. J Infect Dis 2020;222(Suppl 5):S429–36.
27. Jenkins TC, Knepper BC, Jason Moore S, et al. Microbiology and initial antibiotic therapy for injection drug users and non-injection drug users with cutaneous abscesses in the era of community-associated methicillin-resistant Staphylococcus aureus. Acad Emerg Med 2015;22(8):993–7.
28. Passaro DJ, Werner SB, McGee J, et al. Wound botulism associated with black tar heroin among injecting drug users. JAMA 1998;279(11):859–63.
29. Yuan J, Inami G, Mohle-Boetani J, et al. Recurrent wound botulism among injection drug users in California. Clin Infect Dis 2011;52(7):862–6.
30. Sandrock CE, Murin S. Clinical predictors of respiratory failure and long-term outcome in black tar heroin-associated wound botulism. Chest 2001;120(2): 562–6.
31. Hahné S, White JM, Crowcroft NS, et al. Tetanus in injecting drug users, United Kingdom. Emerging Infect Dis 2006;12(4):709–10.
32. Ross JJ, Ard KL, Carlile N. Septic arthritis and the opioid epidemic: 1465 cases of culture-positive native joint septic arthritis from 1990-2018. Open Forum Infect Dis 2020;7(3):ofaa089.
33. Reihsaus E, Waldbaur H, Seeling W. Spinal epidural abscess: a meta-analysis of 915 patients. Neurosurg Rev 2000;23(4):175–204 [discussion 205].

34. Ziu M, Dengler B, Cordell D, et al. Diagnosis and management of primary pyogenic spinal infections in intravenous recreational drug users. Neurosurg Focus 2014;37(2):E3.

35. Rudasill SE, Sanaiha Y, Mardock AL, et al. Clinical outcomes of infective endocarditis in injection drug users. J Am Coll Cardiol 2019;73(5):559–70.

36. Weisse AB, Heller DR, Schimenti RJ, et al. The febrile parenteral drug user: a prospective study in 121 patients. Am J Med 1993;94(3):274–80.

37. Kimmel SD, Walley AY, Li Y, et al. Association of Treatment with medications for opioid use disorder with mortality after hospitalization for injection drug use–associated infective endocarditis. JAMA Netw Open 2020;3(10):e2016228.

38. Marks LR, Munigala S, Warren DK, et al. Addiction medicine consultations reduce readmission rates for patients with serious infections from opioid use disorder. Clin Infect Dis 2019;68(11):1935–7.

39. Ghany MG, Morgan TR, Panel A. Hepatitis C guidance 2019 update: American Association for the Study of Liver Diseases–infectious diseases society of America recommendations for testing, managing, and treating hepatitis C virus infection. Hepatology 2020;71(2):686–721.

40. Norton BL, Fleming J, Bachhuber MA, et al. High HCV cure rates for people who use drugs treated with direct acting antiviral therapy at an urban primary care clinic. Int J Drug Policy 2017;47:196–201.

41. Grady BP, Schinkel J, Thomas XV, et al. Hepatitis C virus reinfection following treatment among people who use drugs. Clin Infect Dis 2013;57(Suppl 2): S105–10.

42. Beieler AM, Dellit TH, Chan JD, et al. Successful implementation of outpatient parenteral antimicrobial therapy at a medical respite facility for homeless patients. J Hosp Med 2016;11(8):531–5.

43. Beieler A, Magaret A, Zhou Y, et al. Outpatient parenteral antimicrobial therapy in vulnerable populations– people who inject drugs and the homeless. J Hosp Med 2019;14(2):105–9.

44. Ho J, Archuleta S, Sulaiman Z, et al. Safe and successful treatment of intravenous drug users with a peripherally inserted central catheter in an outpatient parenteral antibiotic treatment service. J Antimicrob Chemother 2010;65(12):2641–4.

45. Strnad L, Douglass A, Young K, et al. 742. The development, implementation, and feasibility of multidisciplinary treatment planning conference for individuals with unstable substance use disorders and active infections requiring prolonged antimicrobial therapy: the OPTIONS-DC model. Open Forum Infect Dis 2019; 6(Supplement_2):S331–2.

46. Eaton EF, Mathews RE, Lane PS, et al. A 9-point risk assessment for patients who inject drugs and require intravenous antibiotics: focusing inpatient resources on patients at greatest risk of ongoing drug use. Clin Infect Dis 2019;68(6):1041–3.

47. Baddour LM, Wilson WR, Bayer AS, et al. Infective endocarditis in adults: diagnosis, antimicrobial therapy, and management of complications: a scientific statement for healthcare professionals from the American Heart Association. Circulation 2015;132(15):1435–86.

48. Rapoport AB, Fischer LS, Santibanez S, et al. Infectious diseases physicians' perspectives regarding injection drug use and related infections, United States, 2017. Open Forum Infect Dis 2018;5(7):ofy132.

49. Rapoport AB, Fine DR, Manne-Goehler JM, et al. High inpatient health care utilization and charges associated with injection drug use–related infections: a cohort study, 2012–2015. Open Forum Infect Dis 2021;8(3):ofab009.

50. Suzuki J, Johnson J, Montgomery M, et al. Outpatient parenteral antimicrobial therapy among people who inject drugs: a review of the literature. Open Forum Infect Dis 2018;5(9):ofy194.

51. Hurley H, Sikka M, Jenkins T, et al. Outpatient antimicrobial treatment for people who inject drugs. Infect Dis Clin North Am 2020;34(3):525–38.

52. Jafari SJR, Elliot D, Nagji A, et al. A community care model of intravenous antibiotic therapy for injection drug users with deep tissue infection for "Reduce Leaving Against Medical Advice". Int J Ment Heal Addict 2015;13:49–58.

53. Fanucchi LC, Walsh SL, Thornton AC, et al. Outpatient parenteral antimicrobial therapy plus buprenorphine for opioid use disorder and severe injection-related Infections. Clin Infect Dis 2020;70(6):1226–9.

54. Dunne MW, Puttagunta S, Sprenger CR, et al. Extended-duration dosing and distribution of dalbavancin into bone and articular tissue. Antimicrob Agents Chemother 2015;59(4):1849–55.

55. Brade KD, Rybak JM, Rybak MJ. Oritavancin: a new lipoglycopeptide antibiotic in the treatment of gram-positive infections. Infect Dis Ther 2016;5(1):1–15.

56. Morrisette T, Miller MA, Montague BT, et al. Long-acting lipoglycopeptides: "Lineless Antibiotics" for serious infections in persons who use drugs. Open Forum Infect Dis 2019;6(7):ofz274.

57. Krsak M, Morrisette T, Miller M, et al. Advantages of outpatient treatment with long-acting lipoglycopeptides for serious gram-positive infections: a review. Pharmacotherapy 2020;40(5):469–78.

58. Tobudic S, Forstner C, Burgmann H, et al. Dalbavancin as primary and sequential treatment for gram-positive infective endocarditis: 2-year experience at the general hospital of Vienna. Clin Infect Dis 2018;67(5):795–8.

59. Heldman AW, Hartert TV, Ray SC, et al. Oral antibiotic treatment of right-sided staphylococcal endocarditis in injection drug users: prospective randomized comparison with parenteral therapy. Am J Med 1996;101(1):68–76.

60. Iversen K, Ihlemann N, Gill SU, et al. Partial oral versus intravenous antibiotic treatment of endocarditis. N Engl J Med 2019;380(5):415–24.

61. Stamboulian D, Bonvehi P, Arevalo C, et al. Antibiotic management of outpatients with endocarditis due to penicillin-susceptible streptococci. Rev Infect Dis 1991; 13(Suppl 2):S160–3.

62. Li H-K, Rombach I, Zambellas R, et al. Oral versus intravenous antibiotics for bone and joint infection. N Engl J Med 2019;380(5):425–36.

63. Marks LR, Liang SY, Muthulingam D, et al. Evaluation of partial oral antibiotic treatment for persons who inject drugs and are hospitalized with invasive infections. Clin Infect Dis 2020;71(10):e650–6.

64. Spellberg B, Chambers HF, Musher DM, et al. Evaluation of a paradigm shift from intravenous antibiotics to oral step-down therapy for the treatment of infective endocarditis: a narrative review. JAMA Intern Med 2020;180(5):769–77.

65. Englander H, Weimer M, Solotaroff R, et al. Planning and designing the improving addiction care team (IMPACT) for hospitalized adults with substance use disorder. J Hosp Med 2017;12(5):339–42.

# Harm Reduction in Health Care Settings

Carolyn A. Chan, MD[a], Bethany Canver, MD[b], Ryan McNeil, PhD[c],
Kimberly L. Sue, MD, PhD[d],*

## KEYWORDS

- Harm reduction • Substance use • Substance-related disorders • Addiction
- Substance use disorder • Drug overdose • Opioids • Opioid-related disorders

## KEY POINTS

- Harm reduction is an approach to reduce the risk of harms to an individual using substances without requiring abstinence.
- Infection prevention for individuals who use drugs may include counseling, providing resources for safer injection practices, and offering preexposure prophylaxis.
- Naloxone and fentanyl test strips can be strategies used to prevent opioid overdoses.

## INTRODUCTION TO HARM REDUCTION

Harm reduction (HR) in health care settings is a patient-centered approach to reduce the negative health, social, and economic impact of substance use without requiring abstinence.[1] This goal can be achieved through health interventions (eg, syringe exchange), as well as through practical individual strategies (eg, never using substances alone). For clinicians, HR principles help inform our approach to caring for patients who use substances by meeting individuals "where they are at" (**Fig. 1**).

Furthermore, it requires that health care providers express compassion and respect, and use shared decision making for individuals who may continue to use substances, have episodes of drug use reinitiation, or do not seek abstinence as the goal in their interactions with health services. Rather than ignoring substance use or

The authors have nothing to disclose.
[a] Program in Addiction Medicine, Section of General Internal Medicine, Department of Medicine, 367 Cedar Street, Harkness Hall A Suite – Suite 305, New Haven, CT 06510, USA; [b] Section of General Internal Medicine, Department of Medicine, 367 Cedar Street, Harkness Hall A Suite – Suite 305, New Haven, CT 06510, USA; [c] Program in Addiction Medicine, Section of General Internal Medicine, Department of Medicine, 367 Cedar Street, Harkness Hall A, New Haven, CT 06510, USA; [d] Program in Addiction Medicine, Section of General Internal Medicine, Department of Medicine, 367 Cedar Street, Harkness Hall A Suite – Suite 417A, New Haven, CT 06510, USA
* Corresponding author.
*E-mail address:* Kimberly.sue@yale.edu

Med Clin N Am 106 (2022) 201–217
https://doi.org/10.1016/j.mcna.2021.09.002
0025-7125/22/© 2021 Elsevier Inc. All rights reserved.

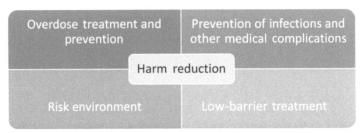

| Overdose treatment and prevention | Prevention of infections and other medical complications |
| --- | --- |
| Harm reduction | |
| Risk environment | Low-barrier treatment |

**Fig. 1.** A variety of approaches can be used to reduce substance-related harm. This figure outlines overarching topics clinicians can address with their patients, including low-barrier treatment, which includes same-day initiation of MOUD, not requiring abstinence to engage in addiction treatment, as well as treating other underlying psychiatric or medical comorbidities.

implementing punitive approaches, the goal is to work with individuals to minimize harms related to substance use. This review discusses substance-specific interventions to lessen harms for individuals who use drugs.

## PATIENT PERSPECTIVES

Understanding the lived experiences of persons who use drugs (PWUD) within health care systems is necessary to engage patients and deliver care that meets their personalized treatment goals. PWUD have described experiences within the hospital, outpatient settings, and across the treatment care cascade including negative interactions with staff and discrimination in care compared with individuals with no substance use[2–4]; particularly persons of color with substance use disorder (SUD) have faced additional forms of discrimination.[5] Furthermore, individuals have reported large barriers to accessing addiction treatment due to cost, lack of insurance coverage, long wait lists, stigma, and distance to clinic.[6] Individuals who have an SUD have a high prevalence of leaving the hospital prematurely (discharge against medical advice).[7] Patient-reported motives leading to premature discharges included negative interactions with hospital staff (including security guards), hospital restrictions regarding substance use, inadequate analgesia, and/or substance withdrawal management, which were further compounded among patients also affected by racial discrimination.[3,8] Health care systems can address these concerns by implementing HR policies aligned with the needs of PWUD, training staff in regard to structural competency and cultural safety, having adequate pain and substance withdrawal management, as well as offering flexible treatment options to patients.[9]

## OPIOID USE

Fentanyl has become the most commonly detected substance in drug-related overdoses in the United States, indicating that illicit fentanyl and fentanyl analogues (FFA) are a key driver in the increase in opioid overdoses.[10] The short half-life of fentanyl may lead to an increased frequency of injections, and thus an increased chance of syringe sharing practices[11]; this consequently places individuals at a higher risk of infectious disease transmissions.[11] Furthermore, there has been an increase in hospital admissions due to injection-related infections (eg, endocarditis, osteomyelitis, soft tissue infections).[12] Whether PWUD are interested in abstinence or not, interactions with the health care system in all clinical settings are an opportunity to build therapeutic relationships with patients, provide education on safe drug use practice, treat substance withdrawal and use disorders, and ultimately reduce opioid-related harms. Practical information on how this can be applied in health care settings is discussed in the next section.

## INFECTION PREVENTION
### Route of Administration

There are various routes of delivery for opioids such as oral, intranasal, injection, rectal, and inhalation among PWUD. Injecting is considered the least safe route of use and is associated with higher rates of blood-borne infections such as hepatitis C (HCV), hepatitis B (HBV), human immunodeficiency virus (HIV), skin and soft tissue infections (SSTI), and endocarditis when compared with noninjection routes of administration.[13,14] Although this section on infection prevention focuses on opioids, it is important to acknowledge that other substances also have various routes of delivery and that the same overarching principles apply. In addition, injection of heroin increases the risk of both fatal and nonfatal overdoses when compared with consuming heroin via intranasal route or inhalation (often heroin or fentanyl can be smoked).[15] Clinicians can counsel patients on safer substance use by discussing with patients that oral, intranasal, and inhalation routes have risks, but are less likely to cause infections or overdoses when compared with injection.

### Injection-Related Practices

Injecting drugs is a multistep process, and clinicians should be knowledgeable on safer injection practices to counsel their patients on approaches to decrease their risk of infections. Peer educators, defined as individuals with lived experience using substances, or who share other common characteristics/experiences with the person they are educating, may be another option if clinicians are not comfortable providing this counseling. We review existing evidence surrounding components of injection-related practices and discuss methods to minimize harms of injection drug use (**Table 1**). When discharging patients from the hospital, or caring for them in the ambulatory setting, we recommend providing PWUD with HR kits that include items outlined in **Fig. 2**.

Drug preparation for injection is variable and depends on multiple factors such as the drug used (eg, black tar heroin commonly found on the west coast of the United States, powdered heroin commonly found on the east coast of the United States, fentanyl, crushed oxycodone) and equipment available. Often, the preparation of drug injections involves the following items: substance, object to mix/heat solutions (cooker), needle, syringe, heat source, water, and occasionally an acidifier like citric acid or ascorbic acid to make substances more soluble for injection use (eg, brown heroin found in Europe or crack cocaine require an acidifier to dissolve substances for injection purposes).[16]

### Injecting conditions

Individuals use drugs in a variety of complex physical, social, economic, and policy circumstances, which can shape harms, also known as a *risk environment*.[17] Harm can be reduced by addressing an individual's environmental circumstances.[18] For example, an individual who is unhoused may lack access to sterile water to dissolve substances, have inadequate syringe access, or experience intimate partner violence that drives unsafe injection practices. We recommend clinicians refer patients to social workers, peer workers, and community resources to reduce the harms related with structural inequities of substance use.

**Table 1**
**Summary of safer injection-related practices and supplies to discuss and personalize for people who inject drugs**

| | Safer Injection-Related Supplies and Practices |
|---|---|
| Sterile equipment | Gold standard: use a new sterile needle and syringe every injection<br>If reusing equipment, clean with undiluted bleach as follows[19]:<br>1. Fill syringe with clean water, shake for 30 s, discard water from syringe<br>2. Fill syringe with bleach, shake for 30 s, discard bleach from syringe<br>3. Fill syringe with clean water, shake for 30 s, discard water from syringe |
| Syringe size | U-100 insulin syringes (0.5 mL–1.0 mL)<br>Tuberculin syringes |
| Needles | Smaller needle gauges (higher number gauge) are preferred because they create a smaller puncture wound and thus a lower infection risk<br>• Needle gauge for IV: 27G or 28G<br>• Needle gauge for IM: 21G or 23G (requires larger gauge needle)<br>Needle length: 1/2 inch (12 mm) or 5/16 inch (8 mm) |
| Cookers and heat | Do not share cookers with others<br>Heat a substance until bubbles form to decrease bacterial and fungal burden |
| Filters | Single-use filters to remove particulates<br>Commercially produced "wheel" filters are preferred and can be purchased online without a prescription or found at local harm reduction agencies<br>Single-use cotton balls when "wheel" filters unavailable |
| Dissolving substances | Use a sterile water supply<br>If not available, use boiled water, bottled or tap water<br>Use a minimal amount of acidifier to decrease risk of venous sclerosis<br>Ascorbic acid (vitamin C) is the preferred acidifier over citric acid, fruit juices, and vinegar |
| Skin cleaning | Disinfect skin with alcohol, soap and water, or iodine before every injection |
| FTS | Test drugs before use (opioids and stimulants)<br>Counsel patients on risk of false-negatives |
| Naloxone and setting | Carry naloxone and never use alone<br>Leave naloxone in a visible location<br>Leave door unlocked<br>Use in location where one is comfortable and can take their time |
| Acidification | Ascorbic acid packets (vitamin C) |

*Abbreviations:* FTS, fentanyl test strips; IM, intramuscular; IV, intravenous.

### Needles/syringes

Encouraging PWUD to use their own sterile syringes and to use one needle for each injection episode is an optimal injection-related practice. Clinicians can prescribe sterile syringes and needles for their patients to pharmacies (see **Table 1**). When sterile equipment is not available, it is important to reduce harm by disinfecting equipment with undiluted bleach, followed by a rinse with clean water. This practice is recommended by Centers for Disease Control and Prevention (CDC) to inactivate HIV and HCV, thus decreasing the risk of these infections.[19] Notably, the World Health Organization does not recommend that syringe disinfection with bleach be used as a primary HIV

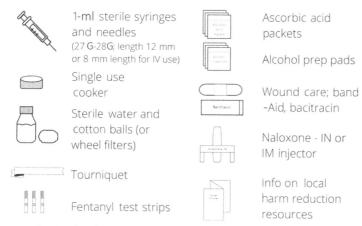

1-ml sterile syringes and needles
(27 G-28G; length 12 mm or 8 mm length for IV use)

Single use cooker

Sterile water and cotton balls (or wheel filters)

Tourniquet

Fentanyl test strips

Ascorbic acid packets

Alcohol prep pads

Wound care; band -Aid, bacitracin

Naloxone - IN or IM injector

Info on local harm reduction resources

**Fig. 2.** Harm reduction kits for injection drug use can be distributed to patients and contain a variety of items for safer substance use. Items that can be included as part of this kit are listed. Depending on local use patterns, ascorbic acid packets may not be applicable. Adding wound care agents should also be considered, such as gauze, topical bacitracin, and Band-Aid. IM, intramuscular; IN, intranasal; IV, intravenous.

prevention strategy, unless syringe exchange programs are inaccessible, due to the lack of evidence of real-world effectiveness.[20] We encourage clinicians to counsel PWUD on the use of a sterile needle/syringe for every injection, but if that is not an option, using bleach as disinfectant to clean needles/syringes can be used as an HR strategy.

Licking needles before injecting drugs is common among people who inject drugs (PWID), and this practice can increase the risk of obtaining SSTIs.[21] Cases of endocarditis and osteomyelitis caused by *Eikenella corrodens,* a bacterium found in human oropharyngeal mucosa among PWID, suggest that this practice can introduce bacteria into the bloodstream.[22] Clinicians should screen and counsel patients against this practice, particularly individuals who are presenting for an SSTI, osteomyelitis, or infective endocarditis.

### Cookers and cooking

PWID should use their own sterile cooking equipment and not share it with others because it may increase their personal risk of acquiring HIV or HCV.[23,24] We recommend the use of sterile commercially produced single-use spoons with handles (eg, Stericups) designed for the preparation of drugs for injection. If those are unavailable a stainless-steel spoon (avoids rust) cleaned after every use with bleach that has depth similar to a ladle spoon to minimize the risk of spilling is another option, although less desirable. Patients who may use bottles caps should be counseled to remove any disposable lining before mixing the substances.

Commonly used techniques to dissolve substances include "hot" and "cold" cooking, each of these methods having their own risk and benefits. "Hot cooking" involves the addition of heat to dissolve the substance. Some evidence exists that heating the drug until bubbles form before aspirating the solution inactivates HIV and decreases the number of existing bacteria in solution.[24,25] A notable harm with hot cooking is that dissolving oral formulations such as pills that contain additives (eg, wax) will be challenging to melt and cause harm through injecting. "Cold cooking" does not add heat to dissolve the substances, and for individuals injecting tablets the benefit is that the fillers/coating will not dissolve and be introduced into the blood vessel, although this method will not reduce bacteria or *Candida*. Providers should counsel patients on the risks of each method, and tailor HR advice to the particular substance.

### Filter

Filters can be placed at the end of a needle or syringe to remove particulates from a drug solution before injection. Numerous types of filter materials have been reported among PWID such as cotton balls, cigarette filters, and commercially produced filters, which may decrease the bacterial burden in the drug solution.[26,27] Commercial wheel filters do not require a prescription and may be available at local HR organizations, syringe exchanges, or can be purchased online without a prescription. We recommend the use of a hierarchy of single-use filters based on their presumed sterility (most safe to least): commercial (wheel) filters, single-use cotton balls, and to avoid the use of cigarette filters.

### Dissolving substances

Fentanyl or white powered heroin may be prepared with only water and heat, otherwise known as "cold cooking."[28] For fentanyl preparation, aseptic techniques should be encouraged among PWID by recommending the use of sterile water, and if this is not available, by recommending the use of boiled water over bottled water or tap water to minimize the risk of infections. In addition, brown heroin (typically found in Europe) requires an acidifier to dissolve. We recommend avoiding the use of lemon juice and vinegar due to their high level of acidity because it has been hypothesized that the use of an acidifier increases the risk of venous sclerosis. Instead, ascorbic acid (vitamin C) is the preferred acidifying agent due its lower level of acidity.[29]

### Skin cleaning

Skin flora may be a leading source of bacterial infections among PWID.[30] A Baltimore survey of PWID found that individuals who reported disinfecting their skin all the time via washing or wiping their skin with alcohol, soap and water, or iodine had a lower frequency of developing abscesses.[31] A recent randomized controlled trial of a brief skin cleaning educational intervention among hospitalized PWID compared with usual care found that those in the brief intervention did reduce the number of uncleaned skin injections at 12-month follow-up, suggesting that a brief intervention can decrease high-risk injection practices.[32] Patients should be encouraged to clean their skin with alcohol or soap before injection and may be prescribed items such as alcohol pads. PWID should also be advised not to lick their needle before or after injection to reduce introduction of oral bacteria into the bloodstream.

## HUMAN IMMUNODEFICIENCY VIRUS PREVENTION: PREEXPOSURE PROPHYLAXIS

Injection drug use can increase the risk of blood-borne infections such has HIV, HCV, and HBV. In 2010, approximately 8% of incident HIV infections were related to injection drug use.[33] Preexposure prophylaxis (PrEP) reduces the transmission rate of HIV for those who inject drugs, as well as reduces the sexual transmission of HIV.[33,34] A randomized placebo controlled trial of PWID found that individuals who received PrEP had a 48.9% reduced risk of HIV and that individuals with tenofovir detected in their blood had a 74% reduced risk of HIV.[34] The CDC recommends offering PrEP to individuals with injection behaviors that places them at an increased risk of acquiring HIV, which includes any sharing of injection or drug preparation equipment in the past 6 months, or risk of sexual acquisition.[33] Clinicians should offer PrEP to qualifying PWID (**Table 2**).

**Table 2**
**The basics of prescribing preexposure prophylaxis for patients**[33]

| | Prescribing PrEP (Once-Daily TDF-FTC 300–200 mg) |
|---|---|
| Indications | People who inject drugs<br>MSM<br>HIV-positive partner<br>Inconsistent condom use<br>Recent sexually transmitted infection<br>Commercial sex work |
| Contraindications | Acute or chronic HIV infection<br>Creatinine clearance <60 mL/min |
| Counsel on side effects | Short term: nausea<br>Long term: potential renal dysfunction, potential bone demineralization |
| Baseline laboratory test results | HIV antigen/antibody test; if symptoms of acute HIV infection test for HIV RNA<br>Creatinine<br>Hepatitis B surface antibody and antigen<br>Hepatitis C antibody<br>Syphilis, gonorrhea, chlamydia (3-site testing at the urethral, rectal, and pharyngeal sites for MSM)<br>Urinalysis for glucose and protein<br>Urine pregnancy test |
| Vaccines | Hepatitis B if not immune |
| Follow-up visits | Every 3 mo |
| Follow-up laboratory test results | HIV antigen/antibody test; every 3 mo; if symptoms of acute HIV infection test for HIV RNA<br>Creatinine clearance at 3 mo and every 6 mo thereafter<br>Sexually transmitted infection screening every 3–6 mo<br>Urine pregnancy test every 3 mo |

*Abbreviations:* MSM, men who have sex with men; TDF-FTC, tenofovir disoproxil fumarate-emtricitabine.

## OPIOID OVERDOSE PREVENTION
### Naloxone

Naloxone is an opioid overdose reversal agent that competitively binds opioid receptors, rapidly displacing opioids from their receptors.[35,36] Naloxone can be given intravenously (0.2–0.6 mg), intramuscularly (0.4 mg/1 mL), intranasally (4–8 mg), or subcutaneously (0.8 mg). In the ambulatory setting, intranasal or intramuscular naloxone is the formulation prescribed in the community. Prehospital administration of naloxone is a life-saving HR tool. Communities where naloxone kits are distributed have fewer opioid overdose deaths,[37–39] as do states where pharmacists can prescribe and dispense naloxone.[40] Naloxone should be distributed to individuals at hospital discharge and prescribed in ambulatory settings.

It is important for clinicians and PWUD to know that naloxone is a safe[35] and effective way to reverse an opioid overdose.[38] In the absence of opioids, naloxone will neither cause harm nor worsen respiratory depression.[35,36] The most common side effect of naloxone is precipitated withdrawal.[35,36] Even in the era of FFA, it is still recommended to use 1 to 2 standardized doses of 4 mg intranasal naloxone or 0.4 mg/1 mL intramuscular naloxone, to reverse an opioid overdose successfully; however, sometimes additional doses might be still necessary.[39,41,42]

Educating PWUD and other nonmedical bystanders is important given a reluctance to call 911 due to fear of invoking police response, which is especially problematic for bystanders with active warrants or on parole.[43] Educating them is also essential for those using nonopioid drugs (cocaine, methamphetamine, pressed pills, counterfeit benzodiazepines), which can unknowingly contain fentanyl, to be aware of the risks of unintentional opioid overdose and to have naloxone on hand.[39,44]

### Fentanyl Test Strips

With the increase in FFA-related fatal overdoses, fentanyl test strips (FTS) have emerged as a potential HR strategy.[45] These rapid (immunoassay or reagent) tests can be used by PWUD to detect FFA in either drug residue or urine. Risk reducing behavior changes if there is a positive result include using smaller amounts or test doses, using around someone else, ensuring availability of naloxone, or injecting slowly.

Despite the potential of FTS as an HR tool, there are concerns regarding test accuracy and the risks associated with false-negative tests.[46] It is uncertain whether FTS can detect other rapidly emerging high-potency synthetic opioids (HPSO) because they are introduced into the drug supply.[46] Analysis of 4 types of FTS showed inconsistent detection of HPSO including the exceptionally potent carfentanil.[47] False-negatives can also occur when the sample tested is too dilute. Because false-negatives put PWUD at increased risk of overdose, there is potential for FTS to cause harm and more rigorous research is necessary.[47] Clinicians should counsel patients on adjusting behavior in the presence of a positive FTS test, as well as the real risk of false-negative tests.

### Low-Barrier Care

In the United States, where most people with Opioid Use Disorder (OUD) are not treated with Medications for OUD (MOUD), low-barrier treatment emerges as a promising vehicle to address this treatment gap. Low-barrier treatment serves to decrease the obstacles to accessing MOUD and minimize treatment interruptions. Key features of low-barrier care include availability of same-day treatment, not requiring concurrent behavioral health treatment, and not mandating complete abstinence from all substances.[48]

Same-day treatment helps mitigate the heightened mortality risk PWUD face while on a treatment waitlist.[49] Reduced wait times also decrease missed appointments and increase treatment initiation.[50] Same-day treatment with buprenorphine is facilitated by the practice of "home-inductions" (unobserved) initiation, which is safe and feasible.[51] In Vancouver, Canada, where methadone is more widely availability in settings like primary care offices and pharmacies, treatment with methadone was associated with decreased HIV seroconversion,[52] improved survival,[53] as well as a decrease in high-risk behaviors like sharing injection equipment.[54]

Low-barrier care can foster ongoing treatment and support adjunctive behavioral health treatment without making it compulsory or required.[51] This pivot away from behavioral health treatment as a requirement of receipt of MOUD is the essence of "medication first," a framework that prioritizes access to medication and absence of punitive policies or perpetual requirements to first facilitate stabilization on medication and minimize harms or ongoing use.[55] Use of a "medication first" approach in Missouri resulted in improved utilization of MOUD, shortened time to starting MOUD, and improved treatment retention.[55]

We recommend rapid access to MOUD without requiring psychosocial treatment as well as avoidance of medication discontinuation unless there is evidence of harm to the patient.[56] Notably, evidence of harm is not inclusive of continued substance use. Finally, low-barrier treatment acknowledges that resumption of use or lack of abstinence does not equal treatment failure. In low-threshold settings, those who resume use are offered additional supports rather than forced cessation of their medication.[51]

## PAIN MANAGEMENT IN THE HOSPITAL

PWUD report inadequate pain or withdrawal management as a reason why they elect to leave the hospital prematurely, thus increasing their risk of readmission, medical complications, or even death.[3,8] In addition, qualitative studies have reported that inadequate pain management resulted in an individual transitioning to heroin injection, a higher-risk form of use.[8] Adequate pain management for individuals with OUD often requires multimodal strategies, and higher amounts of opioids to achieve analgesia due to opioid tolerance for both individuals on MOUD and those who are not on MOUD.[57] Persons with OUD will often require higher, more frequent doses of full agonist opioids for analgesia. Because opioid withdrawal can worsen acute pain, treatment of OUD with methadone and buprenorphine is recommended concurrently with acute pain treatment. Undertreating opioid withdrawal symptoms and acute pain can place individuals at an increased risk of harm, such as using nonregulated forms of opioids.

## HARM REDUCTION FOR ALCOHOL USE

Historically, treatment of alcohol use disorders has focused on abstinence as the only treatment goal. Barriers for individuals to pursue treatment include the perception that seeking treatment required complete abstinence, and people have reported being more open to changes such as decreasing alcohol consumption or drinking in moderation over abstinence.[58] It is known that a reduction in alcohol consumption can improve health outcomes. There is evidence that the benefits of reduced drinking include reduction in all-cause mortality, and decreased severity of psychiatric, family, and social problems.[59,60] Although abstinence may be the safest goal for individuals, minimizing alcohol consumption can result in meaningful health and social outcomes as well and clinicians can help patients understand this.

## MANAGED ALCOHOL PROGRAMS

Managed alcohol programs (MAP) are designed to reduce the harms of alcohol, particularly the risks associated with consuming nonbeverage alcohol (NBA) like rubbing alcohol, hand sanitizer, or other dangerous forms of alcohol.[61] These community-based programs have various eligibility criteria (eg, unhoused). MAPs dispense alcohol every 60 to 90 minutes with limitations on maximum doses a day, and the ability for staff to refuse to provide a drink if an individual is overly intoxicated.[61]

Many MAPs provide additional social services such as food, accommodation, primary care services, or other clinical monitoring.[61] Participants in MAPs have been found to have decreased emergency department visits, have fewer hospital admissions, have reduced NBA consumption, and have fewer police contacts leading to custody.[62] MAPs can create a safer microenvironment to reduce alcohol-related harms.[63]

## HARM REDUCTION FOR STIMULANT USE

Stimulants are often used to increase energy, attention, and alertness. Nonmedical use of substances in the stimulant category, such as cocaine, methamphetamine, and prescription stimulants, can place an individual at risk of adverse health consequences. Stimulant use has been associated with an increase in risky sexual practices, cardiac complications, cerebrovascular accidents, seizures, and psychiatric complications.[64]

"Overamping" is a term frequently used to describe the negative physical and psychological effects of stimulant use, akin to an overdose.[65] This term is not well defined in the literature, and it can imply a wide range of symptoms (stimulant overdose can include cardiovascular collapse and/or death). Further research is needed to improve the definition and develop overamping prevention strategies. In addition, due to FFA detection in the stimulant supply from US drug seizures, all patients with stimulant use should be counseled on the risk of opioid exposure, and should consider the use of FTS in this setting to decrease the risk of an opioid overdose.[66]

For people who use stimulants, clinicians should ask the route of delivery to further tailor HR counseling. Individuals who smoke crack cocaine or methamphetamine via pipes should be instructed to not share their equipment because it could transmit HIV or HCV, particularly in those who may have burns or sores from their pipe use.[67,68] HR kits can be provided to patients who smoke stimulants containing items found in **Fig. 3** that help minimize the risk of burns and infections from pipe use. Rectal use is another route of delivery for stimulants such as methamphetamine.[69] For individuals who use substances rectally, the goal is to prevent infections and to protect the skin from breakdown; we recommend that individuals mix the substance with sterile water, use lubrication, avoid sharing equipment, and use sterile equipment. In addition, all patients should be encouraged to use safe sex practices, such as routine condom use, and offered screening for sexually transmitted infections.

For individuals who inject cocaine, the addition of an acidifier (eg, citric acid, vitamin C) is often required to dissolve the substance.[16] Overacidification of substance preparation has been hypothesized to play a role in venous sclerosis among PWID, causing scarring of small vessels, thereby driving individuals to switch to higher-risk injection site practices (eg, groin, neck vessels).[29] Patients should be counseled on using a

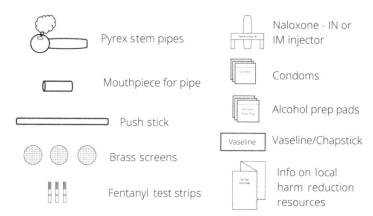

**Fig. 3.** Harm reduction kits for smoking stimulants such as crack cocaine or crystal methamphetamine may include items in this figure. We recommend individuals have their own supplies to decrease risk of infection such as a Pyrex pipe, a personal mouthpiece to prevent burns to lips and oral mucosa, and brass screens with push sticks to insert them into pipes. Owing to fentanyl being found in stimulant supplies we recommend universal fentanyl precautions by carrying naloxone and using fentanyl test strips to test drug supplies. IM, intramuscular; IN, intranasal; IV, intravenous.

minimal quantity of acidifier when dissolving substances and that ascorbic acid may be safer when compared with other acidifiers because of its safer pH.[29]

## CLINICAL CARE POINTS: STIMULANT USE

- Counsel on safer routes of administration, intranasal, insufflation, rectal, over intravenous use.
- Counsel on safer injection and inhalation practices (see **Table 1**, see **Figs. 2** and **3**), not sharing insufflation equipment, and using the minimal needed amount of acidifier to dissolve cocaine and/or certain forms of heroin.
- Carry naloxone and use FTS due to FFA contamination in stimulant supply.[66]

## GENERAL HARM REDUCTION APPROACHES
### Syringe Services Programs

Syringe services programs (SSPs) are community programs that provide access to sterile syringes as well as sterile disposal. Many offer a wide range of additional services such as connection to SUD treatment, condoms, testing for infectious diseases, wound care, and vaccinations. There is extensive evidence that SSPs can prevent transmission of infectious diseases as well as connect individuals to health care services.

Injection drug use can spread viral hepatitis, HIV, and other blood-borne pathogens. Among individuals who elect to not abstain from injection drug use, using sterile injection equipment can reduce the risk of acquiring or transmitting infections. A meta-analysis found that SSP participants had decreased rates of HIV seroconversion compared with nonparticipants.[70] Providing patients with information on how to access nearby SSP programs is important.

SSPs may offer referrals and linkage of care to treatment programs.[71] Individuals who participate in SSP have been found to be 5 times more likely to enter substance use treatment, more likely to report a reduction in injection, and were 3 times more likely to stop using substances completely compared with individuals who never engaged in an SSP.[71]

At this time, there is no evidence that supports that SSPs increase the amount of drug use. SSPs are public health approaches to reducing harm, and we note that these approaches can be adapted within various hospital and legal approaches to reduce harm based on local regulations.

### Housing First

Unhoused (or homeless) individuals with substance use may face additional barriers in obtaining community assistance with housing. The traditional "Treatment First" model supported by communities can require abstinence of drugs, a high degree of motivation for abstinence, or enrollment in SUD treatment program before accessing housing. In contrast, "Housing First" models prioritize housing regardless of the status of an individual's substance use.[63] These programs may decrease the use and cost of community services such as emergency medical services, and lead to fewer hospital days.[72] Frequently housing services are paired with social services to continue to support the individual and can decrease the use of other community services, thus minimizing substance-related harms.

### Overdose Prevention Sites

The first sanctioned overdose prevention site (OPS), also known as safe or supervised injection facilities and safe consumption spaces, in North America was opened in

Vancouver, British Columbia, in 2003.[73] These facilities exist in Canada, and currently are not legal in the United States from the view of federal legislation.[73,74] Rhode Island in July 2021 signed into law a proposal to enact a 2-year pilot of OPSs; the federal stance on this remains unclear because previously federal prosecutors prevented an OPS from being opened in Philadelphia.[75] Most facilities are operated by licensed health professionals, but some sites are peer operated. At these facilities, PWID can consume preobtained drugs under the supervision of medical staff or trained peers.[73] Services include sterile syringes/needles, administration of oxygen or naloxone in the event of an overdose, and linkage to treatment services. Health care professionals do not directly assist with the injection of drugs but may answer questions on safer injection methods or sites as well as monitor for overdose. Peer-assisted injection can now be permitted in some sites. Evidence supports that OPSs reduce the harm of substances use by providing sterile drug equipment, and reduce opioid overdose fatalities.[74,76] In addition, weekly use of an OPS and any contact with the facility's counselors were independently associated with more rapid entry into a detoxification program.[77]

## SUMMARY

HR is an essential component of addiction treatment of individuals with SUDs and those who use substances. Clinicians should be aware of and implement these approaches and refer to local community resources such as SSPs, OPS, and MAPs. Clinicians can play a crucial role in advocating for these interventions in their communities. Clinicians should counsel their patients on methods to reduce harms related to substance use and have resources to minimize complications that are specific to the individual. Prescribing naloxone and sterile syringes are important and feasible. Clinicians should accept that polysubstance use is the norm, and counseling should be tailored to an individual's substance use practices and goals. Applying an HR framework toward patients who use drugs is crucial because it can engage patients who are not seeking abstinence as their treatment goal, and ultimately will improve health outcomes for individuals who use substances.

## CLINICS CARE POINTS

- Infection prevention for PWUD may include referral or integrating local SSP services into a clinical practice, counseling on safer injection practices (see **Table 1**), providing HR kits (see **Figs. 2** and **3**), and offering PrEP (see **Table 2**).
- Prevent opioid overdose fatalities by prescribing naloxone to those who use opioids, stimulants, or any emerging substance at risk of fentanyl contamination.
- Know local and refer individuals to local resources such as SSP, MAP, OPSs, and local HR agencies.
- Refer persons to social workers or community agencies for support in creating individual safer substance use conditions.

## REFERENCES

1. Single E. Defining harm reduction. Drug Alcohol Rev 1995;14(3):287–90.
2. Chan Carusone S, Guta A, Robinson S, et al. "Maybe if I stop the drugs, then maybe they'd care?"—hospital care experiences of people who use drugs. Harm Reduct J 2019;16:16.

3. Simon R, Snow R, Wakeman S. Understanding why patients with substance use disorders leave the hospital against medical advice: a qualitative study. Subst Abuse 2020;41(4):519–25.
4. Cernasev A, Hohmeier KC, Frederick K, et al. A systematic literature review of patient perspectives of barriers and facilitators to access, adherence, stigma, and persistence to treatment for substance use disorder. Explor Res Clin Soc Pharm 2021;2:100029.
5. Fornili KS. Racialized mass incarceration and the war on drugs: a critical race theory appraisal. J Addict Nurs 2018;29(1):65–72.
6. Hall NY, Le L, Majmudar I, et al. Barriers to accessing opioid substitution treatment for opioid use disorder: a systematic review from the client perspective. Drug Alcohol Depend 2021;221:108651.
7. Ti L, Ti L. Leaving the hospital against medical advice among people who use illicit drugs: a systematic review. Am J Public Health 2015;105(12):e53–9.
8. McNeil R, Small W, Wood E, et al. Hospitals as a 'risk environment': an ethno-epidemiological study of voluntary and involuntary discharge from hospital against medical advice among people who inject drugs. Soc Sci Med 2014; 105:59–66.
9. McNeil R, Kerr T, Pauly B, et al. Advancing patient-centered care for structurally vulnerable drug-using populations: a qualitative study of the perspectives of people who use drugs regarding the potential integration of harm reduction interventions into hospitals. Addiction 2016;111(4):685–94.
10. Hedegaard H, Bastian BA, Trinidad JP, et al. Drugs most frequently involved in drug overdose deaths: United States, 2011-2016. Natl Vital Stat Rep 2018; 67(9):1–14.
11. Lambdin BH, Bluthenthal RN, Zibbell JE, et al. Associations between perceived illicit fentanyl use and infectious disease risks among people who inject drugs. Int J Drug Policy 2019;74:299–304.
12. Ronan MV, Herzig SJ. Hospitalizations related to opioid abuse/dependence and associated serious infections increased sharply, 2002–12. Health Aff (Millwood) 2016;35(5):832–7.
13. Vlahov D, Fuller CM, Ompad DC, et al. Updating the infection risk reduction hierarchy: Preventing transition into injection. J Urban Health Bull N Y Acad Med 2004;81(1):14–9.
14. Novak SP, Kral AH. Comparing injection and non-injection routes of administration for heroin, methamphetamine, and cocaine uses in the United States. J Addict Dis 2011;30(3):248–57.
15. Darke S, Hall W. Heroin overdose: research and evidence-based intervention. J Urban Health Bull N Y Acad Med 2003;80(2):189–200.
16. Ponton R, Scott J. Injection preparation processes used by heroin and crack cocaine injectors. J Subst Use 2004;9(1):7–19.
17. Rhodes T. The 'risk environment': a framework for understanding and reducing drug-related harm. Int J Drug Policy 2002;13(2):85–94.
18. Rhodes T. Risk environments and drug harms: a social science for harm reduction approach. Int J Drug Policy 2009;20(3):193–201.
19. Protect yourself if you inject drugs | Prevention | HIV Basics | HIV/AIDS | CDC. 2021. Available at: https://www.cdc.gov/hiv/basics/hiv-prevention/inject-drugs.html. Accessed February 2, 2021.
20. World Health Organization. Effectiveness of sterile needle and syringe programming in reducing HIV/AIDS among injecting drug users. World Health Organization; 2004. Available at: https://www.who.int/hiv/pub/prev_care/effectivenesssterileneedle.pdf.

21. Dahlman D, Håkansson A, Kral AH, et al. Behavioral characteristics and injection practices associated with skin and soft tissue infections among people who inject drugs: a community-based observational study. Subst Abuse 2017;38(1):105–12.

22. Olopoenia LA, Mody V, Reynolds M. Eikenella corrodens endocarditis in an intravenous drug user: case report and literature review. J Natl Med Assoc 1994; 86(4):313–5.

23. Ball LJ, Venner C, Tirona RG, et al. Heating injection drug preparation equipment used for opioid injection may reduce HIV transmission associated with sharing equipment. J Acquir Immune Defic Syndr 2019;81(4):e127–34.

24. Hagan H, Thiede H, Weiss NS, et al. Sharing of drug preparation equipment as a risk factor for hepatitis C. Am J Public Health 2001;91(1):42–6.

25. Kasper KJ, Manoharan I, Hallam B, et al. A controlled-release oral opioid supports S. aureus survival in injection drug preparation equipment and may increase bacteremia and endocarditis risk. PLoS One 2019;14(8):e0219777.

26. Keijzer L, Imbert E. The filter of choice: filtration method preference among injecting drug users. Harm Reduct J 2011;8:20.

27. Ng H, Patel RP, Bruno R, et al. Filtration of crushed tablet suspensions has potential to reduce infection incidence in people who inject drugs. Drug Alcohol Rev 2015;34(1):67–73.

28. Strang J, Keaney F, Butterworth G, et al. Different forms of heroin and their relationship to cook-up techniques: data on, and explanation of, use of lemon juice and other acids. Subst Use Misuse 2001;36(5):573–88.

29. Harris M, Scott J, Wright T, et al. Injecting-related health harms and overuse of acidifiers among people who inject heroin and crack cocaine in London: a mixed-methods study. Harm Reduct J 2019;16(1):60.

30. Stein MD, Phillips KT, Herman DS, et al. Skin-cleaning among hospitalized people who inject drugs: a randomized controlled trial. Addiction 2021;116(5):1122–30.

31. Vlahov D, Sullivan M, Astemborski J, et al. Bacterial infections and skin cleaning prior to injection among intravenous drug users. Public Health Rep 1992;107(5): 595–8.

32. Phillips KT, Stewart C, Anderson BJ, et al. A randomized controlled trial of a brief behavioral intervention to reduce skin and soft tissue infections among people who inject drugs. Drug Alcohol Depend 2021;221:108646.

33. Preventing new HIV infections | Guidelines and recommendations | HIV/AIDS | CDC. 2020. Available at: https://www.cdc.gov/hiv/guidelines/preventing.html. Accessed December 26, 2020.

34. Choopanya K, Martin M, Suntharasamai P, et al. Antiretroviral prophylaxis for HIV infection in injecting drug users in Bangkok, Thailand (the Bangkok Tenofovir Study): a randomised, double-blind, placebo-controlled phase 3 trial. Lancet 2013;381(9883):2083–90.

35. Kim HK, Nelson LS. Reducing the harm of opioid overdose with the safe use of naloxone : a pharmacologic review. Expert Opin Drug Saf 2015;14(7):1137–46.

36. Martin WR. Naloxone. Ann Intern Med 1976;85(6):765–8.

37. Naumann RB, Durrance CP, Ranapurwala SI, et al. Impact of a community-based naloxone distribution program on opioid overdose death rates. Drug Alcohol Depend 2019;204:107536.

38. Walley AY, Xuan Z, Hackman HH, et al. Opioid overdose rates and implementation of overdose education and nasal naloxone distribution in Massachusetts: interrupted time series analysis. BMJ 2013;346:f174.

39. Fairbairn N, Coffin PO, Walley AY. Naloxone for heroin, prescription opioid, and illicitly made fentanyl overdoses: challenges and innovations responding to a dynamic epidemic. Int J Drug Policy 2017;46:172–9.

40. Abouk R, Pacula RL, Powell D. Association between state laws facilitating pharmacy distribution of naloxone and risk of fatal overdose. JAMA Intern Med 2019; 179(6):805–11.

41. Mahonski SG, Leonard JB, Gatz JD, et al. Prepacked naloxone administration for suspected opioid overdose in the era of illicitly manufactured fentanyl: a retrospective study of regional poison center data. Clin Toxicol 2020;58(2):117–23.

42. Bell A, Bennett AS, Jones TS, et al. Amount of naloxone used to reverse opioid overdoses outside of medical practice in a city with increasing illicitly manufactured fentanyl in illicit drug supply. Subst Abuse 2019;40(1):52–5.

43. Kim D, Irwin KS, Khoshnood K. Expanded access to naloxone: options for critical response to the epidemic of opioid overdose mortality. Am J Public Health 2009; 99(3):402–7.

44. Tomassoni AJ, Hawk KF, Jubanyik K, et al. Multiple Fentanyl Overdoses - New Haven, Connecticut, June 23, 2016. MMWR Morb Mortal Wkly Rep 2017;66(4): 107–11.

45. Wilson N. Drug and Opioid-Involved Overdose Deaths — United States, 2017–2018. MMWR Morb Mortal Wkly Rep 2020;69:290–7.

46. McGowan CR, Harris M, Platt L, et al. Fentanyl self-testing outside supervised injection settings to prevent opioid overdose: do we know enough to promote it? Int J Drug Policy 2018;58:31–6.

47. Bergh MS-S, Øiestad ÅML, Baumann MH, et al. Selectivity and sensitivity of urine fentanyl test strips to detect fentanyl analogues in illicit drugs. Int J Drug Policy 2021;90:103065.

48. Jakubowski A, Fox A. Defining low-threshold buprenorphine treatment. J Addict Med 2020;14(2):95–8.

49. Peles E, Schreiber S, Adelson M. Opiate-dependent patients on a waiting list for methadone maintenance treatment are at high risk for mortality until treatment entry. J Addict Med 2013;7(3):177–82.

50. Roy PJ, Choi S, Bernstein E, et al. Appointment wait-times and arrival for patients at a low-barrier access addiction clinic. J Subst Abuse Treat 2020;114:108011.

51. Martin SA, Chiodo LM, Bosse JD, et al. The next stage of buprenorphine care for opioid use disorder. Ann Intern Med 2018;169(9):628–35.

52. Ahamad K, Hayashi K, Nguyen P, et al. Effect of low-threshold methadone maintenance therapy for people who inject drugs on HIV incidence in Vancouver, BC, Canada: an observational cohort study. Lancet HIV 2015;2(10):e445–50.

53. Nolan S, Hayashi K, Milloy M-J, et al. The impact of low-threshold methadone maintenance treatment on mortality in a Canadian setting. Drug Alcohol Depend 2015;156:57–61.

54. Millson P, Challacombe L, Villeneuve PJ, et al. Reduction in injection-related HIV risk after 6 months in a low-threshold methadone treatment program. AIDS Educ Prev 2007;19(2):124–36.

55. Winograd RP, Wood CA, Stringfellow EJ, et al. Implementation and evaluation of Missouri's Medication First treatment approach for opioid use disorder in publicly-funded substance use treatment programs. J Subst Abuse Treat 2020;108:55–64.

56. Winograd RP, Presnall N, Stringfellow E, et al. The case for a medication first approach to the treatment of opioid use disorder. Am J Drug Alcohol Abuse 2019;45(4):333–40.

57. Alford DP, Compton P, Samet JH. Acute pain management for patients receiving maintenance methadone or buprenorphine therapy. Ann Intern Med 2006;144(2): 127–34.

58. Wallhed Finn S, Bakshi A-S, Andréasson S. Alcohol consumption, dependence, and treatment barriers: perceptions among nontreatment seekers with alcohol dependence. Subst Use Misuse 2014;49(6):762–9.

59. Laramée P, Leonard S, Buchanan-Hughes A, et al. Risk of all-cause mortality in alcohol-dependent individuals: a systematic literature review and meta-analysis. EBioMedicine 2015;2(10):1394–404.

60. Kline-Simon AH, Falk DE, Litten RZ, et al. Posttreatment low-risk drinking as a predictor of future drinking and problem outcomes among individuals with alcohol use disorders. Alcohol Clin Exp Res 2013;37(0 1):E373–80.

61. Bernie PB, Vallance K, Wettlaufer A, et al. Community managed alcohol programs in Canada: overview of key dimensions and implementation. Drug Alcohol Rev 2018;37(S1):S132–9.

62. Vallance K, Stockwell T, Pauly B, et al. Do managed alcohol programs change patterns of alcohol consumption and reduce related harm? A pilot study. Harm Reduct J 2016;13(1):13.

63. Bernie PB, Gray E, Perkin K, et al. Finding safety: a pilot study of managed alcohol program participants' perceptions of housing and quality of life. Harm Reduct J 2016;13(1):15.

64. Farrell M, Martin NK, Stockings E, et al. Responding to global stimulant use: challenges and opportunities. Lancet 2019;394(10209):1652–67.

65. What is Overamping? | Harm Reduction Coalition. Available at: https://harmreduction.org/issues/overdose-prevention/overview/stimulant-overamping-basics/what-is-overamping/. Accessed February 6, 2021.

66. Park JN, Rashidi E, Foti K, et al. Fentanyl and fentanyl analogs in the illicit stimulant supply: Results from U.S. drug seizure data, 2011–2016. Drug Alcohol Depend 2021;218:108416.

67. DeBeck K, Kerr T, Li K, et al. Smoking of crack cocaine as a risk factor for HIV infection among people who use injection drugs. CMAJ 2009;181(9):585–9.

68. Fischer B, Powis J, Firestone Cruz M, et al. Hepatitis C virus transmission among oral crack users: viral detection on crack paraphernalia. Eur J Gastroenterol Hepatol 2008;20(1):29–32.

69. Cantrell FL, Breckenridge HM, Jost P. Transrectal methamphetamine use: a novel route of exposure. Ann Intern Med 2006;145(1):78–9.

70. Aspinall EJ, Nambiar D, Goldberg DJ, et al. Are needle and syringe programmes associated with a reduction in HIV transmission among people who inject drugs: a systematic review and meta-analysis. Int J Epidemiol 2014;43(1):235–48.

71. Hagan H, McGough JP, Thiede H, et al. Reduced injection frequency and increased entry and retention in drug treatment associated with needle-exchange participation in Seattle drug injectors. J Subst Abuse Treat 2000; 19(3):247–52.

72. Sadowski LS, Kee RA, VanderWeele TJ, et al. Effect of a housing and case management program on emergency department visits and hospitalizations among chronically ill homeless adults: a randomized trial. JAMA 2009;301(17):1771–8.

73. Hathaway AD, Tousaw KI. Harm reduction headway and continuing resistance: Insights from safe injection in the city of Vancouver. Int J Drug Policy 2008; 19(1):11–6.

74. Kral AH, Lambdin BH, Wenger LD, et al. Evaluation of an unsanctioned safe consumption site in the United States. N Engl J Med 2020;383(6):589–90.

75. Mulvaney K. RI Gov. McKee signs legislation allowing safe-injection sites into law. The Providence J. Available at: https://www.providencejournal.com/story/news/2021/07/07/gov-mckee-signs-legislation-allowing-safe-injection-sites-into-law/7891057002/. Accessed August 7, 2021.
76. Stoltz J-A, Wood E, Small W, et al. Changes in injecting practices associated with the use of a medically supervised safer injection facility. J Public Health 2007;29(1):35–9.
77. Wood E, Tyndall MW, Zhang R, et al. Attendance at supervised injecting facilities and use of detoxification services. N Engl J Med 2006;354(23):2512–4.

# Gender Dynamics in Substance Use and Treatment: A Women's Focused Approach

Miriam T.H. Harris, MD, MSc[a,b],*, Jordana Laks, MD, MPH[a,b],
Natalie Stahl, MD, MPH[c], Sarah M. Bagley, MD, MSc[a,b,d],
Kelley Saia, MD[e], Wendee M. Wechsberg, PhD, MS[f,g,h,i]

## KEYWORDS

- Women • Substance use disorders • Gender • Treatment

## KEY POINTS

- The substance use disorder gap between men and women is narrowing.
- Gender-based differences in substance use disorder development, trajectories, health, and psychosocial consequences exist.
- Gender-responsive care is patient-centered care that considers how gender has affected a woman's experience with drug and alcohol use and treatment.
- There is a need to implement and scale-up gender-responsive addiction programming.
- Advocacy at the policy level to address the root drivers of substance use inequities among women is needed.

Funding: M.T.H. Harris is supported by the Research in Addiction Medicine Fellowship NIDA (R25DA033211-Samet) and the International Collaborative Addiction Medicine Research Fellowship (NIDA R25-DA037756-Fairburn).
[a] Grayken Center for Addiction, Boston Medical Center, 801 Massachusetts Avenue, 1st Floor, Boston, MA 02118, USA; [b] Clinical Addiction Research and Education (CARE) Unit, Section of General Internal Medicine, Department of Medicine, Boston University School of Medicine and Boston Medical Center, 801 Massachusetts Avenue, 2nd Floor, Boston, MA 02118, USA; [c] Yale Program in Addiction Medicine, Yale University School of Medicine, E.S. Harkness Memorial Building A, 367 Cedar Street, Suite 417A, New Haven, CT 06520-8023, USA; [d] Division of General Pediatrics, Department of Pediatrics, 801 Albany Street, Boston, MA 02118, USA; [e] Department of Obstetrics and Gynecology, Boston Medical Center, 850 Harrison Avenue 5th Floor, Boston, MA 02118, USA; [f] Substance Use, Gender, and Applied Research Program, RTI International, Research Triangle Park, NC 27709-2194, USA; [g] Gillings School of Global Public Health, University of North Carolina, Chapel Hill, NC, USA; [h] Department of Psychology, North Carolina State University, Raleigh, NC 27599-7400, USA; [i] Department of Psychiatry and Behavioral Sciences, Duke University School of Medicine, Durham, NC 27701, USA
* Corresponding author. Section of General Internal Medicine, Boston Medical Center, 801 Massachusetts Avenue, 2nd Floor, Boston, MA 02118.
*E-mail address:* Miriam.Harris@bmc.org

Med Clin N Am 106 (2022) 219–234
https://doi.org/10.1016/j.mcna.2021.08.007
0025-7125/22/© 2021 Elsevier Inc. All rights reserved.

## INTRODUCTION

Gender differences exist in the origins, development, course, and treatment of substance use disorders (SUD). Men have historically used alcohol and other substances more than women, and therefore, addiction services, research, and policies have primarily been either tailored to men or designed using a gender-neutral approach.[1] Gender-neutral approaches tend to benefit men over women, as they fail to consider the specific needs of women. This is problematic, as the gender gap in SUD is narrowing.[2,3] Over the past decade in the United States, metrics, such as rates of high-risk drinking and alcohol use disorder,[4] opioid misuse and opioid overdoses rates,[5–7] and methamphetamine-involved overdose rates,[8] have all increased more rapidly in women than men. Given the narrowing gender gap, there have been increasing calls for clinical, public health, and research approaches that comprehensively address women-specific needs.[1,9,10]

Gender-based differences in SUD development, trajectories, health and psychosocial consequences, and treatment outcomes are well documented in the literature.[11–13] Compared with men, women initiate drug and alcohol use at an older age and may exhibit a *telescoping effect*, that is, they more rapidly progress from initiation of substance use to the development of an SUD.[14,15] Research has consistently demonstrated greater physical, psychological, and social harms of drug and alcohol use in women.[16–18] For example, compared with men, women who inject drugs experience higher rates of injection drug use–associated infections, including HIV and hepatitis C.[17,19] Worldwide, women account for approximately one-third of people with SUD but only one-fifth in SUD treatment, highlighting a treatment disparity.[20]

Here, the authors provide a broad overview of critical issues in SUD in women using the biopsychosocial model of addiction.[21] From the wide range of issues relevant to women and SUD, they prioritize the following topics: (1) barriers and facilitators to addiction treatment and harm reduction services; (2) substance use while pregnant and parenting; and (3) gender-responsive addiction care.

## SEX, GENDER, AND THE INTERSECTIONALITY OF RACE

Understanding gender-based differences in substance use requires a comprehensive framework that recognizes the difference between sex and gender and encompasses the full spectrum of gender identity. "Sex" is the biological classification of a human as male or female based on their physical and physiologic attributes.[22] "Gender" refers to socially constructed roles and behaviors that vary across societies and change over time.[22] Gender identity refers to one's internal sense of being a woman, man, or anywhere along the gender spectrum, including transgender, nonbinary, and genderqueer identities.[23] In this article, "women" refers to all individuals who identify as a woman, regardless of their sex. However, it is recognized that compared with cisgender women, transgender and genderqueer individuals experience enhanced marginalization and discrimination based on their gender identity.[18] Transgender and genderqueer women are twice as likely to misuse alcohol and other drugs compared with cisgender women.[24] They also experience heightened risk for other SUD-related comorbidities, gender-based violence, suicide, and murder compared with cisgender women.[25]

There is also a need for a comprehensive and intersectional perspective that recognizes that women's experiences with substance use are not homogeneous. Intersectionality affirms that sex and gender interact with race/ethnicity, class, sexual orientation, and other social categories to shape human experiences (**Fig. 1**).[26] In particular, structural racism enhances stigma, discrimination, gender-based violence,

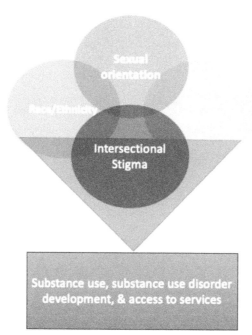

**Fig. 1.** Intersectionality of sex, gender, race/ethnicity, and substance use.

and treatment barriers for Black, Indigenous, and other Women of Color compared with White women with SUD.[27,28] Racism is a primary driver of drug law enforcement and public conceptions of drug use, and in the United States, Black Women are disproportionately targeted by laws and policies that reinforce racial inequities in the consequences of substance use.[29,30]

## THE BIOPSYCHOSOCIAL MODEL OF ADDICTION

The authors use the biopsychosocial model of addiction that roots SUD as a product of the genetic, neurobiological, and social environment.[21] This framework orients women's experiences with substance use and addiction treatment across 4 dimensions: biological, psychological, social, and system structures (**Fig. 2**). The authors provide a high-level overview of each dimension. It is beyond the scope of the article to explore each dimension fully.

### Biological

Sex differences exist in how men versus women respond biologically to alcohol and drugs in both the short and the long term.[11] Different alcohol metabolism in men compared with women is the most consistent and well-understood finding. Women develop higher blood alcohol levels after drinking equivalent amounts of alcohol compared with men and are at higher risk of cirrhosis than men.[31–33] The evidence on effects of sex hormones on subjective drug experiences is equivocal with no consistent differences found.[11] In addition, associations between sex and neural responses to substances are not well studied, as most structural brain studies on addiction and substance use do not evaluate sex differences.[34] Ongoing research to better understand the intersection of sex, genetics, and risks of substance use and addiction is needed.[1]

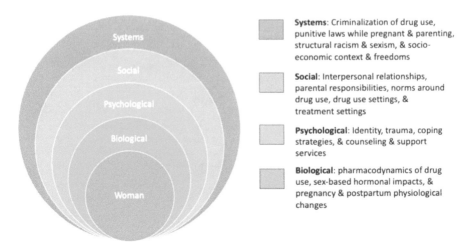

**Fig. 2.** Biopsychosocial model of addiction and gender.

## Psychological

In the psychological realm, women with SUD have higher rates of cooccurring psychiatric disorders, including mood disorders, posttraumatic stress disorder, and eating disorders.[35,36] Women are also disproportionately affected by trauma and abuse.[37,38] These experiences drive substance use initiation and persistent use.[13,39]

## Social

Interpersonal relationships and communities substantially influence women's substance use patterns. For example, women are more likely to start using substances if their intimate partner does so.[40] Male-dominated street cultures influence women's drug injection practices, whereby women are more likely than men to use assisted injection methods.[41] Women who use drugs are also more likely than men to engage in sex work.[42] Because of structural factors, such as the criminalization of sex work, sex work environments increase the risk of violence, trauma, and sexually transmitted infections.[16]

## Systems

The criminalization of some substance use and sex work, and stigma surrounding these while pregnant and parenting disproportionately impact women.[43,44] Women face increased policing and police violence while using illegal drugs and doing sex work that limits harm reduction behaviors and service utilization.[45,46] Current punitive legal and child welfare approaches to substance use while pregnant and parenting reinforce stigma, discourage health care access, and perpetuate substance use among women.[47,48]

## BARRIERS TO ADDICTION AND HARM REDUCTION SERVICES

Women are less likely to enter substance use treatment compared with men relative to the prevalence of SUD in the general population.[12] However, once in treatment, gender has not consistently been associated with differences in retention or substance use, suggesting women can and do benefit from treatment.[12,49] Therefore, examining psychological, social, and systems barriers to treatment is critical to reducing disparities for women.

### Psychological Barriers

Psychological factors, such as high rates of cooccurring trauma and severe mental illness, among women with SUDs can influence engagement with care.[49,50] At least half of the women seeking treatment for SUD have experienced trauma and have a cooccurring mental illness.[49] Women who use drugs and have experienced abuse are reluctant to seek care and have more unmet and complex health care needs when they present to care compared with those who have not experienced abuse.[51,52] Nevertheless, SUD treatment services do not universally address trauma or have mental health services. The US 2019 National Survey of Substance Abuse Treatment Services found that only 70% of SUD treatment facilities offered some degree of mental health treatment services (**Table 1**).[53] As defined in this survey, mental health services could be counseling alone and did not necessarily include access to psychiatric evaluation and vice versa. Unaddressed trauma and untreated mental illness reduce attendance and retention in SUD care.[12]

### Social Barriers

Harm reduction and other low-barrier treatment programs can become male-dominated, reproducing street-gendered relations and inequalities that limit women's access to services.[54] Women who use drugs are also more likely than their male counterparts to enter dependent and/or violent relationships dominated by their partner, hindering their economic freedom and autonomy to seek treatment.[11,40] Substance use services often fail to take sufficient steps to counteract these gendered barriers. For example, despite evidence that gender-concordant providers improve entry into and continuation in treatment,[55,56] 1 national study of 108 methadone programs found that only 9% offered and matched clients to gender-concordant clinicians,[51] and another study showed only 38% provided domestic violence services.[53] Work force challenges, namely fewer women practicing addiction medicine, likely limit programs' abilities to offer gender-concordant clinicians.

### Systems Barriers

Enhanced surveillance and punitive policies for pregnant and parenting women increase stigma and disincentivize women from accessing treatment.[48,57] Women

Table 1
**Availability of gender-responsive services among substance use disorder treatment programs, United States 2019[a]**

| Ancillary Services | Percent of Facilities Offering Services |
| --- | --- |
| Case management | 96 |
| Mental health | 75 |
| Transportation assistance | 46 |
| Domestic violence | 38 |
| Childcare for client's children | 6 |
| Residential bed for client's children | 3 |

[a] Data derived from the Substance Abuse and Mental Health Services Administration 2019 National Survey of Substance Abuse Treatment Services.[53]

also cite limited treatment options while pregnant, difficulty accessing childcare, and difficulty balancing rigid treatment schedules while fulfilling caretaking obligations as barriers to SUD treatment.[48] The same 2019 US survey of SUD programs found that 24% offered treatment for pregnant or postpartum women, 6% provided child care for clients' children, and 3% had residential beds for families (see **Table 1**).[53] In addition, other structural determinants of health, such as housing instability, legal issues, and lack of transportation, disproportionately reduce women's access to services compared with men.[58] SUD services do not universally prioritize addressing these social determinants, for example, by paying for transportation to and from treatment, thereby reducing access for women.[53,59]

## FACILITATORS TO ADDICTION TREATMENT AND HARM REDUCTION SERVICES

Although there is robust literature documenting the gendered barriers to SUD treatment that women encounter, less research has focused on facilitators to treatment among women compared with men. The strengths-based approach, most notably used by social workers, highlights competencies, motivations, and social/environmental supports that facilitate engagement with care.[60] A strengths-based approach recognizes that gender also positively influences women's treatment engagement and outcomes.

### Biological Facilitators

From a biological standpoint, women are more likely than men to engage in the health care system when they are young and healthy for preventive, sexual, and reproductive health needs.[61] Women are more likely to have a regular clinician from whom they seek routine care and medical advice, which improves trust in the health care system.[61] Regular engagement in medical services could facilitate screening for high-risk substance use, SUD diagnosis, and linkage to treatment for both SUD and psychiatric disorders.

### Psychological Facilitators

Concerning psychological differences, the higher prevalence of cooccurring mood and anxiety disorders in women with SUD can present challenges, but also opportunities for engagement in mental health therapies that simultaneously improve SUD outcomes (eg, cognitive-behavioral therapy).[62] Studies show women are more likely to seek and receive medical treatment for underlying psychiatric disorders than men, in part because of conventional gender norms that make it more acceptable for women to express strong emotions and engage in counseling.[63,64] Use of antidepressants is more common in women than men.[65] Engagement with mental health services and openness to treatment present opportunities to address substance use in women.

### Social Facilitators

Socially, women's recreational and community activities are less likely to center on alcohol or drug use, thus reducing their exposure to habitual substance use early in life.[11] Women tend to form more intimate, supportive relationships with both friends and romantic partners.[66] The ability to sustain relationships and mobilize social support is positively associated with individuals' psychological well-being and capacity to cope with adverse events.[67] In addition, although women's role as caregivers can serve as a barrier to seeking SUD treatment, it can also be a facilitator; research has consistently demonstrated that the desire to maintain or regain child custody is a strong motivator for SUD treatment in women.[12,68] Engaging and leveraging women's community support networks provides an opportunity to increase treatment success.

### System Facilitators

Finally, system-level factors can also facilitate SUD treatment among women. Women-led policy and community efforts that seek to reduce substance use harm inequities have a long and strong history in many communities. Women-led community organizations designed for women who use drugs and women engaged in sex work improve health outcomes and engagement in care, as they are perceived as safe and welcoming spaces for women.[69,70] Thoughtful policies and programs that prioritize the well-being of the fetus and parent-infant dyad provide investment opportunities to expand women-only and family-based treatment programming.[71]

## SUBSTANCE USE AMONG PREGNANT AND PARENTING WOMEN
### Pregnancy

The 2019 National Survey of Drug Use and Health data found, in the last month, 5.8% of pregnant women reported illicit substance use, 9.6% reported tobacco product use, and 9.5% reported alcohol use.[72] Although pregnant women report less substance use than nonpregnant women, the medical risks are greater. For example, women who use illicit drugs, alcohol, and tobacco are at greater risk of miscarriage and preterm delivery.[73,74] Stimulant and alcohol use are associated with medical complications of pregnancy, such as gestational hypertension and preeclampsia.[74] The consequences of cannabis use during pregnancy are less understood, but a large 2019 retrospective study found cannabis use was associated with an increased risk of preterm labor and placental abruption.[75] Substance use during pregnancy also impacts the health of the developing fetus, which is well described elsewhere.[74]

Although pregnancy can be a strong motivator for treatment among women with SUD, punitive laws and practices regulating substance use during pregnancy are major barriers to accessing care. Thirty-six states recognize fetuses as potential victims of crime, and, in 2014, Tennessee became the first state to explicitly criminalize drug use during pregnancy.[76] Data from 2021 show that 23 states and the District of Columbia classify drug use during pregnancy as child abuse; 3 states find drug use during pregnancy as grounds for civil commitment, and 25 states and the District of Columbia mandate reporting of prenatal drug use to child welfare services.[77] Many of the mandated reporting laws include medications prescribed during pregnancy to treat opioid use disorder as a reason to file a report to child welfare.[77] Such mandates alienate pregnant women from seeking care, and among those that do, discourage them from accepting lifesaving pharmacologic treatment for SUD.[78,79] For Black, Indigenous, and pregnant Women of Color, the punitive nature of these mandates is compounded by institutional racism resulting in significantly more report filings and custody disruptions.[80,81]

Despite these barriers, pregnancy is a powerful catalyst for change and engagement with SUD treatment among women with SUD. A 2016 survey found 88% of pregnant women self-disclosed their substance use to their obstetric provider.[82] SUD treatment that is individualized, responsive to the women's context, and integrated with mental health and postpartum care is critical. However, many SUD treatment programs for pregnant women are not integrated with postpartum or pediatric care.[68] The postpartum period can be particularly challenging for women with SUD given high rates of postpartum depression, fragmented transitions of care, lapses in insurance after delivery, physiologic changes impacting SUD treatment, and stress and shame related to neonatal withdrawal syndromes or loss of child custody.[83,84] A 2019 study found that overdose risk was greatest 7 to 12 months following delivery compared with all other prenatal and postpartum periods.[85]

### Breastfeeding

Breastfeeding is an important aspect of the postpartum period for women with SUD. There are specific advantages of breastfeeding for substance-exposed mother-infant dyads; for example, breastfeeding reduces the severity of neonatal-opioid withdrawal syndrome and decreases the need for pharmacologic treatment.[86] Despite this, breastfeeding rates among women with SUD vary widely, in part because of restrictive breastfeeding guidelines.[87] Current recommendations from the American Academy of Breastfeeding Medicine stipulate that in addition to women being engaged in prenatal care and stable in recovery, they should also have no record of substance use (by urine drug testing) 90 to 30 days before delivery.[88] Such policies reduce the number of women who are supported in breastfeeding initiation.[89]

Although there are clear harms to breastfeeding by women with active substance use, substance use in the third trimester should not disqualify women who are not using substances at delivery and are motivated from initiating breastfeeding. A retrospective cohort study from 2020 showed that the predictive value for postpartum substance use based on urine drug testing from the third trimester was only 36%.[90] Most substances are eliminated in hours to days rather than days to weeks from the maternal system.[91] Therefore, women who discontinue substance use before delivery or during the delivery hospitalization could be supported to initiate breastfeeding. Women-centered recommendations paired with ongoing screening, home lactation visiting programs, and SUD treatment support could facilitate successful breastfeeding among substance-exposed mother-infant dyads.

### Parenting

In the United States, between 55% and 70% of women in substance use treatment programs have children.[72] The same stressors leading to drug and alcohol use and SUD development among women can be exacerbated when parenting. Namely, parents experience increases in stress, sleep deprivation, and economic responsibilities and often need to prioritize their children's needs over their own SUD treatment and other health care needs.[92]

Integrated treatment programs are critical to supporting parenting women with SUD. Different models exist, but dyadic models, or programs that provide care to both parents and children, offer several advantages. Examples of such programs include the FOCUS program at the University of New Mexico and the FIR Square and Sheway programs in Vancouver, Canada.[93,94] Both programs are medical homes for families that provide wrap-around services to women and their children up to ages 3 to 5. These programs focus on interdisciplinary care delivery, case management, community outreach, housing, and legal services.[93] Integrated programs have been shown to increase treatment retention, reduce parenting stress, decrease substance use and relapse, increase self-esteem, and improve parenting knowledge.[95]

## GENDER-RESPONSIVE ADDICTION CARE

Given the differences in the impact and patterns of substance use between women and men, it follows that clinical programs providing care for women who use drugs should reflect those differences. This can be called "gender-responsive care," and for this review, is defined as patient-centered care that considers how gender has affected a woman's experience with drug and alcohol use and treatment (**Fig. 3**).

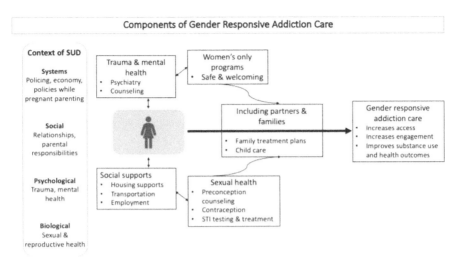

**Fig. 3.** Gender-responsive care.

Even when clinical programs are not exclusively focused on women, any addiction treatment provider or program can ensure women receive care tailored to their needs by adopting specific approaches described in later discussion.

### Specific Components of Gender-Responsive Care

### Trauma and mental health
As discussed earlier, cooccurring mental health disorders and trauma are high among women with SUDs. Programs should offer trauma-informed integrated treatment for cooccurring mental health disorders, including considering single-gender group therapy, which some women report creates a safer environment.

### Sexual health
If available, programs should offer comprehensive reproductive and sexual health care. In addition to routine screening for sexually transmitted infections, age-appropriate cervical cancer screening, assessing pregnancy timing goals, and providing appropriate counseling for contraception or preconception should be offered. Addressing the sexual and reproductive health needs of women increases engagement with addiction treatment.[96]

### Social needs
Different clinical programs will have varying capacities to respond to social needs affecting women. However, having the capacity to refer to clinical and community supports, such as housing services, life skills programs, and recovery management, is necessary. Wherever possible, providing childcare, transportation, and cell phones for those who need them can concretely increase access to care for women.

### Women's only programs
Women's only treatment offers a safe environment that women may be more comfortable accessing. Programs unable to offer women's only spaces all the time could alternatively offer select women's only groups, days, or times for treatment or harm reduction services.[97]

### Including partners and families

Data demonstrate the importance of including families and partners in treatment.[98] Families can provide critical support for women outside of the clinical setting at home and in the community. When possible, this includes providing childcare services for parenting women.

Overall, gender-responsive care can mitigate many of the barriers to care described earlier. By acknowledging gender-based differences and tailoring care, treatment programs can provide care that meets women's unique needs and improves their outcomes.

## SUMMARY

Women have unique, currently unmet, needs that impact their substance use initiation, SUD development trajectories, and harms related to drug and alcohol use. Implementing and scaling up gender-responsive addiction programming is critical given the evolving epidemiology of substance use among women, and evidence that shows gender-responsive services improve treatment outcomes.[99] Additional investments in research to maintain and build multidisciplinary research programs that seek to address all aspects of the consequences of substance among women are needed.[100] In addition, advocacy at the policy level to expand postpartum Medicaid coverage, expand funded parental leave, expand childcare benefits, and dismantle punitive policies that target pregnant and parenting women are needed to address the root drivers of substance use inequities and barriers to care among women.

## ACKNOWLEDGMENTS

The authors acknowledge that the land where we work, live, teach, learn, and gather is the traditional territory of Massachusetts and their neighbors, the Wampanoag and Nipmuc Peoples, who have stewarded this land for hundreds of generations and continue to do so today.

## CONFLICT OF INTEREST

None to declare.

## REFERENCES

1. Meyer JP, Isaacs K, El-Shahawy O, et al. Research on women with substance use disorders: reviewing progress and developing a research and implementation roadmap. Drug Alcohol Depend 2019;197:158–63.
2. Keyes KM, Grant BF, Hasin DS. Evidence for a closing gender gap in alcohol use, abuse, and dependence in the United States population. Drug Alcohol Depend 2008;93(1):21–9.
3. Seedat S, Scott KM, Angermeyer MC, et al. Cross-national associations between gender and mental disorders in the World Health Organization World Mental Health Surveys. Arch Gen Psychiatry 2009;66(7):785–95.
4. Grant BF, Chou SP, Saha TD, et al. Prevalence of 12-month alcohol use, high-risk drinking, and DSM-IV alcohol use disorder in the United States, 2001-2002 to 2012-2013: results from the National Epidemiologic Survey on Alcohol and Related Conditions. JAMA Psychiatry 2017;74(9):911–23.
5. Jones C, Logan J, Gladden M, et al. Vital signs: demographic and substance use trends among heroin users — United States, 2002–2013. MMWR Morb Mortal Wkly Rep 2015;64(26):719–25.

6. VanHouten JP. Drug overdose deaths among women aged 30–64 years — United States, 1999–2017. MMWR Morb Mortal Wkly Rep 2019;68:1–5.

7. Vital signs: overdoses of prescription opioid pain relievers — United States, 1999–2008. Available at: http://www.cdc.gov/mmwr/preview/mmwrhtml/mm6043a4.htm. Accessed February 28, 2021.

8. Han B, Cotto J, Etz K, et al. Methamphetamine overdose deaths in the US by sex and race and ethnicity. JAMA Psychiatry 2021. https://doi.org/10.1001/jamapsychiatry.2020.4321.

9. Meyers SA, Smith LR, Werb D. Preventing transitions into injection drug use: a call for gender-responsive upstream prevention. Int J Drug Policy 2020;83:102836.

10. Collins AB, Bardwell G, McNeil R, et al. Gender and the overdose crisis in North America: moving past gender-neutral approaches in the public health response. Int J Drug Policy 2019;69:43–5.

11. McHugh RK, Votaw VR, Sugarman DE, et al. Sex and gender differences in substance use disorders. Clin Psychol Rev 2018;66:12–23.

12. Greenfield SF, Brooks AJ, Gordon SM, et al. Substance abuse treatment entry, retention, and outcome in women: a review of the literature. Drug Alcohol Depend 2007;86(1):1–21.

13. Ait-Daoud N, Blevins D, Khanna S, et al. Women and addiction: an update. Med Clin North Am 2019;103(4):699–711.

14. Hernandez-Avila CA, Rounsaville BJ, Kranzler HR. Opioid-, cannabis- and alcohol-dependent women show more rapid progression to substance abuse treatment. Drug Alcohol Depend 2004;74(3):265–72.

15. Lewis B, Hoffman LA, Nixon SJ. Sex differences in drug use among polysubstance users. Drug Alcohol Depend 2014;145:127–33.

16. Park JN, Footer KHA, Decker MR, et al. Interpersonal and structural factors associated with receptive syringe-sharing among a prospective cohort of female sex workers who inject drugs. Addiction 2019;114(7):1204–13.

17. El-Bassel N, Strathdee SA. Women who use or inject drugs: an action agenda for women-specific, multilevel and combination HIV prevention and research. J Acquir Immune Defic Syndr 2015;69(Suppl 2):S182–90.

18. Pinkham S, Malinowska-Sempruch K. Women, harm reduction and HIV. Reprod Health Matters 2008;16(31):168–81.

19. Degenhardt L, Peacock A, Colledge S, et al. Global prevalence of injecting drug use and sociodemographic characteristics and prevalence of HIV, HBV, and HCV in people who inject drugs: a multistage systematic review. Lancet Glob Health 2017;5(12):e1192–207.

20. United Nations Office on Drugs and Labor. World drug report 2020 (Set of 6 booklets). Geneva, Switzerland: United Nations; 2021.

21. Buchman DZ, Skinner W, Illes J. Negotiating the relationship between addiction, ethics, and brain science. AJOB Neurosci 2010;1(1):36–45.

22. Government of Canada CI of HR. What is gender? What is sex? - CIHR. 2014. Available at: https://cihr-irsc.gc.ca/e/48642.html. Accessed March 5, 2021.

23. General definitions. LGBT resource center. Available at: https://lgbt.ucsf.edu/glossary-terms. Accessed March 5, 2021.

24. Connolly D, Gilchrist G. Prevalence and correlates of substance use among transgender adults: a systematic review. Addict Behav 2020;111:106544.

25. Boyer TL, Youk AO, Haas AP, et al. Suicide, homicide, and all-cause mortality among transgender and cisgender patients in the Veterans Health Administration. LGBT Health 2021.

26. Hankivsky O. Women's health, men's health, and gender and health: implications of intersectionality. Soc Sci Med 2012;74(11):1712–20.

27. Waltermaurer E, Watson C-A, McNutt L-A. Black women's health: the effect of perceived racism and intimate partner violence. Violence Women 2006; 12(12):1214–22.

28. Center for Substance Abuse Treatment. Substance abuse treatment: addressing the specific needs of women. Substance Abuse and Mental Health Services Administration (US); 2009. Available at: http://www.ncbi.nlm.nih.gov/books/ NBK83252/. Accessed November 16, 2020.

29. Race & the war on drugs. American civil liberties union. Available at: https:// www.aclu.org/other/race-war-drugs. Accessed March 5, 2021.

30. Knight KR. Structural factors that affect life contexts of pregnant people with opioid use disorders: the role of structural racism and the need for structural competency. Womens Reprod Health 2020;7(3):164–71.

31. Chrostek L, Jelski W, Szmitkowski M, et al. Gender-related differences in hepatic activity of alcohol dehydrogenase isoenzymes and aldehyde dehydrogenase in humans. J Clin Lab Anal 2003;17(3):93–6.

32. Rehm J, Taylor B, Mohapatra S, et al. Alcohol as a risk factor for liver cirrhosis: a systematic review and meta-analysis. Drug Alcohol Rev 2010;29(4):437–45.

33. Tapper EB, Parikh ND. Mortality due to cirrhosis and liver cancer in the United States, 1999-2016: observational study. BMJ 2018;362:k2817.

34. Lind KE, Gutierrez EJ, Yamamoto DJ, et al. Sex disparities in substance abuse research: evaluating 23 years of structural neuroimaging studies. Drug Alcohol Depend 2017;173:92–8.

35. Conway KP, Compton W, Stinson FS, et al. Lifetime comorbidity of DSM-IV mood and anxiety disorders and specific drug use disorders: results from the National Epidemiologic Survey on Alcohol and Related Conditions. J Clin Psychiatry 2006;67(2):247–57.

36. Mergler M, Driessen M, Havemann-Reinecke U, et al. Differential relationships of PTSD and childhood trauma with the course of substance use disorders. J Subst Abuse Treat 2018;93:57–63.

37. Hien D, Cohen L, Campbell A. Is traumatic stress a vulnerability factor for women with substance use disorders? Clin Psychol Rev 2005;25(6):813–23.

38. Back SE, Payne RL, Wahlquist AH, et al. Comparative profiles of men and women with opioid dependence: results from a national multisite effectiveness trial. Am J Drug Alcohol Abuse 2011;37(5):313–23.

39. Mburu G, Ayon S, Mahinda S, et al. Determinants of women's drug use during pregnancy: perspectives from a qualitative study. Matern Child Health J 2020; 24(9):1170–8.

40. Mburu G, Limmer M, Holland P. Role of boyfriends and intimate sexual partners in the initiation and maintenance of injecting drug use among women in coastal Kenya. Addict Behav 2019;93:20–8.

41. Boyd J, Collins AB, Mayer S, et al. Gendered violence and overdose prevention sites: a rapid ethnographic study during an overdose epidemic in Vancouver, Canada. Addict Abingdon Engl 2018;113(12):2261–70.

42. Chettiar J, Shannon K, Wood E, et al. Survival sex work involvement among street-involved youth who use drugs in a Canadian setting. J Public Health 2010;32(3):322–7.

43. Goldenberg S, Watt S, Braschel M, et al. Police-related barriers to harm reduction linked to non-fatal overdose amongst sex workers who use drugs: results of

a community-based cohort in Metro Vancouver, Canada. Int J Drug Policy 2020; 76:102618.

44. Duff P, Shoveller J, Chettiar J, et al. Sex work and motherhood: social and structural barriers to health and social services for pregnant and parenting street and off-street sex workers. Health Care Women Int 2015;36(9):1039–55.

45. Goldenberg S, Liyanage R, Braschel M, et al. Structural barriers to condom access in a community-based cohort of sex workers in Vancouver, Canada: influence of policing, violence and end-demand criminalisation. BMJ Sex Reprod Health 2020;46(4):301–7.

46. Odinokova V, Rusakova M, Urada LA, et al. Police sexual coercion and its association with risky sex work and substance use behaviors among female sex workers in St. Petersburg and Orenburg, Russia. Int J Drug Policy 2014;25(1): 96–104.

47. Patrick SW, Schiff DM, Prevention C on SUA. A public health response to opioid use in pregnancy. Pediatrics 2017;139(3):e20164070.

48. Stone R. Pregnant women and substance use: fear, stigma, and barriers to care. Health Justice 2015;3(1):1–15.

49. Greenfield SF, Pettinati HM, O'Malley S, et al. Gender differences in alcohol treatment: an analysis of outcome from the COMBINE Study. Alcohol Clin Exp Res 2010;34(10):1803–12.

50. Huhn AS, Berry MS, Dunn KE. Review: sex-based differences in treatment outcomes for persons with opioid use disorder. Am J Addict 2019;28(4):246–61.

51. Zule WA, Lam WKK, Wechsberg WM. Treatment readiness among out-of-treatment African-American crack users. J Psychoactive Drugs 2003;35(4): 503–10.

52. Substance Abuse and Mental Health Services Administration. Trauma-informed care in behavioral health services. Rockville, MD: Substance Abuse and Mental Health Services Administration; 2014.

53. Substance Abuse and Mental Health Services Administration. National survey of substance abuse treatment services (N-SSATS): 2019. Data on substance abuse treatment facilities. Rockville, MD: Substance Abuse and Mental Health Services Administration; 2020. Available at: https://www.samhsa.gov/data/data-we-collect/n-ssats-national-survey-substance-abuse-treatment-services.

54. Fairbairn N, Small W, Shannon K, et al. Seeking refuge from violence in street-based drug scenes: women's experiences in North America's first supervised injection facility. Soc Sci Med 2008;67(5):817–23.

55. Marsh JC, Miller NA. Female clients in substance abuse treatment. Int J Addict 1985;20(6–7):995–1019.

56. Wechsberg W, Suerken C, Crum L, et al. Availability of special services for women in methadone treatment: results from a national study 2001. Atlanta, GA: The 129th Annual Meeting of the American Public Health Association; 2001.

57. Roberts SC, Pies C. Complex calculations: how drug use during pregnancy becomes a barrier to prenatal care. Matern Child Health J 2011;15(3):333–41.

58. Miguel AQC, Jordan A, Kiluk BD, et al. Sociodemographic and clinical outcome differences among individuals seeking treatment for cocaine use disorders. The intersection of gender and race. J Subst Abuse Treat 2019;106:65–72.

59. Grella CE, Greenwell L. Substance abuse treatment for women: changes in the settings where women received treatment and types of services provided, 1987-1998. J Behav Health Serv Res 2004;31(4):367–83.

60. Shaima N, Narayanan G. A glass half full not empty: strength-based practice in persons with substance use disorders. Psychol Stud 2018;63(1):19–24.

61. Women and health care in the early years of the ACA: key findings from the 2013 Kaiser Women's Health Survey. KFF. 2014. Available at: https://www.kff.org/womens-health-policy/report/women-and-health-care-in-the-early-years-of-the-aca-key-findings-from-the-2013-kaiser-womens-health-survey/. Accessed March 5, 2021.

62. Horsfall J, Cleary M, Hunt GE, et al. Psychosocial treatments for people with co-occurring severe mental illnesses and substance use disorders (dual diagnosis): a review of empirical evidence. Harv Rev Psychiatry 2009;17(1):24–34.

63. Wendt D, Shafer K. Gender and attitudes about mental health help seeking: results from national data. Health Soc Work 2016;41(1):e20–8.

64. Pattyn E, Verhaeghe M, Bracke P. The gender gap in mental health service use. Soc Psychiatry Psychiatr Epidemiol 2015;50(7):1089–95.

65. Brody DJ. Antidepressant use among adults: United States, 2015–2018. NCHS Data Brief 2020;(377):8.

66. Umberson D, Chen MD, House JS, et al. The effect of social relationships on psychological well-being: are men and women really so different? Am Sociol Rev 1996;61(5):837–57.

67. Southwick SM, Sippel L, Krystal J, et al. Why are some individuals more resilient than others: the role of social support. World Psychiatry 2016;15(1):77–9.

68. Sword W, Jack S, Niccols A, et al. Integrated programs for women with substance use issues and their children: a qualitative meta-synthesis of processes and outcomes. Harm Reduct J 2009;6:32.

69. Deering KN, Kerr T, Tyndall MW, et al. A peer-led mobile outreach program and increased utilization of detoxification and residential drug treatment among female sex workers who use drugs in a Canadian setting. Drug Alcohol Depend 2011;113(1):46–54.

70. Kim SR, Goldenberg SM, Duff P, et al. Uptake of a women-only, sex-work-specific drop-in center and links with sexual and reproductive health care for sex workers. Int J Gynaecol Obstet 2015;128(3):201–5.

71. Niv N, Hser Y-I. Women-only and mixed-gender drug abuse treatment programs: service needs, utilization and outcomes. Drug Alcohol Depend 2007;87(2–3):194–201.

72. Substance Abuse and Mental Health Services Administration. Key substance use and mental health indicators in the United States: results from the 2019 national survey on drug use and health. Rockville, MD: Center for Behavioral Health Statistics and Quality, Substance Abuse and Mental Health Services Administration; 2020. Available at: https://www.samhsa.gov/data/.

73. Pineles BL, Park E, Samet JM. Systematic review and meta-analysis of miscarriage and maternal exposure to tobacco smoke during pregnancy. Am J Epidemiol 2014;179(7):807–23.

74. Louw K-A. Substance use in pregnancy: the medical challenge. Obstet Med 2018;11(2):54–66.

75. Corsi DJ, Walsh L, Weiss D, et al. Association between self-reported prenatal cannabis use and maternal, perinatal, and neonatal outcomes. JAMA 2019;322(2):145–52.

76. Murphy AS. A survey of state fetal homicide laws and their potential applicability to pregnant women who harm their own fetuses. Indiana Law J 2014;89:847.

77. Guttmacher Institute. New York, NY: Substance use during pregnancy. Guttmacher Institute; 2021. Available at: https://www.guttmacher.org/print/state-policy/explore/substance-use-during-pregnancy. Accessed April 1, 2021.

78. Kozhimannil KB, Dowd WN, Ali MM, et al. Substance use disorder treatment admissions and state-level prenatal substance use policies: evidence from a national treatment database. Addict Behav 2019;90:272–7.

79. Hui K, Angelotta C, Fisher CE. Criminalizing substance use in pregnancy: misplaced priorities. Addiction 2017;112(7):1123–5.

80. Harp KLH, Bunting AM. The racialized nature of child welfare policies and the social control of black bodies. Soc Polit 2020;27(2):258–81.

81. Harp KLH, Oser CB. A longitudinal analysis of the impact of child custody loss on drug use and crime among a sample of African American mothers. Child Abuse Negl 2018;77:1–12.

82. McCarthy JJ, Leamon MH, Finnegan LP, et al. Opioid dependence and pregnancy: minimizing stress on the fetal brain. Am J Obstet Gynecol 2017; 216(3):226–31.

83. Chapman SLC, Wu L-T. Postpartum substance use and depressive symptoms: a review. Women Health 2013;53(5):479–503.

84. Pace CA, Kaminetzky LB, Winter M, et al. Postpartum changes in methadone maintenance dose. J Subst Abuse Treat 2014;47(3):229–32.

85. Schiff DM, Nielsen T, Terplan M, et al. Fatal and nonfatal overdose among pregnant and postpartum women in Massachusetts. Obstet Gynecol 2018;132(2): 466–74.

86. Welle-Strand GK, Skurtveit S, Jansson LM, et al. Breastfeeding reduces the need for withdrawal treatment in opioid-exposed infants. Acta Paediatr 2013; 102(11):1060–6.

87. Tsai LC, Doan TJ. Breastfeeding among mothers on opioid maintenance treatment: a literature review. J Hum Lact 2016;32(3):521–9.

88. Reece-Stremtan S, Marinelli KA. ABM clinical protocol #21: guidelines for breastfeeding and substance use or substance use disorder, revised 2015. Breastfeed Med 2015;10(3):135–41.

89. Wachman EM, Saia K, Humphreys R, et al. Revision of breastfeeding guidelines in the setting of maternal opioid use disorder: one institution's experience. J Hum Lact 2016;32(2):382–7.

90. Harris M, Joseph K, Hoeppner B, et al. A retrospective cohort study examining the utility of perinatal urine toxicology testing to guide breastfeeding initiation. J Addict Med 2020. https://doi.org/10.1097/ADM.0000000000000761.

91. D'Apolito K. Breastfeeding and substance abuse. Clin Obstet Gynecol 2013; 56(1):202–11.

92. Barlow J, Sembi S, Parsons H, et al. A randomized controlled trial and economic evaluation of the parents under pressure program for parents in substance abuse treatment. Drug Alcohol Depend 2019;194:184–94.

93. Stulac S, Bair-Merritt M, Wachman EM, et al. Children and families of the opioid epidemic: under the radar. Curr Probl Pediatr Adolesc Health Care 2019;49(8): 100637.

94. Marshall SK, Charles G, Hare J, et al. Sheway's services for substance using pregnant and parenting women: evaluating the outcomes for infants. Can J Commun Ment Health 2005;24(1):19–34.

95. Moreland AD, McRae-Clark A. Parenting outcomes of parenting interventions in integrated substance-use treatment programs: a systematic review. J Subst Abuse Treat 2018;89:52–9.

96. Wright TE. Integrating reproductive health services into opioid treatment facilities: a missed opportunity to prevent opioid-exposed pregnancies and improve the health of women who use drugs. J Addict Med 2019;13(6):420–1.

97. Greenfield SF, Sugarman DE, Freid CM, et al. Group therapy for women with substance use disorders: results from the Women's Recovery Group Study. Drug Alcohol Depend 2014;142:245–53.

98. Bagley SM, Ventura AS, Lasser KE, et al. Engaging the family in the care of young adults with substance use disorders. Pediatrics 2021;147(Suppl 2): S215–9.

99. Ashley OS, Marsden ME, Brady TM. Effectiveness of substance abuse treatment programming for women: a review. Am J Drug Alcohol Abuse 2003; 29(1):19–53.

100. Wechsberg WM. Promising international interventions and treatment for women who use and abuse drugs: focusing on the issues through the InWomen's Group. Subst Abuse Rehabil 2012;3(Suppl 1):1–4.

# Moving?

## Make sure your subscription moves with you!

To notify us of your new address, find your **Clinics Account Number** (located on your mailing label above your name), and contact customer service at:

**Email: journalscustomerservice-usa@elsevier.com**

**800-654-2452** (subscribers in the U.S. & Canada)
**314-447-8871** (subscribers outside of the U.S. & Canada)

**Fax number: 314-447-8029**

**Elsevier Health Sciences Division**
**Subscription Customer Service**
**3251 Riverport Lane**
**Maryland Heights, MO 63043**